Palgrave Studies in Public Health Policy Research

Series Editors
Patrick Fafard, University of Ottawa, Ottawa, ON, Canada
Evelyne de Leeuw, University of New South Wales, Liverpool, NSW,
Australia

Public health has increasingly cast the net wider. The field has moved on from a hygiene perspective and infectious and occupational disease base (where it was born in the 19th century) to a concern for unhealthy lifestyles post-WWII, and more recently to the uneven distribution of health and its (re)sources. It is of course interesting that these 'paradigms' in many places around the world live right next to each other. Hygiene, lifestyles, and health equity form the complex (indeed, wicked) policy agendas for health and social/sustainable development. All of these, it is now recognized, are part of the 'social determinants of health'.

The broad new public health agenda, with its multitude of competing issues, professions, and perspectives requires a much more sophisticated understanding of government and the policy process. In effect, there is a growing recognition of the extent to which the public health community writ large needs to better understand government and move beyond what has traditionally been a certain naiveté about politics and the process of policy making. Public health scholars and practitioners have embraced this need to understand, and influence, how governments at all levels make policy choices and decisions. Political scientists and international relations scholars and practitioners are engaging in the growing public health agenda as it forms an interesting expanse of glocal policy development and implementation.

Broader, more detailed, and more profound scholarship is required at the interface between health and political science. This series will thus be a powerful tool to build bridges between political science, international relations and public health. It will showcase the potential of rigorous political and international relations science for better understanding public health issues. It will also support the public health professional with a new theoretical and methodological toolbox. The series will include monographs (both conventional and shorter Pivots) and collections that appeal to three audiences: scholars of public health, public health practitioners, and members of the political science community with an interest in public health policy and politics.

More information about this series at
https://link.springer.com/bookseries/15414

Patrick Fafard · Adèle Cassola ·
Evelyne de Leeuw
Editors

Integrating Science and Politics for Public Health

palgrave
macmillan

Editors
Patrick Fafard
Global Strategy Lab; Faculty of Social
Sciences, Faculty of Medicine
University of Ottawa
Ottawa, ON, Canada

Adèle Cassola
Global Strategy Lab
York University
Toronto, ON, Canada

Evelyne de Leeuw
University of New South Wales
Sydney, NSW, Australia

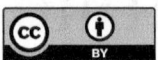

Palgrave Studies in Public Health Policy Research
ISBN 978-3-030-98984-2   ISBN 978-3-030-98985-9   (eBook)
https://doi.org/10.1007/978-3-030-98985-9

Cover credit: Richard Drury

This Palgrave Macmillan imprint is published by the registered company Springer Nature Switzerland AG
The registered company address is: Gewerbestrasse 11, 6330 Cham, Switzerland

FOREWORD

My work with the World Health Organization and national governments over many years has provided a constant reminder of how politics shapes what we do and do not do in public health. This led me to make the case for using the tools and insights of political science to better understand the inherently political nature of public health and the political determinants of health.

The editors of this important book have assembled an impressive group of experts who understand the worlds of both public health, policy theory, and political science. They offer important insights into the challenges and opportunities of integrating these disciplines to the benefit of both. Furthermore, this book highlights the role that scientific evidence does or does not play in creating public health policies, and the need to better understand the interaction of evidence and politics to improve the public health policy and, ultimately, the health of the population overall.

This book will be enormously useful to students, academics, and professionals in the fields of public health, political science, and public policy. Furthermore, this may appeal to public health advocates who are interested in developing a more nuanced understanding of the political nature of public health policy making.

Ilona Kickbusch
Graduate Institute of International
and Development Studies
Geneva, Switzerland

ACKNOWLEDGEMENTS

Patrick Fafard
This book originated in an international workshop held at York University in July 2019, I wish to thank colleagues in the Global Strategy Lab, especially Brooke Campus, Isaac Weldon, and Lathika Laguwaran, for making this workshop possible. I also want to thank Steven Hoffman who contributed to this project in numerous ways, large and small. I also want to acknowledge the financial support of the Canadian Institutes of Health Research for the workshop. This book would not have been possible without the wisdom and enthusiasm of Evelyne de Leeuw. Most importantly, it reflects the patience, the intellectual creativity, and the strategic insights of Adèle Cassola. I also wish to acknowledge the good cheer and diligent efforts of Elizabeth Mebrahtu, who played a key role to bringing this project to a conclusion. Finally, my deepest thanks to Katherine for her ongoing love, support, and patience.

Adèle Cassola
It has been a privilege to contribute to the development of this book and the larger intellectual project behind it over the past several years. I am grateful to the workshop participants and book contributors for many stimulating conversations, to my co-editors for their wisdom and generosity, and to my Global Strategy Lab colleagues for their creativity and support in bringing this project to fruition.

Evelyne de Leeuw
Against many odds, I found a great political and health equity home in Sydney. I wish to thank both my global scholarly and activist support network at CHETRE and HUE for believing in my rants. I also acknowledge the global friendships and collegiality of colleagues in—and beyond—this book, especially Patrick Fafard. During the challenging pandemic months, a shred of sanity was preserved by my dearest Lynne—in a way she made this book.

Praise for Integrating Science and Politics for Public Health

"This volume is a welcome and timely contribution to our understanding of the realities of public health policy making as an essentially political endeavour. Its sophisticated mix of theoretical, conceptual and empirical analysis can serve as a guide to the complicated challenges inherent in making public policy that accounts for and improves population health."
—Tom McIntosh, Ph.D., *Professor, Politics and International Studies and Co-Director, Saskatchewan Population Health and Evaluation Research Unit, University of Regina, Canada*

"The editors of this important book have assembled an impressive group of experts who understand the worlds of both public health, policy theory, and political science. They offer important insights into the challenges and opportunities of integrating these disciplines to the benefit of both."
—Ilona Kickbusch, Ph.D., *Professor, Graduate Institute of International and Development Studies, Geneva, Switzerland; Founder and Chair, Global Health Centre, Graduate Institute of International and Development Studies, Geneva, Switzerland; Director, Kickbusch Health Consult, Brienz, Switzerland*

CONTENTS

Part I   Public Health Political Science: Prospects for
        Partnership

1   Introduction: Virchow Revisited on the Importance
    of Public Health Political Science   3
    Patrick Fafard, Evelyne de Leeuw, and Adèle Cassola

2   Political Science In, Of, and With Public Health   15
    Patrick Fafard, Adèle Cassola, and Isaac Weldon

3   Professions, Data, and Political Will: From
    the Pandemic Toward a Political Science with Public
    Health   33
    Scott Greer

4   Public Health Policymaking, Politics, and Evidence   59
    Anita Kothari and Maxwell J. Smith

Part II   Politics, Evidence, and Policymaking: A Public
          Health Political Science Approach

5   How Policy Appetites Shape, and Are Shaped
    by Evidence Production and Use   77
    Kathryn Oliver

6   Sidestepping the Stalemate: The Strategies of Public
     Health Actors for Circulating Evidence into the Policy
     Process   103
     Carole Clavier, France Gagnon, and Blake Poland

7   Beyond the Public Health/Political Science Stalemate
     in Health Inequalities: Can Deliberative Forums Help?   127
     Katherine E. Smith, Anna Macintyre, and Sarah Weakley

8   Is Local Better? Evolving Hybrid Theorising for Local
     Health Policies   153
     Evelyne de Leeuw

9   Select Committee Governance and the Production
     of Evidence: The Case of UK E-cigarettes Policy   187
     Benjamin Hawkins and Kathryn Oliver

Part III   Making Public Health Policy: Insights from
            Political Science

10   The Policy and Politics of Public Health in Pandemics   211
     Katherine Fierlbeck, Kevin McNamara,
     and Maureen MacDonald

11   How Can Policy Theory Help to Address
     the Expectations Gap in Preventive Public Health
     and 'Health in All Policies'?   239
     Paul Cairney, Emily St. Denny, and Heather Mitchell

12   Moving Beyond Health in All Policies: Exploring
     How Policy Could Front and Centre the Reduction
     of Social Inequities in Health   267
     Ditte Heering Holt and Katherine L. Frohlich

13   Mechanisms to Bridge the Gap Between Science
     and Politics in Evidence-Informed Policymaking:
     Mapping the Landscape   293
     Adèle Cassola, Patrick Fafard, Michèle Palkovits,
     and Steven J. Hoffman

14   Conclusion: The Added Value of Political Science in,
     of, and with Public Health   329
     Evelyne de Leeuw, Patrick Fafard, and Adèle Cassola

Index   341

LIST OF CONTRIBUTORS

Paul Cairney Division of History, Heritage, and Politics, University of Stirling, Stirling, Scotland, UK

Adèle Cassola Global Strategy Lab, York University, Toronto, ON, Canada

Carole Clavier Department of Political Science, Université du Québec à Montréal, Montréal, QC, Canada

Emily St. Denny Department of Political Science, University of Copenhagen, Copenhagen, Denmark

Evelyne de Leeuw University of New South Wales, Sydney, NSW, Australia

Patrick Fafard Global Strategy Lab; Faculty of Social Sciences, Faculty of Medicine, University of Ottawa, Ottawa, ON, Canada

Katherine Fierlbeck McCulloch Chair of Political Science, Dalhousie University, Halifax, NS, Canada

Katherine L. Frohlich Département de médecine sociale et préventive, École de Santé Publique, Université de Montréal, Montreal, QC, Canada

France Gagnon School of Administration Sciences, Université TÉLUQ, Quebec City, QC, Canada;
Quebec Population Health Research Network, Quebec City, QC, Canada

Scott Greer School of Public Health, University of Michigan, Ann Arbor, MI, USA

Benjamin Hawkins MRC Epidemiology Unit, University of Cambridge, Cambridge, UK

Steven J. Hoffman Global Strategy Lab; Global Health, Law, and Political Science, York University, Toronto, ON, Canada

Ditte Heering Holt National Institute of Public Health, University of Southern Denmark, Copenhagen, Denmark

Anita Kothari School of Health Studies, Faculty of Health Sciences, Western University, London, ON, Canada

Maureen MacDonald Halifax, NS, Canada

Anna Macintyre School of Social Work and Social Policy, University of Strathclyde, Glasgow, UK

Kevin McNamara Halifax, NS, Canada

Heather Mitchell Institute for Social Marketing, University of Stirling, Stirling, Scotland, UK

Kathryn Oliver Faculty of Public Health and Policy, London School of Hygiene and Tropical Medicine, London, UK

Michèle Palkovits Global Strategy Lab, York University, Toronto, ON, Canada

Blake Poland Dalla Lana School of Public Health, University of Toronto, Toronto, ON, Canada

Katherine E. Smith School of Social Work and Social Policy, University of Strathclyde, Glasgow, UK

Maxwell J. Smith School of Health Studies, Faculty of Health Sciences, Western University, London, ON, Canada

Sarah Weakley College of Social Sciences, University of Glasgow, Glasgow, UK

Isaac Weldon Department of Politics, York University, Toronto, ON, Canada

LIST OF FIGURES

Chapter 8

Fig. 1 Current WHO/EURO Healthy City priorities (cf http://
        www.euro.who.int/en/health-topics/environment-and-hea
        lth/urban-health/who-european-healthy-cities-network/hea
        lthy-cities-vision)   161
Fig. 2 Seven categories of theories and conceptual frameworks
        that explain what happens between research, policy
        and practice for health   165
Fig. 3 Graphical representation of seven categories of acting
        at the nexus between research, policy and practice   166

Chapter 11

Fig. 1 Key elements of the policy process (Cairney, 2017a)   249

Chapter 13

Fig. 1 Examples of typology dimensions in relation to mechanism
        selection and design   314

LIST OF TABLES

Chapter 2

Table 1   Political science for, of, and with public health   20

Chapter 7

Table 1   Average public support for policy proposals for tackling health inequalities according to the national sample survey (from most to least popular)   136

Table 2   Citizen juries sample description ($n = 56$)   138

Table 3   Average public support for policy proposals for national survey and average public support and group voting for citizens' juries   139

Table 4   The top ranked proposals in each jury in final group voting round   140

Table 5   Three intersecting factors that appeared to reduce (the relatively high) support for macro-level policy responses to health inequalities   145

Chapter 8

Table 1   Cobb & Elder agenda-setting parameters against their operations at local level   157

Table 2   Hancock and Duhl (1986) evidence-based recommendations for the values of a healthy city   159

Chapter 12

Table 1   Definitions   272

Chapter 13

Table 1   Mechanisms identified in the literature to bridge the gap
           between science and politics in public health policymaking   299
Table 2   Proposed typology of mechanisms to bridge the gap
           between science and politics in public health policymaking   313

PART I

Public Health Political Science: Prospects for Partnership

Introduction: Virchow Revisited on the Importance of Public Health Political Science

Patrick Fafard, Evelyne de Leeuw, and Adèle Cassola

Early in the study of public health, most students come across the famous quote from the nineteenth-century German pathologist and social reformer Ruddolf Virchow: 'Medicine is a social science and politics is nothing else but medicine on a large scale' (Aston, 2006). The phrase has been used and abused many times since but is usually invoked to draw a link between medicine and public health on the one hand and politics on the other hand. The coronavirus 2019 (COVID-19) pandemic that

P. Fafard (✉)
Global Strategy Lab; Faculty of Social Sciences, Faculty of Medicine, University of Ottawa, Ottawa, ON, Canada
e-mail: patrick.fafard@globalstrategylab.org

E. de Leeuw
University of New South Wales, Sydney, NSW, Australia

A. Cassola
Global Strategy Lab, York University, Toronto, ON, Canada

© The Author(s) 2022
P. Fafard et al. (eds.), *Integrating Science and Politics for Public Health*,
Palgrave Studies in Public Health Policy Research,
https://doi.org/10.1007/978-3-030-98985-9_1

3

ravaged the world and the efforts to address it have made the link between public health and politics very visible to all. Specifically, the pandemic has demonstrated that the choices that governments make to address infectious disease threats are necessarily and inherently informed by both scientific evidence and a host of other economic, social, and ethical considerations. Reconciling these sometimes-conflicting imperatives is the stuff of politics.

But Virchow's understanding of politics was very particular, as revealed in the second and less well-known part of his statement. After characterizing politics as medicine on a larger scale, Virchow went on to write, 'Medicine as a social science, as the science of human beings, has the obligation to point out problems and to attempt their theoretical solution; the politician, the practical anthropologist, must find the means for their actual solution' (Aston, 2006). For Virchow, indeed for many in public health, politics is a practical matter, something that is done by politicians, and something that can and should be informed by the insights of medicine and, by extension, public health sciences such as epidemiology. Unfortunately, translating scientific evidence into public policy is a messy business indeed. Moreover, medicine and public health have few effective tools for systematically understanding the choices governments make, much less the broader complexities of politics.

It is for this reason that, over the last 25 years or so, there has been a growing interest among public health scholars and practitioners in what political science—the systematic study of politics and government—can offer. Simply put, if public health is political, it only makes sense to draw on the insights of efforts to systematically understand how politics and government work. This has led to the proliferation of research that draws on concepts and theories from political science to better understand the public health policy and programme choices that governments make at all levels—global, national, regional, and local. However, a nascent 'public health political science' is both an analytical and a normative project. It is analytical insofar as scholars deploy theories and concepts from political science to better understand not only what governments choose to do, but why and how they do it. It is normative insofar as scholars also draw on political science to explain how the public health enterprise (Tilson & Berkowitz, 2006) can more effectively make claims about what governments should do and investigate the normative underpinnings of disagreements, often quite profound, about what constitutes good public health policy.

Public health political science is, however, a relatively underdeveloped cross-disciplinary effort. It arises as a response to the realization from researchers in both disciplines that despite the political nature of public health, work in political science and public health research typically unfolds within 'disciplinary silos' (Fafard & Cassola, 2020, p. 108). For example, the inherently political nature of public health has been much discussed in the public health literature including, for example, by Nancy Milio (Cohen et al., 2000; Milio, 1981, 1986, 1987), Amy Fairchild (Fairchild et al., 2007, 2010), and Nancy Krieger (Beckfield & Krieger, 2009; Krieger & Birn, 1998). Similarly, but much more rarely (at least before the COVID-19 pandemic), political science occasionally took note of public health (Alley, 2012; Asare et al., 2009; Axelrod, 2008; Fox et al., 2012; Givel, 2006; Marmor & Weale, 2012; Studlar, 2002). However, these literatures do not tend to overlap. Political science engagement with public health published in political science journals is most often written for a political science audience and is a political science *of* public health (see Chapter 2, Fafard et al., 2022).

Certain structural barriers have, to date, hindered productive partnerships between the two disciplines. Some of these barriers involve engrained differences in disciplinary identities, methodologies, and knowledge processes, including an enduring professional distinction between politics and science in public health, which leads many to see their mandate as chiefly technical; the divergence between clinical and policy-related needs and processes when it comes to integrating scientific evidence; and a gap in the traditional level of analysis, with political science typically focused on macro-level processes and public health often focused on micro-level interventions (reflecting the field's biomedical origins) (Bernier & Clavier, 2011; Breton & de Leeuw, 2011; Golden & Wendel, 2020; Greer et al., 2017). In addition, the system of incentives in the respective disciplinary research communities—particularly as they relate to funding and publishing—also creates key structural barriers to effective partnerships.

To bring these two bodies of research and thought together, an intellectual conversation has begun that is designed to bridge the gap between public health and political science. The volume and intensity of the conversation has grown over the past decade or so, and many of the editors and contributors to this volume have been at the centre of it (Bernier & Clavier, 2011; Breton & de Leeuw, 2011; Cairney & Oliver,

2017; de Leeuw et al., 2014; Fafard, 2015; Greer et al., 2017; Hawkins & Parkhurst, 2016; Smith, 2013).

1   Introducing This Book

The book you are currently reading is a continuation and a consolidation of this conversation about the interconnections of political science and public health. It began with an international invitation-only workshop at York University in Toronto in June 2019 (Fafard & Cassola, 2020). Since then, the importance of building a robust public health political science has become more salient. High-profile scholarly outlets like *The Lancet* and *Nature* have started to recognize the political nature of public health and as an issue of both scholarly and practical interest (Editor, 2020; Horton, 2020).

With this context in mind, the book has three ambitious goals. First, it provides direct examples of how political science perspectives (broadly defined) can inform public health research and practice with a view to, ultimately, improving the overall health of the population. In doing so, it aims to address and ameliorate the current underutilization of political science tools, theories, and knowledge within the public health field, particularly as they relate to the policymaking process and the role of science and evidence within it.

Second, this book is designed to demonstrate that there is also much that political science can gain from a deeper engagement with public health (Fafard & Cassola, 2020; Lynch, 2019). In particular, there is a need for political science to consider the full scope of the public health enterprise and pursue truly interdisciplinary work that goes beyond positioning public health simply as a case subject or a target for critique (Fafard & Cassola, 2020). Amid calls for scientific advice and modelling to become more transparent, it is critical for political scientists to learn from and engage with public health researchers' understanding of evidence generation and use.

Third, this book is intended to advance the interconnection of public health and political science as scholarly disciplines. Here, we tackle a long-standing intellectual stalemate arising from different conceptions of the relationship between evidence and policy. The premise that policy decisions should be 'evidence-based' or at the very least, evidence-informed is commonplace in the field of public health, and efforts to achieve a better relationship between science and public health policy are ubiquitous. Perspectives from political science do not discount the value of scientific knowledge, but highlight the political nature of evidence and emphasize that policy choice is a negotiated reality (Fafard & Cassola, 2020; see Chapter 13, Cassola et al., 2022). A central focus of this book is to bridge these two perspectives, towards a more fulsome understanding of the relationship among evidence, policy, and institutions of representative democracy.

2   Conceptual Ground Clearing

Before moving on, it is important to specify what we mean by 'public health' and 'political science'. First, we are using these terms to describe academic disciplines. In most high-income countries,[1] this is straightforward at least insofar as in most universities, the study and teaching of each are done in separate places. Public health is typically the purview of a faculty of medicine or a faculty of applied health sciences or is a stand-alone faculty. Political science, by contrast, is usually a department or school in a faculty of social sciences or arts and humanities. In some places, schools of public policy or international relations also are home to large numbers of political scientists. However, unlike political science, public health is an inherently interdisciplinary academic exercise, and some 'atypical' formats for the institutional presence of research, development, teaching, and learning have been identified (de Leeuw, 1995). Typically, a school of public health will have experts in disciplines closely identified with or unique to public health (such as epidemiology and biostatistics), faculty with expertise in other medical and health disciplines, and faculty trained in bodies of knowledge that inform public health practice, such as economics and psychology. It is much less common for schools and departments of public health to have faculty who self-identify as political scientists and bring to bear political science theory and concepts.

Second, unlike political science, the term 'public health' is used to describe not only an academic discipline but also an area of applied practice and institutional grounding. Public health is routinely characterized

---

[1] The pattern is Latin America, Asia, and Africa is sometimes quite different. For example, in Latin America, a long-standing tradition of social medicine (Porter, 2006) shapes how public health is understood and practised.

as an 'applied' discipline designed to train students to take jobs in public health, usually but not always in government (be it local, state/provincial, national, or global) or the not-for-profit sector (e.g. health charities that seek to influence public policy).[2] The chapters in this book are meant to be of interest to both public health scholars and public health practitioners. In fact, it is the latter who, absent formal training in political science and government, may find themselves having to 'learn on the job' and work hard to better understand how government works and how policy choices are made. Over time they often develop a keen understanding of politics and the policy process but may lack the conceptual language needed to articulate this understanding. Public health practitioners are thus arguably the largest part of the public health enterprise who could benefit from the insights of political science or, at least, particular forms of applied political science (Cairney, 2015).

Third, it is important to clarify that only particular dimensions of political science and public health, of necessity, emphasized in this book. In the case of political science, we focus those parts of the discipline focused on policy making and, by extension, the role of scientific evidence in the making of public policy. There is some discussion of the closely linked political science sub-discipline of public administration or public management. This emphasis reflects the book's goal of reconciling public health and political science conceptions of evidence and policy as well as the disciplinary background of the editors and authors, which is disproportionately in political science or social policy. As a result, this volume does not engage explicitly with sub-disciplines such as international relations, various forms of political economy, and political theory, despite the relevance of these fields to public health governance and practice more broadly. In addition, this book is primarily about public health *policy* not public health *politics*. Consequently, partisan politics, political culture, social movements, interest group lobbying, and other expressly political questions that are the central preoccupation of much research and teaching in political science come up obliquely in the chapters of this book insofar as they are part of the story of the making of public health policy. Others have pursued this linkage more directly (Greer et al., 2017). In the case of public health, this book does not directly address a host of contemporary challenges in public health such as the health impact of

---

[2] This pattern can be found in political science (e.g. schools of public policy or public administration) but is, relatively speaking, a much smaller part of the discipline.

climate change; the securitization of public health; global health equity; and various aspect of chronic disease prevention and health promotion. Finally, the book draws on the expertise of the authors and editors with public health policy in high-income countries with only passing references to the challenges in low- and middle-income countries.

3   This Book in Detail

The central theme of this volume concerns how the different perspectives on scientific evidence and policymaking from public health and political science can be reconciled towards more effective public health policy and practice. The chapters approach this theme from different angles, use a variety of methodologies, and address diverse areas of public health policy.

The three remaining chapters in Part I are designed to set the stage and investigate the relationship between public health and political science and consider how the two fields can work productively in partnership. In Chapter 2, Fafard, Cassola, and Weldon propose a framework for understanding the different forms of interaction between public health and political science and address their implications for the way questions of evidence and policy are tackled. This is then followed in Chapter 3 by a consideration by Greer of key areas of tension and misunderstanding between public health and political science and associated research pathways to address them. Of note is his effort to rescue the oft-used concept of 'political will'. In Chapter 4, Kothari and Smith introduce the interrelationships among evidence, policymaking, and politics from a public health perspective, elucidate how these conceptions tie in with the field's community orientation, and consider potential areas of engagement between public health and political science.

In Part II, a set of empirical chapters use a public health political science approach to focus specifically on the evidence-policy stalemate and examine processes of knowledge production, evidence circulation, and policy learning. In Chapter 5, Oliver analyses the reciprocal relationship between processes of evidence production, mobilization, and use on the one hand, and the types of knowledge that are valued and sought out by policymakers on the other. Chapter 6 by Clavier, Gagnon, and Poland examines the ways in which local public health actors in the Canadian cities of Toronto and Montréal engage with the policymaking process and use evidence strategically within it and investigates what this engagement reveals about these actors' conception of the role of evidence in policy.

In Chapter 7, Smith uses the case of health inequalities in England and Scotland to provide an in-depth look at the potential for one such mechanism—deliberative citizens' juries—to overcome the 'stalemate' between science and politics. In Chapter 8, de Leeuw describes the ever-evolving research journey of local health policymaking and analysis associated with the global network of 'Healthy Cities'. She argues that for both the study of health policy processes and policy impact, 'local is better'. Finally, using the e-cigarette debate as a launching point, in Chapter 9 Hawkins and Oliver examine the role of Parliamentary Select Committees in the United Kingdom as producers and synthesizers of evidence for policy and highlight the implications of the governance of these committees for the influence of corporate actors on regulatory debates.

In Part III, a series of chapters analyse different aspects of public health evidentiary systems or policymaking processes more broadly and the politics and intersectoral complexities of public health policymaking. Fierlbeck, McNamara, and MacDonald take an in-depth look in Chapter 10 at the political dynamics of pandemic decision-making about vaccines and antivirals in the context of the H1N1 crisis in the Canadian province of Nova Scotia. In Chapter 11, Cairney, St. Denny, and Mitchell draw on public policy theories to explain the gap between public health commitment, policy, and policy outcomes. They examine these themes in the context of a qualitative systematic review of 'Health in All Policies' (HiAP) research. HiAP is also the focus of Chapter 12, where Holt and Frohlich argue that these approaches have been ineffective at reducing social inequities in tobacco use and make the case for a distinct policy framework based on the capabilities approach to address social inequities in health. Finally, in Chapter 13, Cassola and her co-authors describe and categorize mechanisms that aim to reconcile scientific considerations and democratic politics in evidence-informed policymaking and develop an analytical typology that identifies salient dimensions of variation in their selection and design. In their concluding chapter, the editors review the stated ambitions of this volume and provide an overview of the chapters to make the case that political science perspectives do, in fact, add value to the public health enterprise but that many challenges remain.

Closing the gap and breaking the stalemate, between public health and political science, is not only a lofty intellectual pursuit. It is a necessary endeavour. With this book, we intend to offer strong, evidence-informed views on policy processes to enhance population health. Although the public health realm, at least rhetorically, has embraced the need for good policy processes since the writings of Villermé and Virchow, the COVID-19 pandemic more than anything else has demonstrated the urgency of embracing the complex nature of policymaking and its drivers. It is time to leave naïve allusions of the impenetrable nature and yet necessity of good policymaking behind us and argue health to policy and policy for health.

REFERENCES

Alley, D. (2012). Providing science to improve the public's health: A fellow's view from the office of the US surgeon general. *PS: Political Science & Politics, 45*(3), 580–581. https://doi.org/10.1017/S1049096512000601

Asare, B., Cairney, P., & Studlar, D. T. (2009). Federalism and multilevel governance in tobacco policy: The European Union, the United Kingdom, and devolved UK Institutions. *Journal of Public Policy, 29*(1), 79–102. https://doi.org/10.1017/S0143814X09000993

Aston, J. (2006). Virchow misquoted, part-quoted, and the real McCoy. *Journal of Epidemiology and Community Health,60*(8), 671.

Axelrod, R. (2008). Political science and beyond: Presidential address to the American Political Science Association. *Perspectives on Politics, 6*(1), 3–9. https://doi.org/10.1017/S153759270808002X

Beckfield, J., & Krieger, N. (2009). Epi + demos + cracy: Linking political systems and priorities to the magnitude of health inequities—Evidence, gaps, and a research agenda. *Epidemiologic Reviews, 31*(1), 152–177. https://doi.org/10.1093/epirev/mxp002

Bernier, N. F., & Clavier, C. (2011). Public health policy research: Making the case for a political science approach. *Health Promotion International, 26*(1), 109–116. https://doi.org/10.1093/heapro/daq079

Breton, E., & de Leeuw, E. (2011). Theories of the policy process in health promotion research: A review. *Health Promotion International, 26*. https://doi.org/10.1093/heapro/daq051

Cairney, P. (2015). How can policy theory have an impact on policy making? The role of theory-led academic-practitioner discussions. *Teaching Public Administration, 33*(1), 22–39. https://doi.org/10.1177/0144739414532284

Cairney, P., & Oliver, K. (2017). Evidence-based policymaking is not like evidence-based medicine, so how far should you go to bridge the divide between evidence and policy? *Health Research Policy and Systems, 15*(1). https://doi.org/10.1186/s12961-017-0192-x

Cassola, A., Fafard, P., Palkovits, M., & Hoffman, S. J. (2022). Mechanisms to bridge the gap between science and politics in evidence-informed policymaking: Mapping the landscape. In P. Fafard, A. Cassola, & E. De Leeuw (Eds.), *Integrating science and politics for public health.* Palgrave Springer.

Cohen, J. E., Milio, N., Rozier, R. G., Ferrence, R., Ashley, M. J., & Goldstein, A. O. (2000). Political ideology and tobacco control. *Tobacco Control, 9*(3), 263–267. https://doi.org/10.1136/tc.9.3.263

de Leeuw, E. (1995). European schools of public health in state of flux. *Lancet, 345*(8958), 1158–1160.

de Leeuw, E., Clavier, C., & Breton, E. (2014). Health policy—Why research it and how: Health political science. *Health Research Policy and Systems, 12*(1), 55. https://doi.org/10.1186/1478-4505-12-55

Editor. (2020). Science and politics are inseparable. *Nature, 586*(7828), 169–170. https://doi.org/10.1038/d41586-020-02797-1

Fafard, P. (2015). Beyond the usual suspects: Using political science to enhance public health policy making. *Journal of Epidemiology and Community Health, 69*(11), 1129–1132. https://doi.org/10.1136/jech-2014-204608

Fafard, P., & Cassola, A. (2020). Public health and political science: Challenges and opportunities for a productive partnership. *Public Health, 186*, 107–109. https://doi.org/10.1016/j.puhe.2020.07.004

Fafard, P., Cassola, A., & Weldon, I. (2022). Political science in, of, and with public health: Implications for the role of evidence. In P. Fafard, A. Cassola, & E. De Leeuw (Eds.), *Integrating Science and Politics for Public Health.* Palgrave Springer.

Fairchild, A. L., Bayer, R., Colgrove, J., & Wolfe, D. (2007). *Searching eyes: Privacy, the state, and disease surveillance in America* (1st ed.). University of California Press.

Fairchild, A. L., Rosner, D., Colgrove, J., Bayer, R., & Fried, L. P. (2010). The EXODUS of public health. *American Journal of Public Health, 100*(1), 54–63.

Fox, D. M., Day, P., & Klein, R. (2012). The power of professionalism: Policies for AIDS in Britain, Sweden, and the United States. In T. R. Marmor & R. Klein (Eds.), *Politics, health, and health care: Selected essays* (pp. 464–480). Yale University Press.

Givel, M. (2006). Punctuated equilibrium in Limbo: The tobacco lobby and U.S. state policymaking from 1990 to 2003. *Policy Studies Journal, 34*(3), 405–418. https://doi.org/10.1111/j.1541-0072.2006.00179.x

Golden, T. L., & Wendel, M. L. (2020). Public health's next step in advancing equity: Re-evaluating epistemological assumptions to move social determinants from theory to practice. *Frontiers in Public Health, 8*. https://doi.org/10.3389/fpubh.2020.00131

Greer, S. L., Bekker, M., de Leeuw, E., Wismar, M., Helderman, J.-K., Ribeiro, S., & Stuckler, D. (2017). Policy, politics and public health. *European Journal of Public Health, 27*(suppl_4), 40–43. https://doi.org/10.1093/eurpub/ckx152

Hawkins, B., & Parkhurst, J. (2016). The "good governance" of evidence in health policy *Evidence & Policy: A Journal of Research. Debate and Practice, 12*(4), 575–592. https://doi.org/10.1332/174426415X14430058455412

Horton, R. (2020). Offline: Science and politics in the era of COVID-19. *The Lancet, 396*(10259), 1319. https://doi.org/10.1016/S0140-6736(20)322 21-2

Krieger, N., & Birn, A. E. (1998). A vision of social justice as the foundation of public health: Commemorating 150 years of the spirit of 1848. *American Journal of Public Health, 88*(11), 1603–1606.

Lynch, J. (2019). What can political science learn from public health? Reflections on epidemiology and methodology. *EuropeNow*. https://www.europenowjou rnal.org/2019/06/10/what-can-political-science-learn-from-public-health-reflections-on-epidemiology-and-methodology%EF%BB%BF/

Marmor, T., & Weale, A. (2012). A new perspective on health: Learning from Lalonde? In T. R. Marmor & R. Klein (Eds.), *Politics, health, and health care: Selected essays* (pp. 507–520). Yale University Press.

Milio, N. (1981). *Promoting Health through Public Policy*. FA Davis Company.

Milio, N. (1986). Pressure groups and Australian health policymaking in the 1980s. *Politics, 21*(2), 51–61.

Milio, N. (1987). Making healthy public policy; developing the science by learning the art: An ecological framework for policy studies. *Health Promotion International, 2*(3), 263–274.

Porter, D. (2006). How did social medicine evolve, and where is it heading? *PLOS Medicine, 3*(10), e399. https://doi.org/10.1371/journal.pmed.003 0399

Smith, K. (2013). *Beyond evidence based policy in public health*. Palgrave Macmillan.

Studlar, D. (2002). *Tobacco control: Comparative politics in the United States and Canada*. Broadview Press.

Tilson, H., & Berkowitz, B. (2006). The public health enterprise: Examining our twenty-first-century policy challenges. *Health Affairs (project Hope), 25*(4), 900–910. https://doi.org/10.1377/hlthaff.25.4.900

Villermé, L.-R. (1840) *Tableau de l'état physique et moral des ouvriers employés dans les manufactures de coton, de laine et de soie* (Study of the Physical Condition of Cotton, Wool and Silk workers). Forgotten Books Classic Reprin

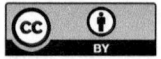

CHAPTER 2

Political Science In, Of, and With Public Health

Patrick Fafard, Adèle Cassola, and Isaac Weldon

1   Introduction

The continuing importance of public health is not hard to see. Even before the COVID-19 pandemic, the continuing challenge of the Ebola virus in sub-Saharan Africa, measles outbreaks around the world, divisive debates about the role of vaping as an alternative to combustible tobacco products, the looming crisis of bacteria resistant to existing antibiotics; these and other issues point to the fact that public health is a critical

P. Fafard (✉)
Global Strategy Lab; Faculty of Social Sciences, Faculty of Medicine, University of Ottawa, Ottawa, ON, Canada
e-mail: patrick.fafard@globalstrategylab.org

A. Cassola
Global Strategy Lab, York University, Toronto, ON, Canada

I. Weldon
Global Strategy Lab, Department of Politics, York University, Toronto, ON, Canada

© The Author(s) 2022   15
P. Fafard et al. (eds.), *Integrating Science and Politics for Public Health*,
Palgrave Studies in Public Health Policy Research,
https://doi.org/10.1007/978-3-030-98985-9_2

policy challenge for governments around the world. The pandemic has served to magnify many times over the critical importance of public health, However, precisely because the response to a pandemic and other public health challenges require action by governments and the closely associated reality that citizens often disagree on whether and what to do, public health is inherently political. This is well understood by actors within public health and has been for a long time. Thus, it is both appropriate and indeed essential that the tools and insights of political science be applied to public health. In fact, over the past decade there has been a slow and steady increase in the amount of interaction between disciplines. Political scientists have begun to pay close attention to public health and, in parallel, public health scholars and actors have slowly begun to appreciate the contribution of political science.

The result, alas, has been a less than ideal partnership and something of stalemate. If nothing else, the public health enterprise (Tilson & Berkowitz, 2006) continues to be unduly concerned with the ways in which "politics," understood as a largely negative influence, interferes with or otherwise distorts the making of scientifically based public health policy. For political scientists, by contrast, politics and political conflict are endemic and the task at hand is not how to eliminate or contain political influence but rather to understand it. Conversely, all too often the political science of public health does not fully engage with the ongoing public health research that offers rich insights into a myriad of policy and political questions, even if this is not done in ways familiar to political scientists and, by extension, readily accessible to a political science audience. To explore and hopefully get past this stalemate, in this exploratory essay, we propose a typology of the possible interactions between political science and public health. In addition to the common pattern of public health without political science, we suggest there are three broad patterns to describe the intersection between the two disciplines. Drawing on earlier work in sociology (Mykhalovskiy et al., 2018), we suggest that what some have called health political science (de Leeuw et al., 2014; Kickbusch, 2015) can be divided into four broad categories: political science *without* public health political science *in* public health, political science *of* public health, and political science *with* public health. Each has different implications for what role political science can play in better understanding the public health enterprise and, by extension, what role scientific evidence does and does not play in the making of public health policy. The essay is divided into three parts. The first briefly sketches the original typology drawn from sociology. The second part offers an application of this model to political science and public health. The third section explores the implications of this typology for the place of scientific evidence in the making of public health policy. A short conclusion ends the essay.

2 FROM A SOCIOLOGY OF MEDICINE TO A SOCIOLOGY OF PUBLIC HEALTH

As well described in a recent paper by Mykhalovskiy and colleagues (Mykhalovskiy et al., 2018), in 1957 the American sociologist Robert Straus introduced the distinction between sociology *in* medicine and a sociology *of* medicine (Straus, 1957). He distinguished between an applied sociology in medicine where scholars with a background in sociology worked with health professionals in a health sciences setting. This is in marked contrast with a sociology of medicine, a more basic and much less applied exercise which was, and presumably still is, the preoccupation of scholars working largely outside of medicine. For this latter group medicine is an institution and as he put it, "a behaviour system" that is an object of inquiry, something to be understood from without. In this same era, sociologists in other countries, including Canada, began to pay closer attention to public health (Badgley et al., 1963).

In their highly original (if somewhat overstated)[1] paper, Mykhalovskiy and his colleagues build on this approach in medical sociology to develop a framework for understanding the relationship between sociology and public health.[2] They extend the original distinction and offer an account of a sociology that is neither *in* or *of*, but rather is a sociology *with* public health. In their view, a critical sociology *with* public health is a set of research practices that recognizes the epistemological and other

---

[1] While the article speaks of "social science" and public health, for the most part social science is used synonymously with sociology. There is no real engagement with the diversity of disciplines with social science and no mention of the differences that might exist between public health and political science, economics, social psychology, criminology, and other social science disciplines.

[2] Note that for both sociology and political science the dance partner, public health, is at times hard to define. As we suggested in the introduction to this volume, public health is simultaneously an academic discipline, an organization (often, but not always, conceived of as part of government), a profession, and finally, what amounts to a social movement. Nor is it a unitary enterprise and what constitutes the core values of public health are often contested.

differences between sociology and public health but seeks to turn these differences into productive opportunities.

On this account, a sociology *in* public health is one where scholars trained in sociology find themselves working closely with public health scholars and especially practitioners. The task at hand is to use the tools and insights of sociology to address public health challenges and problems. The downside risk is that sociologists lose their unique status qua sociologists and focus almost exclusively on the preoccupations and concerns, not of sociology, but of public health. Pushed to an extreme, this becomes a "service relation" where sociological "theories, concepts and methods are used to support public health aims" (Mykhalovskiy et al., 2018, p. 3). In this situation, the scholarly autonomy of the social sciences is weakened in support of "applied public health reasoning and objectives" (Mykhalovskiy et al., 2018, p. 3). Using the example of population health intervention research (PHIR) (Bärnighausen, 2017; Hawe & Potvin, 2009) they suggest that sociology might become nothing more than "a kind of conceptual handmaiden – a reservoir of concepts that might fix a public health research problem" (Mykhalovskiy et al., 2018, p. 4).

In contrast, a sociology *of* public health retains far more critical distance from the public health enterprise. Mykhalovskiy and colleagues cite the work of Levinson (2005), for example, who sought to understand why there is often a tendency in public health (or at least applied public health policy making) to emphasize individual risk behaviors as opposed to the more structural causes of the health of populations. In this same vein, they go on to cite the examples of applications of the work of Bourdieu, Foucault, and Science and Technology Studies to a variety of public health issues where the emphasis is increasingly on offering a rather fundamental critique of some of the basic foundations of the public health enterprise (Mykhalovskiy et al., 2018, pp. 4–5). They raise concerns that, when pushed too far, the critique can become "a tendency to take pleasure in pointing out the failings of public health, while remaining relatively unencumbered by an obligation to help produce something that might work differently" (Mykhalovskiy et al., 2018, p. 5).

As an alternative to sociology in service of public health or a sociology that is hypercritical of public health, they then sketch a sociology *with* public health that draws on similar efforts to develop a sociology *with* medicine. They emphasize that this requires recognizing and addressing epistemological and ideational sources of difference and tension between public health and sociology. To oversimplify a complex argument, they draw simultaneously on Chantal Mouffe's work on agonism (Mouffe, 2000) and the applied case of tobacco control, Mykhalovskiy and colleagues explore the possibilities of a sociology *with* public health.

In summary, a sociology *in* public health puts the former in a service relationship with the latter and theories, concepts, and research methods of sociology are used instrumentally to address public health challenges. A sociology *of* public health, in contrast, is far more focused on public health as an object of study and, quite often, offering rather fundamental critiques of the failings of the public enterprise. A sociology *with* public health seeks to strike a new path that respects and engages with the epistemological foundations of each partner. In what follows, we will argue that much the same situation exists with respect to the relationship between political science and public health. Our goal is to situate the growing body of political science research on public health issues before moving on to consider the implications of this typology for debates about the role of scientific evidence in the making of public health policy.

3   A Typology of the Interaction of Public Health and Political Science

Despite the inherently political nature of public health and the fact that government action of all kinds (e.g., regulation, taxation, exhortation) is critical to addressing public health challenges, there are relatively few examples that suggest that public health scholars have a good understanding of how the insights of political science can shed light on the perennial challenges of public health. Similarly, even though they often develop a deep practical understanding of the realities of politics, most public health practitioners (or what has been described as the "government arm" of public health [Contandriopoulos, 2021]) have little or no formal training that is rooted in political science. Thus, the dominant trend is public health *without* political science (even as the public health workforce often seems to have an insatiable appetite for in-service learning opportunities on how government and politics work (Cairney, 2015)).

To make sense of the various possible relationships between political science and public health, Table 1 offers a preliminary overview of a political science in, of, and with public health as well as the status quo where public health is understood with little or no reference to political science.

Table 1 Political science for, of, and with public health

	Public health without political science	Political science in public health	Political science of public health	Political science with public health
Goals	Advance public health	Advance public health by instrumentally using political science concepts	Advance political science theory building and conceptual development	Advance both political science and public health with mutual learning
Accept the inherent legitimacy of politics	No	Partially	High	High
Deploy the range of political science theory and research	No	Instrumental to explain public health policy outcomes	Empirically to explain lack of public health progress	Collaborative and integrated
Public health as a case study	NA	NA	High	Possible
Commitment to the broader public health project	High	High	Unlikely/Low	Medium–High
Embrace of core themes of public health:				
policy must be based on scientific evidence	High	Medium	Low	Low
primacy of health	High	High	Low	Low
social justice	High	High	Low	Medium
Research will appear:	Public health journals	Public health journals	Political science journals	Both public health and political science journals

The first point of comparison is the extent to which theory and concepts from political science are used instrumentally (see Chapter 11 [Cairney et al., 2022]) to better understand public health, or to borrow from Mykhalovskiy et al., political science is nothing more than a "conceptual handmaiden" to public health. The second point of comparison is whether and to what extent the research accepts the inherent legitimacy and autonomy of politics. The third point of comparison is one of breadth: Following Greer and colleagues (S. L. Greer et al., 2017), does the relationship consider the depth and breadth of theorizing and empirical research in political science? The fourth comparator is whether and to what extent public health and issues arising in public health are the raw material for a case study of a broader theoretical, conceptual, or empirical concern of political science. The fifth comparator is the extent of the shared commitment to the core principles that inform the public health enterprise. Public health scholarship and practice are built on the foundation of science, the primacy of health, and social justice. The first of these refers to a deep commitment to the primacy of science and scientific evidence. The second refers to the pattern of asserting that population health is the most important goal of a society, a form of health essentialism, or what Coggon refers to as "health theocracy" (Coggon, 2012, pp. 193–200) that is to say the deep-rooted conviction that the most important goal of a good society is and must be the protection and promotion of health. On this view when, inevitably, there is a conflict between health and other societal goals (e.g., freedom, economic growth, national security), health should prevail. The third core principle refers to the oft-repeated commitment of public health to some overarching vision of social justice which, more recently, has become a deep-rooted commitment to health equity. The final point of comparison is a more pragmatic one that is about the intended audience for scholarly work produced in each category, as described by the forum where the research from each perspective is likely to appear.

3.1 Public Health *Without* Political Science

It is critical to emphasize that much theoretical, conceptual, and practical work in public health is done with no reference to political science in general or its various sub-disciplines and approaches. While there is a widespread acceptance that there is a political dimension to public health (this is where Virchow is usually quoted (see Chapter 1 in this volume

[Fafard et al., 2022])), there is typically little perceived need to draw on the systematic study of politics (and by extension, no need to try and draw on the full range of tools and insights of political science). This may be because the dominant view of politics in public health (or at least in academic public health) does not accept the inherent legitimacy and autonomy of politics. Typically, in public health scholarship "politics" and "ideology" or a "lack of political will" (see Chapter 3 [S. Greer, 2022]) are the enemies of the public health enterprise. Politics thus becomes a problem to be solved. While this is a common view among public health practitioners and scholars alike, the latter, as they gain experience and seniority, often develop an appreciation of the necessity and utility of politics and how to advance public health goals in ways that accept if not embrace political realities (see Chapter 13 [Cassola et al., 2022]).

For public health researchers, on the other hand, it is quite common to continue to see politics as nothing more than something that gets in the way of evidence-based or at least evidence-informed decision making. On this account, the making of public policy is like other forms of decision making and the knowledge translation or knowledge transfer tools that are useful in medicine and public health practice can easily be repurposed for making public policy (for a contrasting view see Fafard & Hoffman, 2018). In this space the commitment to the broader public health project is very high as is the embrace of the core themes of public health: scientific primacy, health essentialism, and social justice. Of necessity, the only possible venue for scholarly research in this tradition is public health journals.

3.2   Political Science *in* Public Health

To the extent that there is within academic public health a recognition of political science, often the relationship is one of a political science *in* public health. As with a sociology *in* public health, the goal of studies in this tradition is to shed light on the challenges facing public health per se. They do not seek to advance political science as a discipline or, more precisely, test or at least refine political science theories. While this is not, in of itself, a problem, it also means that political science concepts and theories are used in a rather naïve, instrumental manner. They are invoked almost tactically to try and explain how and why politics and ideology get in the way of a proper, evidence-based policy process. Moreover, the use of political science is often quite "loose"—concepts and theories are referred to almost metaphorically. So, for example, while Kingdon's multiple streams theory is very popular in the public health literature, researchers often pay little or no attention to the role of policy entrepreneurs, and few studies examine the evolution of the theory over time. Yet for others, Kingdon is popular because, as Greer and colleagues have noted, the multiple streams approach is one of the few that allows for agency and allows analysts to position public health actors to imagine themselves as skilled policy entrepreneurs (S. L. Greer et al., 2017). In their words, "Despite the empirical power of multiple streams analysis, excessive use of it risks reinforcing the focus on heroism and voluntarism in the public health literature by suggesting that sheer will, sufficiently adept framing or policy entrepreneurship leads to the adoption of policies" (S. L. Greer et al., 2017, p. 42). Kingdon is also commonly used in public health to try and understand why "politics" is getting in the way of evidence-based policy and program change. The politics stream is identified but is perceived as an impediment as opposed to a necessary part of representative democracy.

However, even when there is selected reference to political science theory, too little attention is paid to more basic but powerfully important features of policymaking at all levels. Again, see Greer and colleagues for a discussion of the need to consider the powerful shaping roles of federalism and other basic features of how power is shared (e.g., Westminster vs. congressional systems) (S. L. Greer et al., 2017). Thus, as with sociology, in a political science in public health, political science as a discipline risks being not much more than a source of concepts (e.g., policy cycle, policy window, securitization) or theories (e.g., multiple streams; policy transfer) that are deployed instrumentally to, again, fix a public health research problem (Mykhalovskiy et al., 2018).

3.3   Political Science *of* Public Health

Of course, the salience and importance of many of the core issues facing the public health enterprise—think COVID-19, Ebola, tobacco control—means that there is an independent body of scholarship and analysis that is rooted, not in public health per se, but in political science. The most common form of this is public health as case study. In this case, to advance research on a concern of political science there is a case study drawn from public health. The primary focus of the research is not necessarily public health per se, it is advancing our collective political science understanding of politics and government. This includes, for example, electoral studies (Mattila et al., 2013; Zeitoun et al., 2019), the policymaking process (see, e.g., Givel, 2006; Pacheco, 2017), the changing nature of international relations, or the capability approach to social justice (see Chapter 12; Holt & Frohlich, 2022; Prah Ruger & Mitra, 2015; Saith, 2011). Of course, this perspective rarely exists in its pure form—in many cases there is some degree of concern with advancing public health scholarship if not public health goals. This approach to a public health political science has dramatically increased since 2020 as political science seeks to make sense of the politics and governance of the COVID-19 pandemic.

3.4   *Political Science with Public Health*

The final approach, a political science *with* public health, is, we would submit, the dominant one among political science scholars who do research on public health subjects (at least before the COVID-19 pandemic). Political science theories, concepts, and tools are not simply used instrumentally to inform some broader public health goals. It is taken as axiomatic that there is an inherent legitimacy to politics and political institutions. Politics is much more than something that gets in the way of doing good (public health) policy. However, unlike a simple political science critique of public health, a political science with public health tries to find ways to reconcile the realities of politics with the goals of public health.

What perhaps distinguishes a political science *with* from a political science simply *of* public health is the commitment to the broader public health project. Research that is meant to be political science *with* public health must, necessarily, have some minimal degree of interest in, if not commitment to, the broad goals of the public health enterprise. A political science *with* public health will also be interested in the core themes of public health—use of scientific evidence, social justice, health essentialism—but will take a variable and often critical perspective. For example, one can be sympathetic to the desire to ensure that public health policy is informed by the best available scientific evidence but for this to happen a sophisticated conception of the nature and role of evidence in representative democracies is required (see the chapters in Part II of this volume). Similarly, while it is likely that a political science with public health will be based in a broad agreement on the importance of health as an overriding societal goal, the approach will be critical and self-aware. In this case, a critical contribution of political science might be to emphasize and explain what health essentialism entails, why it is a matter of considerable philosophical debate, and critically consider the many practical implications for what governments do and do not do when it comes to making policy and program choices. To take one concrete example, a political science with public health will seek to draw attention to the fact that much of the academic public health critique of how governments have responded to the COVID-19 pandemic assumes shared agreement that maximizing population health is the most important goal for governments when, in fact, inside government and in civil society more generally, this is a matter for debate and discussion.

A political science *with* public health is most clearly prominent in international relations where there is an important and growing body of research on global health governance and global health security (see, e.g., Hindmarch, 2016; Lee & Kamradt-Scott, 2014; McInnes, 2020; Parker & García, 2018; Rushton & Youde, 2014). One can also find examples of a political science *with* public health for selected public health issues including tobacco control (Breton et al., 2006; Cairney, 2007; Studlar & Cairney, 2014), health promotion, (Clavier & de Leeuw, 2013), so-called health in all or joined up policies (Baum et al., 2013; see Chapter 11 [Cairney et al., 2022]; Carey, 2016; Chapter 12 [Holt & Frohlich, 2022]) and collaboration more generally (Fierlbeck, 2010). More recently, there are studies of pandemic response that are broadly consistent with a political science *with* public health (S. Greer et al., 2021).

4 IMPLICATIONS FOR THINKING ABOUT THE ROLE OF EVIDENCE IN THE MAKING OF PUBLIC HEALTH POLICY

In a public health *without* political science, there is a tendency emphasize the baseline proposition that public health policy should be evidence-based or, at least, evidence-informed. Of course, senior public health officials learn from experience the limits of what can be accomplished by relying too heavily on the "best available evidence" as the sole or at least the primary tool to make the case for policy and program change. However, this can often give rise to conflict within public health organizations as highly trained staff at the lower levels becomes frustrated that senior executives or the minister does not pay sufficient heed to what the evidence says the government should do. Moreover, in a public health *without* political science, the lack of evidence-based public policy is often explained by invoking a rather pejorative view of politics or making more and less sophisticated references to "political will," "ideology," or neoliberalism (Bell & Green, 2016; Fishbeyn, 2015; Fox et al., 2017). For example, Brownson et al. refer to politics, a lack of political will, and special interests as barriers to evidence-based policymaking (Brownson et al., 2009). Similarly, in a study on the taxation of sugary beverages in the USA asked "why is this policy not supported by several States even though it is underpinned by evidence?" (Roberto et al., 2015). A public health *without* political science is also likely to preoccupy with conventional approaches to knowledge translation that emphasize process (e.g., plain-language summaries, knowledge brokers, bringing public health scientific expertise inside government, etc.). However, the premise often remains one of a knowledge deficit, that governments would act differently and make different choices if they were fully aware of the best available scientific evidence.

In marked contrast, in a political science *in* public health, while there will be more critical perspective on the role that scientific evidence does and does not play in the making of public health policy, it may be restricted to pointing out how evidence is but one factor among many that influences public health policy. This is one of the core messages of the papers in Part II of this volume. Note, however, there is a risk is that the role of political science, or at least a political science perspective, is reduced to explaining how to be ever more sophisticated in giving the best available science some influence on policymaking or in how governments and international organizations can organize science advice (Gluckman & Wilsdon, 2016; Wilsdon, 2014). Alternatively, when we are talking about non-state actors who wish to influence public policy, the role of political science is reduced to an offering an instrumental guide to how politics and government work. At worst, this becomes political science as lobbying advice.

A political science *with* public health is arguably one that joins a strong commitment to the broader public health project with a sophisticated account of the role that scientific evidence does and does not play in the making of public health policy. This is by far the dominant perspective in the public policy literature on public health particularly that which deals with the role of evidence in the making of public health policy.

5   CONCLUSION

In the necessary and inevitable post-mortem on the government response to the COVID-19 pandemic, there are calls to get "politics" out of evidence-based public health policy. From the perspective of political science, this is both impossible and undesirable. While the senior public health leaders in government understand this by virtue of experience, public health scholars are slower to accept this as demonstrated by both what is so often taught in schools of public health and their interventions in the public square. There is thus something of a stalemate between competing views about the role that politics and evidence in the making of public health policy. To foster a rapprochement between the two disciplines this essay proposes a typology of the possible interactions between political science and public health: political science *without, in, of,* and ideally *with* public health. Each interaction has often distinct assumptions about the goal of studying public health policy, the legitimacy of politics, the commitment to the core themes of public health that focus on science, the primacy of health, and the importance of health equity if not social justice. We make the case for a political science *with* public health that, as others have argued for sociology, recognizes the epistemological and ideational sources of difference and tension between public health and political science. Rather than asking public health leaders to learn about politics on the job, the goal is to foster a new, more integrated account of public health policy that can be shared with students who will be the public health leaders of tomorrow.

REFERENCES

Badgley, R. F., Mitton, G. T., Carpenter, H., Robinson, C. E. A., Robertson, E. C., Goodacre, R. H., Jones, T. L., Doughty, J. H., & Osborne, J. E. (1963). Social sciences and public health. *Canadian Journal of Public Health / Revue Canadienne de Sante'e Publique, 54*(4), 147–163.

Bärnighausen, T. (2017). Population health intervention research: Three important advancements. *International Journal of Public Health, 62*, 841. https://doi.org/10.1007/s00038-017-0985-2

Baum, F., Lawless, A., & Williams, C. (2013). Health in all policies from international ideas to local implementation: Policies, systems, and organizations. In C. Clavier & E. de Leeuw (Eds.), *Health promotion and the policy process* (pp. 189–217). Oxford University Press.

Bell, K., & Green, J. (2016). On the perils of invoking neoliberalism in public health critique. *Critical Public Health, 26*(3), 239–243. https://doi.org/10. 1080/09581596.2016.1144872

Breton, E., Richard, L., Gagnon, F., Jacques, M., & Bergeron, P. (2006). Fighting a tobacco-tax rollback: A political analysis of the 1994 cigarette contraband crisis in Canada. *Journal of Public Health Policy, 27*(1), 77–99. https://doi.org/10.1057/palgrave.jphp.3200060

Brownson, R. C., Fielding, J. E., & Maylahn, C. M. (2009). Evidence-based public health: A fundamental concept for public health practice. *Annual Review of Public Health, 30*(1), 175–201. https://doi.org/10.1146/annurev. publhealth.031308.100134

Cairney, P. (2007). A 'multiple lenses' approach to policy change: The case of tobacco policy in the UK1. *British Politics, 2*(1), 45–68. https://doi.org/10. 1057/palgrave.bp.4200039

Cairney, P. (2015). How can policy theory have an impact on policy making? The role of theory-led academic-practitioner discussions. *Teaching Public Administration, 33*(1), 22–39. https://doi.org/10.1177/0144739414532284

Cairney, P., Mitchell, H., & St Denny, E. (2022). Addressing the expectations gap in preventative public health and 'health in all policies': How can policy theory help? In P. Fafard, A. Cassola, & E. De Leeuw (Eds.), *Integrating science and politics for public health*. Palgrave Springer.

Carey, G. (2016). *Grassroots to government: Creating joined-up working in Australia*. Melbourne University Press.

Cassola, A., Fafard, P., Nagi, R., & Hoffman, S. J. (2022). Tensions and opportunities in the roles of senior public health officials. *Health Policy*.

Clavier, C., & De Leeuw, E. (Eds.). (2013). *Health promotion and the policy process*. Oxford University Press.

Coggon, J. (2012). *What makes health public? A critical evaluation of moral, legal, and political claims in public health*. Cambridge University Press.

Contandriopoulos, D. (2021). The year public health lost its soul: A critical view of the COVID-19 response. *Canadian Journal of Public Health, 112*(6), 970–972. https://doi.org/10.17269/s41997-021-00583-8

de Leeuw, E., Clavier, C., & Breton, E. (2014). Health policy—Why research it and how: Health political science. *Health Research Policy and Systems, 12*(1). https://doi.org/10.1186/1478-4505-12-55

Fafard, P., de Leeuw, E., & Cassola, A. (2022). Introduction: Virchow revisited on the importance of public health political science. In P. Fafard, A. Cassola, & E. De Leeuw (Eds.), *Integrating science and politics for public health*. Palgrave Springer.

Fafard, P., & Hoffman, S. J. (2018). Rethinking knowledge translation for public health policy. *Evidence & Policy: A Journal of Research, Debate and Practice*. https://doi.org/10.1332/174426418X15212871808802

Fierlbeck, K. (2010). Public health and collaborative governance. *Canadian Public Administration, 53*(1), 1–19. https://doi.org/10.1111/j.1754-7121. 2010.00110.x

Fishbeyn, B. (2015). When ideology trumps: A case for evidence-based health policies. *The American Journal of Bioethics, 15*(3), 1–2. https://doi.org/10. 1080/15265161.2015.1019781

Fox, A. M., Feng, W., & Yumkham, R. (2017). State political ideology, policies and health behaviors: The case of tobacco. *Social Science & Medicine, 181,* 139–147. https://doi.org/10.1016/j.socscimed.2017.03.056

Givel, M. (2006). Punctuated equilibrium in Limbo: The tobacco lobby and U.S. state policymaking from 1990 to 2003. *Policy Studies Journal, 34*(3), 405–418. https://doi.org/10.1111/j.1541-0072.2006.00179.x

Gluckman, P., & Wilsdon, J. (2016). From paradox to principles: Where next for scientific advice to governments? *Palgrave Communications, 2,* 16077.

Greer, S. (2022). Professions, data, and political will. In P. Fafard, A. Cassola, & E. De Leeuw (Eds.), *Integrating science and politics for public health.* Palgrave Springer.

Greer, S., King, E., Massard da Fonseca, E., & Peralta-Santos, A. (2021). Coronavirus politics: The comparative politics and policy of COVID-19. *University of Michigan Press.* https://doi.org/10.3998/mpub.11927713

Greer, S. L., Bekker, M., de Leeuw, E., Wismar, M., Helderman, J.-K., Ribeiro, S., & Stuckler, D. (2017). Policy, politics and public health. *European Journal of Public Health, 27*(suppl_4), 40–43. https://doi.org/10.1093/eurpub/ ckx152

Hawe, P., & Potvin, L. (2009). What is population health intervention research? *Canadian Journal of Public Health, 100*(1), I8–I14.

Hindmarch, S. (2016). *Securing health: HIV and the limits of securitization.* Routledge, Taylor & Francis Group.

Holt, D., & Frohlich, K. L. (2022). Moving beyond health in all policies: Exploring how policy could front and centre the reduction of social inequities in health. In P. Fafard, A. Cassola, & E. De Leeuw (Eds.), *Integrating science and politics for public health.* Palgrave Springer.

Kickbusch, I. (2015). The political determinants of health—10 years on. *BMJ, 350*(jan08 2), h81–h81. https://doi.org/10.1136/bmj.h81

Lee, K., & Kamradt-Scott, A. (2014). The multiple meanings of global health governance: A call for conceptual clarity. *Globalization and Health, 10*(1), 28. https://doi.org/10.1186/1744-8603-10-28

Levinson, R. (2005, August 19). *Issues at the interface of medical sociology and public health.* Modernity, Medicine and Health. https://doi.org/10.4324/ 9780203980651-9

Mattila, M., Söderlund, P., Wass, H., & Rapeli, L. (2013). Healthy voting: The effect of self-reported health on turnout in 30 countries. *Electoral Studies, 32*(4), 886–891.

McInnes, C. (2020). Global health governance. In C. McInnes, K. Lee, & J. Youde (Eds.), *The Oxford handbook of global health politics* (pp. 263–279). Oxford University Press. https://doi.org/10.1093/oxfordhb/978019 0456818.013.17

Mouffe, C. (2000). *The democratic paradox.* Verso.

Mykhalovskiy, E., Frohlich, K. L., Poland, B., Di Ruggiero, E., Rock, M. J., & Comer, L. (2018). Critical social science *with* public health: Agonism, critique and engagement. *Critical Public Health,* 1–12. https://doi.org/10.1080/ 09581596.2018.1474174

Pacheco, J. (2017). Free-riders or competitive races? Strategic interaction across the American states on tobacco policy making. *State Politics & Policy Quarterly, 17*(3), 299–318. https://doi.org/10.1177/1532440017705150

Parker, R., & García, J. (Eds.). (2018). *Routledge handbook on the politics of global health* (1st ed.). Routledge. https://doi.org/10.4324/9781315297255

Prah Ruger, J., & Mitra, S. (2015). Health, disability and the capability approach: An introduction. *Journal of Human Development and Capabilities, 16*(4), 473–482. https://doi.org/10.1080/19452829.2015.1118190

Roberto, C. A., Swinburn, B., Hawkes, C., Huang, T., Costa, S. A., Ashe, M., Zwicker, L., Cawley, J. H., & Brownell, K. D. (2015). Patchy progress on obesity prevention: Emerging examples, entrenched barriers, and new thinking. *The Lancet, 385*(9985), 2400–2409. https://doi.org/10.1016/ S0140-6736(14)61744-X

Rushton, S., & Youde, J. (Eds.). (2014). *Routledge handbook of global health security.* Routledge.

Saith, R. (2011). A public health perspective on the capability approach. *Journal of Human Development and Capabilities, 12*(4), 587–594.

Straus, R. (1957). The nature and status of medical sociology. *American Sociological Review, 22*(2), 200. https://doi.org/10.2307/2088858

Studlar, D. T., & Cairney, P. (2014). Conceptualizing punctuated and non-punctuated policy change: Tobacco control in comparative perspective. *International Review of Administrative Sciences.* https://doi.org/10.1177/002 0852313517997

Tilson, H., & Berkowitz, B. (2006). The public health enterprise: Examining our twenty-first-century policy challenges. *Health Affairs (project Hope), 25*(4), 900–910. https://doi.org/10.1377/hlthaff.25.4.900

Wilsdon, J. (2014). The past, present and future of the chief scientific advisor. *European Journal of Risk Regulation, 5*(3), 293–299.

Zeitoun, J.-D., Faron, M., de Vaugrigneuse, S., & Lefèvre, J. H. (2019). Health as an independent predictor of the 2017 French presidential voting behaviour: A cross-sectional analysis. *BMC Public Health, 19*(1), 1–10.

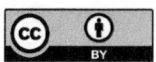

CHAPTER 3

Professions, Data, and Political Will: From the Pandemic Toward a Political Science with Public Health

Scott Greer

1 Prologue: Fermentation and Science

Early in the bleak month of July 2020, a team of researchers lightened the mood when they published "Association between consumption of fermented vegetables and Coronavirus 2019 (COVID-19) mortality at a country level in Europe" (Fonseca et al., 2020). The manuscript, a preprint, claimed to find that fermented food consumption predicted lower COVID-19 mortality.

There was much to criticize about this article. Even the title is wrong, given that its independent variables included fermented dairy as well as vegetable products. Country-level analysis obscured within-country heterogeneity. Its dependent variable was endogenous to the political

S. Greer (✉)
School of Public Health, University of Michigan, Ann Arbor, MI, USA
e-mail: slgreer@umich.edu

© The Author(s) 2022
P. Fafard et al. (eds.), *Integrating Science and Politics for Public Health*,
Palgrave Studies in Public Health Policy Research,
https://doi.org/10.1007/978-3-030-98985-9_3

system since COVID-19 mortality data is a function of testing avail-ability and reporting policies. Its sparse controls entirely excluded politics and policy (there were stringent lockdowns in a number of central and eastern European countries with high consumption of fermented foods, but once those countries eased their non-pharmaceutical interventions, their second wave mortality in autumn was horrific) (Löblovà et al., 2021). Fermented food never gained much attention as an explanation for COVID-19 mortality, though the authors at least got their journal publication (Bousquet et al., 2021).

The reason to discuss this paper, one small flake in a blizzard of COVID-19 preprints, is that it is a memorable caution. It reminds us all just how wrong research can go when it crosses into new areas, and thereby gives us all a teachable moment: how can researchers avoid the kinds of traps that the fermented food researchers fell into? (de Leeuw, 2009) The outlandish hypothesis might seem easy enough to avoid, but before we dismiss it, consider the amount of political science scholarship on COVID-19 that pays too little attention to the fact that COVID-19 data are endogenous to the political outcomes they putatively measure. Before dismissing its lack of policy variables, consider the amount of public health scholarship that simply neglects well-established political variables, including social policy measures and elite cueing, in explana-tions of COVID-19 outcomes. And consider the risk that in something as complex as the pandemic, it could be possible that a powerful expla-nation of mortality might be an immunological pattern entirely outside the scope of social sciences (e.g., [Pretti et al., 2020], the plausibility of which I cannot judge, argues that the distribution of certain characteristics of immune systems explains differential mortality).

2   Introduction

The global pandemic that began in 2020 promised to teach us many things. One of the things it can help to teach us is about ways to do political science *with* public health. Put another way, how can we avoid political and public health equivalents of the fermented food hypothesis?

A political science with public health can work best if informed by a broad social-scientific understanding of both fields. This chapter, there-fore, takes its inspiration from not just political science but also sociology and Science and Technology Studies, a field which focuses on the social construction of facts and their flow through society (a good introduction to the field can be found in [Vinck, 2010]). In particular, focusing on the small-p politics of knowledge and scientific enterprise complements political scientists' preferred focus of the big-p politics of institutions, parties, and voters.

The chapter focuses on three issues that seem to be particular causes of disciplinary misunderstanding and potentially fruitful research. The first is the *professional authority of public health*, including the extent to which it has a clear domain of expertise that others in government and academia respect. How do we understand the political process by which public health policymakers or scholars try to establish an identified area of expertise which they dominate and which generalist policymakers respect? The second is the *politics of data*. Many political scientists discussing COVID-19 showed their poor preparation in epidemiology, which was not surprising or objectionable in itself. What was surprising was how frequently they failed to recognize that data are endogenous to the political process because the collection and coding of data of any kind are political decisions. The pandemic showed the potential value of viewing statistics as a dependent variable of the political process. Political scientists have given the politics of health data very little attention but could shed light on the topic by treating data as indicators of politics as well as whatever they are supposed to represent. The third is of the most contested concepts that can be found at the border of public health and political science: *political will*. "Political will" can seem to political scientists like a simple call for voluntarism without reference to incentives and constraints, but it might be that we can synthesize the practical public health search for a champion or advocate with the extensive political science research on the ways institutions locate and shape agency.

The chapter draws on our recent work on COVID-19 politics, in particular; that work is informed by a longer history of research on the politics of public health and communicable disease control (Greer, 2017a; Greer & Jarman, 2020; Greer & Kurzer, 2013; Greer & Mätzke, 2012) as well as new comparative research on the politics of the pandemic (Greer, Jarman, et al., 2020; Greer, King, et al., 2020; Greer et al., 2021).

3 THE POLITICAL STATUS OF THE PUBLIC HEALTH PROFESSION: ON TOP OR ON TAP?

Political science literature, to the limited extent that it engages with professionals, professionalism, and organized professions, tends to focus only on their operation as interest groups. But professionalism is one of the key tools used in modern society to "depoliticize" an area by taking it out of partisan politics, and thereby more fully institutionalizing it in some different arena of politics with its own distinctive behavior and sets of actors.

We can view professions, for the purposes of understanding public health politics, as groups of people engaged in an effort to institutionalize a domain of action and expertise as theirs to define. This domain is intellectual as well as practical and can also be certified by law, so while it is possible for non-lawyers to appear in court in many countries, the intellectual and social dominance of lawyers means such people will probably fare poorly, and it is normally illegal in most jurisdictions for non-surgeons to perform surgery.

Since the political science literature on professions in politics is so sparse, it is reasonable to borrow from the much better entrenched field of the sociology of the professions. Viewing public health as a profession, using literature from the sociology of the professions, might help us to understand some of the much-lamented challenges faced in improving the connection between political and public health thought.

It is axiomatic in sociological studies of the professions that they—and their individual members—tend to fall into hierarchical relationships. Equality between professions that have much to do with each other is rare and produces friction; law and medicine might be a good example. Professions and professionals' typical relationship is summarized by the phrase "on top or on tap."[1] On top means that the members of that profession decide what kind of situation they are in and what action and expertise is needed. On tap means that they are available to help. A doctor orders a test, a treatment, and a prescription; the technician does the test, the nurse does the treatment, and the pharmacist delivers the prescription. The doctor is on top and the others on tap. Being on top is about having the right to define the nature of the situation and the allocation of skills. This tendency to seek hierarchy, born of an entirely natural professional perspective and socialization, means that interprofessional work on a basis of equality is famously difficult (e.g., [Bridges et al., 2011]).

---

[1] The phrase seems to have its origins with Irish writer George William Russell and, unsurprisingly, ended up attributed to Winston Churchill. Many of its uses have apparently been a dictum that experts *should* be on tap vis-a-vis politicians, not on top. See: https://quoteinvestigator.com/2019/01/26/expert/.

Andrew Abbott created a sophisticated and more formal version of this insight in his *System of Professions* (Abbott, 1994). In his model, professions are not so much characterized by formal institutions (education, certification, self-government) as by their ability to sustain a claim to expertise over a given domain of activity. Sustaining a claim requires a system of abstract thought, since abstraction is what allows professions and professionals to adapt and maintain their claim to expertise even as problems, context, and technology change. Over time they can expand the domain of their members, whether through entrenching professional activities in law, advising government, or incorporating fields of research previously occupied by others. They can also acquire dominance over policy areas not strictly related to their expertise. One salient example is the justifiably contested extent to which pregnancy and childbirth is a suitable area for medicalization (Wagner, 1997). Another is the way medical associations in many countries have leveraged their public credibility and professional power into influence over topics like payment systems that do not, strictly speaking, require a medical degree to understand (for two excellent US studies with general applicability[Laugesen, 2016; Patashnik et al., 2020]).

Professions and specialties or disciplines within them are constantly engaged in border wars, such as economists' regular invasions of the domains of other social sciences. Border conflicts are thus endemic to the system of professions and between specialists within a profession (e.g., between medical specialists) (Rozier et al., 2020; Zetka, 2003). Successful professions (and specialties within them, e.g., medical specialties or academic disciplines) nonetheless have a core domain within which they are largely untouchable, with efforts to occupy that domain not ratified by legal, scholarly, or bureaucratic actors. Political scientists and economists both write about all sorts of topics, but in areas such as electoral behavior and political institutions, political scientists dominate while economists dominate macroeconomic discussions.

Some professions—which Glazer called the "minor professions"—are structurally subordinate (as with pharmacy or nursing) and frequently feminized, while leaders and practitioners of others, such as public health or education, are constantly engaged in disputes about the nature and scope of their professional authority (Glazer, 1974). The status of profession tails off into occupations, but it is noteworthy how many and how often organized occupations try to stake out a professional domain. Studies of all sorts of occupations regularly note their efforts to establish both the formal accoutrements of a profession (licensing, postgraduate degrees, accreditation) and a claim to both a domain of expertise and an abstract body of knowledge.

Framing public health as a profession—and political science as a field within an established profession, academia—helps to highlight some of the barriers to collaboration and thereby points out possible routes. In *intellectual and academic* terms, public health is an interdisciplinary enterprise. While epidemiology is largely native to public health, other fields found in public health schools, from economics to toxicology to medicine, are simultaneously institutionalized elsewhere. As Glazer notes, and Rojas neatly demonstrated decades later, leading scholars of the minor fields will frequently have their terminal degrees in some more prestigious field and frequently publish there (Glazer, 1974; Rojas, 2010). To some extent this is a useful division of labor. Higher-status disciplinary researchers such as political scientists develop theoretical and empirical tools for understanding politics, while researchers in public health develop tools for making and implementing public health policies. But in a system of hierarchical professions, the result is a fault line through public health education. The status and intellectual drive points to doing political science *of* public health even if the whole point of a School of Public Health, its students, and its funding is probably to do political science *in* public health. The resulting tensions are part of everyday life for people who work anywhere near the nexus of political science, or any social science, and public health. We can, however, give thanks that the weakly disciplinary nature of public health admits social scientists. Political scientists or any other non-medical field can have a much harder time in medical schools, where they are inevitably very subordinate (political science *in* medicine).

In *formal and legal terms* public health's professional closure varies around the world but is usually low. In the UK, for example, at the core of public health is a medical subspecialty, one that is not especially well regarded, but a large part of the public health workforce, including people at the relatively significant level of Directors of Public Health, does not have medical training. Arguments about whether public health's professional bodies should specify a particular kind of training are a long-standing and tiresome feature of England's public health history. France has a similar story: the elite of the public health workforce are medical doctors, but public health doctors are so few as to leave much of the system staffed by non-doctors. In the US public health is not a medical field; a doctor can pursue a Master's in Public Health (MPH) but that is no different from a doctor who pursues a degree in public policy or history. Lack of professional closure means that an MPH does not provide access to any particular kind of job or power in the way that a social work, law, or medical degree does. Most of the US public health workforce does not have any formal public health training, let alone an MPH (Leider et al., 2020).

The upshot is that public health has a very small domain and a huge area of ambition. Activities that were bundled with public health at the turn of the twentieth century, meanwhile, have often moved off into other professional domains such as social work, and low-status ones such as restaurant inspection, water quality inspection, and health education have in various places been cut away from formal public health agencies with no apparent loss to the status of public health. For example, in the UK, social work split off from the responsibilities of Medical Officers of Health and "environmental health" took over sanitarian work in local government in 1974 with no apparent damage to food safety or even the prestige of its academic public health. What we might, following Patrick Fafard, call the "public administration of public health" and its relationships to other areas of public health such as policymaking and academia merits more, comparative and historical as well as contemporary, research.

The synthesis that has been most widely proposed worldwide in recent years focuses on establishment of a central public health agency which can advise policymakers and selectively reinforce other parts of government (there is even an association to promote such "Public Health Institutes," headquartered in Atlanta and supported by the Bill & Melinda Gates Foundation). This internationally advocated model, which has echoes in many traditions, is of an elite set of disease detectives trained in some combination of microbiology and epidemiology whose expertise is the control of communicable and perhaps the prevention of noncommunicable diseases (Binder et al., 2008; Frieden & Koplan, 2010; Myhre et al., 2020). A public health institute is loosely modeled on the US CDC and in country after country has "CDC" in its initials. It is a small body of highly trained people who can strengthen capacity (design surveillance systems), advise government, communicate, and do both science and field epidemiology when there is a crisis. It is akin to a fire department for public health—even if actually addressing a pandemic turns out to require something more like a bucket brigade, as Mätzke points out (Mätzke,

2012), with groups from police to doctors to the army involved in often improvised responses.

The problem for the professional and institutional project of public health is that the core of its domain since its modern foundation early in the twentieth century is the control of communicable diseases through non-pharmaceutical interventions such as masking or closures, and to some extent vaccination (Markel et al., 2007). Yet in a paradigmatic communicable disease outbreak that required NPIs, COVID-19, the striking thing we found in our cross-national study of 34 countries was the weakness of any claimed intellectual or formal monopoly of public health decision-making (Greer et al., 2021). Perhaps the fates of Public Health England (whose reorganization was brusquely announced in August 2020) or the US CDC (humbled by Donald Trumps' political appointees and blamed for confusing guidance under Joseph Biden) are especially humiliating. In country after country, though, the formal public health apparatus turned out to have nothing approaching dominance of science and public advice on communicable disease control. Top scientific or medical advisors were frequently prominent, but it seems that in most cases they were not formally trained or employed in public health and were far from being seen to dominate the definition of relevant knowledge.

It is easier to mention the exceptions to this broad pattern of sidelining. In a few counties, such as South Korea (Park 2021) and Colombia (Acosta et al., 2021), politicians made a very clear decision to gain authority and credibility precisely by standing behind their communicable disease control agency leaders. In Sweden, politicians respected the deeply entrenched autonomy of that country's agencies, in this case the state public health agency, and found themselves on an internationally unusual and much-debated course that might explain why Sweden had substantially higher excess mortality than its neighbours (Baldwin, 2021; Irwin, 2020). That was close to the whole list, though some subnational leaders did the same (e.g., British Columbia and Nova Scotia). In most countries, heads of government initially centralized power unto themselves, convening ad hoc committees for advice (Greer, et al., 2022; Jarman, et al., 2020; Greer, King, et al., 2020). In most places public health officials and researchers did not enjoy any kind of specialist monopoly or even dominance of a domain in the eyes of practitioners of other disciplines or heads of government, and were relegated to part of the answer and solution. Intellectually, legally, and organizationally, public health was sidelined by top politicians when they sought advice, frequently replaced by a mixture of more prestigious medical and scientific experts and administrative figures (Rozenblum, 2021).

We might expect this. Fox divides government into generalists and specialists (Fox, 2017). Generalists are the politicians, especially heads of government and executives, and their core staff, who typically cluster around the head of government and perhaps the finance ministry. They specialize in running the country—and in staying in office by winning elections. Good senior staff will usually support politicians in making policies that win elections. This means allocating time, energy, and money between priorities. Everybody else is a specialist, whether they work in public health or any other field. Establishing professional dominance over government activity is hard because it requires that generalist government cede its core power, which is the power to decide priorities between specialists. An independent central bank is a perfect example of a high level of formal autonomy for specialists (Adolph, 2013); the military is often an interesting case because of high esteem for its leaders and expertise combined with an urgent constitutional case for civilian, generalist, oversight of its activities. Professionalism is a way to buttress a claim to a putatively depoliticized area of domination—a claim that the profession, added to institutional frameworks, will produce consistent enough policy to justify a loss of generalist power and a displacement of politics into a distinctive professional realm. (Adolph shows that central bank appointments are highly political, but the politics look different because of the autonomy of central banking.) Put another way, it is a claim that the professions will do a good enough and predictable enough job to merit autonomy. It turns out that public health agencies did not manage to establish enough of a domain of professional expertise to persuade generalists to let them lead or even dominate advice and communications in most countries.

For developing a political science with public health, the suggestion is that we need a research agenda on how and why public health took the intellectual, professional, legal, and bureaucratic form it took in different countries—a comparative politics of public health (for an effort in the EU context, see [Greer & Jarman, 2020]). That would give us a sense of the value and likely outcome of, for example, the "health security" movement or the Gates-led push for Public Health Institutes, and a better understanding of the interplay of generalist government, public health researchers and practitioners, and other professions such as medicine, and thereby show what might work to strengthen public health as an actor or policy goal.

4   THE POLITICS OF DATA

One of the most striking things about the interface between political science and public health in the 2020 pandemic was the extent to which it revealed the limits of empirical political science scholarship. Basic epidemiological data turned out to be not just new to political scientists but difficult to understand.

For example, test positivity should be easy to understand in the terms of political science: it is an indicator of a sampling problem. Test positivity reports the number of tests administered and reported that are positive. If it is above three or five percent, then it is likely that the test data is unreliable because testing is conditional on something else, such as a likely diagnosis. That might make the tests useful in clinical settings, but it means that the testing is not useful as a random sample that would give us population-level information. Test positivity was data about the test, not about the virus (Trump et al., 2020).

For a more serious problem, efforts to compare country outcomes were often hampered by using COVID-19 test data, whether it was case numbers, COVID-19 attributed mortality, or something similar. The problem is that *data are endogenous to politics*. Testing and surveillance systems of any kind are expensive, require resources and infrastructure, and can influence public behavior and political debate (Greer, 2017a). Not only do they require complex bureaucracies and data management systems, but they can also tread on the autonomy of individual doctors by inserting a public health rule on issues such as determining cause of death (e.g., if a patient with COVID-19 dies of a heart attack, attributing the death involves a decision that doctors might regard as part of their clinical decision space). Home testing gives individuals autonomy over data reporting and many public health systems might not even ask the public about at-home test results. The decisions to test, to gather data, and to report it are all political and therefore are dependent variables in themselves. Donald Trump certainly knew that.[2] Political scientists trying to understand COVID-19 ought to know it as well.

Thus, COVID-19 data for the United States for most of the pandemic were unreliable, as we can see from test positivity that was often above 5% and frequently in the double digits. At-home testing, a very useful tool for managing risk, also reduced the usefulness of case counts in any jurisdiction where they were common. As a result, the scale and patterns of the US outbreak were at best hazily understood. Meanwhile, there was no consistent rule in most states, let alone the country, for attribution of deaths (Rocco et al., 2021). It would therefore be hazardous, for example, to use COVID-19 infections or COVID-19 attributed deaths as dependent variables for studies of policy effects or behavior.[3] Instead, the behavior of governments, statistical agencies, health care organizations, and individual doctors signing death certificates is the right dependent variable. Data from testing are a clue for that study, not an indicator of government success or failure. The question should be why the United States' public health surveillance system, and its broader public health system, collapsed so dramatically, not what unreliable testing data says about the difference between two places in August or October. The further question might be: why didn't more countries invest in better surveillance and data presentation during the pandemic?

The logical extension is that COVID-19 data are no exception to what we might call Trench's Law, coined by Alan Trench in the context of comparative federalism: *data are useful or comparable but not both* (Greer, 2019). As a look at any existing data project, or a scan of the Science and Technology Literature will show, data are a political project and outcome. Data are expensive to gather, organize, and maintain. They require not just resources and money, but also a variety of forms of compliance, as

---

[2] There were multiple reported occasions when he explicitly tried to slow testing because he regarded reports of positive cases as bad for his political position. For one example, the *New York Times* reported him as saying that "I want to do what Mexico does. They don't give you a test till you go to the emergency room and you're vomiting" (Shear et al., 2021).

[3] For a particularly striking example of bad practice that somehow was published, and in a public health journal no less, consider this remark in an article on the politically salient topic of the epidemiologically consequences of Black Lives Matter protests in the United States in 2020: "Data for each parameter were readily available on the Google search engine by entering the name of the city and the parameters studied" (Valentine et al., 2020).

simple as people agreeing to response to surveys or as complex as agreeing to code complex clinical procedures, lab findings, and patient outcomes. A national rule for coding deaths took discretion away from individual doctors, with costs and benefits in terms of data quality.

For a good outcome variable, instead, we can use excess mortality. Excess mortality is calculated by taking an average of mortality—the deaths on a given day or week over the last five or ten years—and comparing it to mortality on that day in 2020. The spike in mortality would likely be attributable to the pandemic. Excess mortality might *understate* COVID-19 deaths, in fact, because nonpharmaceutical interventions such as business closures might reduce other causes of death such as drunken driving and construction work. Mortality and natality data are among the statistics that states are most likely to collect consistently and competently because they are enormously useful for taxation, conscription, disbursements such as pensions or conditional cash transfers, and all manner of government databases from driving licenses to passport issuance. That many states do not reliably collect them is interesting, but they are more likely to be reliably collected than most other data.

Excess mortality data are not perfect. It is slow. In most countries a death report must travel up a long chain, from a doctor's signature on a death certificate, through local government, figures such as coroners who might review deaths before reporting them, and then different levels of government that collect and collate death data. As a result, excess mortality is not widely reported in the popular media. It is a poor real-time guide to the progress of the pandemic or relevant policy. For a mixture of inevitable statistical and frustrating bureaucratic reasons, it will often lack detailed geographic or subgroup information. It also fails to reflect improving COVID-19 treatment and differential risks among infected people which meant that over the course of the pandemic the case fatality ratio and infection fatality ratios clearly changed. There is no fixed relationship between the number of people with the virus and the number of deaths. It is, however, probably the best statistic for political scientists to use in gauging the success or failure of pandemic response policies.

Beyond using excess mortality or other indicators to gauge the effects of government decisions, something that political scientists might wish to leave to epidemiologists, the problems with testing raise a series of important political science questions. Above all, what are the politics of surveillance? This is a topic on which remarkably little is known (Greer,

2017a). Why do governments collect the health data that they collect, what are the political forces for and against collection of such data, and how does data collection interact with practice? The effects of introducing electronic health records (EHRs), for example, are very well documented. They change practice in the service of managers and researchers who seek more information about clinical practice even if the results are unsatisfying to clinicians (Timmermans & Berg, 2003). An even better empirical issue is the collection, or non-collection, of information about racial and other disparities in COVID-19 infection and mortality. On one hand, the story of COVID-19 is in many ways a story of inequalities, but on the other hand it highlighted the politics of collecting data on inequality. The politics of racial data on every level are fraught. Not only do we have well-known cases such as what amounts to a ban on such data collection in France (Fredette, 2014), but on the individual level doctors' decisions about when to mention race reflects deep and often racist structures (Balderston et al., 2021).

Data and metrics shape perceptions of reality and all kinds of practice by making some things tangible and apparently manipulable—"what's measured is what's managed," as the dictum goes. In other words, what is measured is what is going to be managed. Once the measurement is good enough for managers, then it will be used even if, or because, it distorts reality and norms as perceived on the ground. This is why so many EHRs around the world are effectively billing systems that are hard to use for public health, research, or quality improvement. Those who can muster the monetary and organizational effort to impose EHRs are usually those interested above all in budgets. Likewise, part of the appeal of syndromic surveillance (such as testing wastewater for COVID or monitoring internet searches) is that it requires less bureaucratic investment because it draws on data that is easily collected (wastewater sampling) or already exists for another purpose (internet searches) (Fearnley, 2008a, 2008b; Ziemann, 2015).

Public health and medical researchers and leaders will often naturalize these data, partly through familiarity and partly because data shape theories and concepts (consider GDP, or unemployment, data full of value judgments, politics, and bureaucratic oddities which have nonetheless shaped the whole field of academic economics). It is also because of the determinedly apolitical style and culture of public health research. Pointing out the extent to which public health data is politically constructed is not part of the conventional public health style of apolitical expertise. For decades, historians and activists have documented and fought over surveillance (Fairchild, 2015; Fairchild & Bayer, 2015; Fairchild et al., 2007). The HIV pandemic, naturally, created enormous political contests about testing and privacy, with different jurisdictions creating very divergent testing and privacy regimes (Baldwin, 2005; Berridge, 1996). The public health literature nonetheless presents antiseptic and apolitical "good practice" as if surveillance systems were not in the middle of a hurricane of privacy, practice, legal, and coercive issues (Lee et al., 2010).

In short, a great many political scientists in 2020 and 2021 were floating empirical studies based on grievously flawed data. It might be frustrating that COVID-19 data are endogenous to politics—but we should really embrace that. Rather than competing with observational epidemiology to identify the effects of policies, it might be useful to look at how governments and others gathered and processed the data they had. The picture of the world that policymakers and researchers used throughout the pandemic was one shaped by expensive, flawed, and political data collection and management systems. The fact that so few countries meaningfully improved surveillance over a long pandemic is a political science puzzle. Data are a valuable object of political study in itself; rather than bemoaning data problems or pushing on regardless of data problems, we might study them. The data problem is the puzzle, and one that political scientists, with colleagues in sociology and STS, might explain.

Part of the contribution of political science with public health could be precisely in explaining why and how decisions about surveillance are inherently political. A political science with public health would share the overall goal of good surveillance data but would help model the proverbial hurricane of issues and tease out that issues and help identify which are real issues (e.g., privacy) and which are more in the order of pretexts for inaction or avoiding politically difficult issues (Patrick Fafard, personal communication, 2021).

5   Political Will and the Politics of Agency

"Political will" might be the phrase that most neatly marks the division between public health and political science researchers. To most public health researchers, it is crucial to making policy, and much of the practical education in politics that can be had in public health is geared toward finding and creating it. To most political scientists, it is wormwood. It seems to be a voluntaristic concept that ignores politicians' incentives and actual ability to act.

One way to approach this debate is to point out that some of the problem is terminological. Is it really that contrary to political science findings to point out that policies are more likely to be adopted and implemented when they have entrepreneurs and politicians *willing* to promote them? To simply call for political will, outside of an analysis of what is possible and desirable from the perspective of working politicians, is indeed quixotic. But is that what is really happening when public health practitioners are being taught advocacy and policy skills? Is it really fair to imply that advocacy classes for public health practitioners aren't discussing political incentives and constraints when they tutor students about ways to identify interested politicians and tailor the case to their situation? Kingdon's multiple streams analysis might be taught too often and unreflectively, and with too much attention to the policy entrepreneurs, but it is still a good theory (Greer, 2015; Kingdon, 2003). There is good applied political science *in* public health, and concepts like political will might often just be teaching tools. The problem that arises with simplifying teaching tools, of course, is that they might persist in people's heads—an analogy might be the simple and easily refutable models taught in introductory economics which no working economist would endorse but which pollute analysis of economies.

A more productive way to think about the problem might be in terms of the politics of agency. How is the ability to have political will distributed? Structurally, who has agency and how are they selected? Whose political will matter and why? This is a way to approach and synthesize an enormous volume of political science, especially the study of formal and informal institutions.

Thus, for example, presidentialism creates a distinctive politics of agency. A presidentialist system has, in Linz's definition, "an executive with considerable constitutional powers—generally including full control of the composition of the cabinet and administration—is directly elected by the people for a fixed term and is independent of parliamentary votes of confidence. [The president] is not only the holder of executive power but also the symbolic head of state and can be removed between elections only by the drastic step of impeachment. In practice...presidential systems may be more or less dependent on the cooperation of the legislature; the balance between executive and legislative power in such systems can thus vary considerably." Linz continued that "two things about presidential government stand out. The first is the president's strong claim to democratic, even plebiscitarian, legitimacy; the second is [the president's] fixed term in office" (Linz, 1990, pp. 52–53).

Linz's interest was in democratic stability, and of all the thousands of publications his insight inspired, most are likewise about regime stability and transitions rather than public policy (though public policy and domestic politics researchers are quite aware of the impact of presidents on public policy, e.g., [Skowronek, 1982]). Subsequent scholarship has qualified Linz's point by emphasizing the extent to which party systems and electoral rules change presidential powers, accountability, and incentives (Elgie, 2005; Mainwaring & Shugart, 1997). But Linz's point has power for understanding who mattered in COVID-19 response. The analysis above suggests that presidents as diverse as Jair Bolsonaro, Emmanuel Macron, Joe Biden, and Donald Trump would wield tremendous power during the emergency of the pandemic. They would have concentrated agency with limited accountability and use it for better or for worse—whether to act, to not act, or to shift credit and blame.

Presidents in presidentialist systems have not been the only leaders whose leadership counted in the pandemic. We can rescue another hoary and much-debated concept: majoritarianism (Lijphart, 1984, 1999). Without endorsing all of Lijphart's coding decisions and his particular construction of the index, we can define majoritarianism in politics as a high score on two axes: the ease with which a single party can take control of government; and its ability to act once it has. Thus, for example, presidentialist France is very majoritarian. Emmanuel Macron's career demonstrates it. Consider the ease with which Macron could constitute a political party almost out of thin air, take the presidency and legislature a short time later, and make nearly unilateral decisions for the country. But other, especially Westminster political systems, are also highly majoritarian. A plurality of voters empowered Conservative governments to not just govern but take the UK out of the EU on very hard terms in Brexit. It is reasonable to argue that the Canadian prime minister is the most powerful executive in the west, constrained only by negotiations with provincial premiers who are equally dominant in their provinces.

Majoritarianism would mean, then, that agency lies in the central executive. The agency given to Boris Johnson, Scott Morrison, and Justin Trudeau meant that, like their presidential colleagues, their leadership and behavior were extremely important because they could be elected on a thin majority and make major changes.

This is not to say that majoritarian systems did better or worse in excess mortality during the crisis, though a number of the most flamboyantly questionable COVID-19 responses were majoritarian leaders—Jair Bolsonaro, Boris Johnson, Andrej Babiš, Narendra Modi, or Donald Trump. For each of them, there were in parallel (or "also") strongly empowered leaders who did not become known worldwide for ineffective responses—Justin Trudeau and Scott Morrison were highly empowered individual leaders who did not make strikingly bad policy, while a number of consensus democracies such as Sweden produced strikingly high excess mortality.

Federalism also redistributes agency by creating powerful elected general governments with constitutional status. They can create coordination problems and veto points, as much literature laments, but they can also create resilience by creating a second line of governments which can supplant a negligent or destructive federal government (as happened during the pandemic in Brazil, India, and the United States).

For our purposes, it simply means that the leaders of state or regional governments matter. This can be further divided by following Elazar's distinction between self-rule and shared rule in federalism (Elazar, 1987; Hooghe et al., 2010) (Greer et al., 2015). In federations with a high level of regional self-rule (autonomy), such as Brazil and the United States, they have spheres in which they can take their own actions, complicating and perhaps diversifying responses. High levels of shared rule, such as in Germany, create more consensual democracies since regional or state governments can shape the federal government's action.

Leadership clearly mattered during the COVID-19 pandemic, but it did not matter consistently because leaders do not matter consistently. More consensual democracies, even Westminster -descended ones with coalitions (e.g., Ireland, New Zealand), have leaders subject to more constraints who must aggregate interests within complex coalitions. *The importance of leadership is a dependent variable of formal and informal rules.* Thus, the behavior of some leaders mattered more than others. The hazard of leadership literature, like the hazard of writing about political will, is that it concentrates on the leader (in many cases because the target audience is would-be leaders). Both can perhaps be recovered by examining the circumstances under which political will and leadership matter, thereby creating a possible middle ground between political science theories, which tend to infer action from structure, and leadership theories, which tend to pay too much attention to the leaders at the expense of their circumstances.

One of the more successful political concepts in public health is that of the "decision space," which demarcates what governments can do in light of all their different constraints (Bossert, 1998; Greer, 2017b; Koivusalo, 2015). Its value is in its ability to synthesize political science findings into an immediately valuable concept that tells us what is possible, what the problems are, and what might be improved. The politics of agency might be a similarly useful concept. It is a tool for synthesizing vast amounts of political science, most of it developed for different purposes (e.g., understanding democratic stability and regime transitions) for identifying who can do what in different political systems and how that might change.

6   Conclusion

As the editors' introduction to this volume made clear, political science and public health scholarship can stand in different relationships to each other, with more or less productive results. A failure to connect clearly impairs both (Carpenter, 2012; de Leeuw, 2016; Fafard & Cassola, 2020; Gagnon et al., 2017; Gore & Parker, 2019). Part of the solution can lie in greater use of insights from STS and sociology about the ways that small-p politics and the construction and contestation of knowledge work and shape the priors of people focused on the big-p politics political scientists study.

This chapter set out to use the COVID-19 pandemic experience to think about three issues that might help in developing a public health with political science: the nature of public health's intellectual and professional status; the politics of public health data; and the nature of leadership and political will. In each case, the hope was to at least reduce misunderstanding, and to perhaps identify a productive research direction.

Public health, even among the "lesser professions," has an unusually small core domain (much of it low status and variable from country to country, e.g., restaurant inspection or health care for the indigent) combined with a tendency to intellectual imperialism. A field with an often-narrow set of bureaucratic responsibilities and political role has an intellectual superstructure of great ambition. The core of its domain, furthermore, is communicable disease control. In the pandemic, generalist policymakers showed little respect for public health claims to a monopoly in even that domain. In country after country, they sidelined or subordinated public health agencies and researchers, listening instead to ad hoc groups which often had limited public health representation.

Data preoccupy both political science and public health researchers, but this often means a focus on trying to work with imperfect data or bemoaning imperfections in available data. I suggest that what we need is research in political science, with public health, on the politics of data. Analyses of how data are generated and used have done much to illuminate the politics of different policy areas. Understanding the politics of data and surveillance might improve data as well as our understanding of politics and public administration.

Finally, political analysis within public health has a tendency that political scientists find frustrating to urge political will, as if finding a legislative champion is all one needs. I argue that a search for a champion, a leader, or for that matter a policy entrepreneur is a very rational advocacy strategy. Further, the COVID-19 pandemic reminds us that leadership matters in a way that sits badly with political science's structuralist tendencies. Much political science, particularly institutionalist research, can be read as study of the allocation of agency. Rather than thinking that political will or leadership is a property of the person, we might better think of it as a use of agency, which is unevenly distributed within and between political systems, and regard the distribution of agency as part of the explanation of when leadership mattered and what happened during the pandemic.

I opened this chapter with reference to a particularly unfortunate piece of health research. It is a cautionary tale; in that it reminds us just how badly wrong research can go. The risk of interdisciplinary inquiry is that political scientists and public health researchers will, through lack of knowledge of each other's achievements, do something similar—reinvent the wheel, at best, or end up with the intellectual equivalent of fermented foods. The hope is that we can avoid these problems by not just good scholarship and exchange, but by attention to the conditions under which the different disciplines operate and interact.

Acknowledgements This chapter relies on discussions with Holly Jarman, Elizabeth J. King, Julia Lynch, Elize Massard, Margitta Mätzke, Phil Rocco, Sarah Rozenblum, and my other collaborators in the HMP Governance Lab at the University of Michigan and the European Observatory on Health Systems and

Policies. I am very grateful to Patrick Fafard and Evelyn de Leeuw for comments on a draft, and to Adèle Cassola.

REFERENCES

Abbott, A. (1994). *The system of professions: An essay on the division of expert labor*. University of Chicago Press.

Acosta, C., Uribe Gómez, M., & Velandia-Naranjo, D. (2021). Colombia's response to COVID-19: Between pragmatic command, social contention and political challenges. In S. L. Greer, E. J. King, E. Massard da Fonseca, & A. Peralta-Santos (Eds.), *Coronavirus politics: The comparative politics and policy of COVID-19* (pp. 511–520). University of Michigan Press. https://www.press.umich.edu/11927713/coronavirus_politics

Adolph, C. (2013). *Bankers, bureaucrats, and central bank politics: The myth of neutrality*. Cambridge University Press.

Balderston, J. R., Gertz, Z. M., Seedat, R., Rankin, J. L., Hayes, A. W., Rodriguez, V. A., & Golladay, G. J. (2021). Differential documentation of race in the first line of the history of present illness. *JAMA Internal Medicine*. https://doi.org/10.1001/jamainternmed.2020.5792

Baldwin, P. (2005). *Disease and democracy: The industrialized world faces AIDS*. University of California Press.

Baldwin, P. (2021). *Fighting the first wave: Why the Coronavirus was tackled so differently across the globe*. Cambridge University Press.

Berridge, V. (1996). *AIDS in the UK: The making of policy, 1981–1994*. Oxford University Press.

Binder, S., Adigun, L., Dusenbury, C., Greenspan, A., & Tanhuanpaa, P. (2008). National public health institutes: Contributing to the public good. *Journal of Public Health Policy, 29*, 3–21.

Bossert, T. (1998). Analyzing the decentralization of health systems in developing countries: Decision space, innovation and performance. *Social Science and Medicine, 47*(10), 1513–1527. http://ac.els-cdn.com/S02779536980 02342/1-s2.0-S0277953698002342-main.pdf?_tid=1b03f5a2-6dfa-11e4-80e2-00000aab0f02&acdnat=1416188349_b243366b872c19accc1930f5a b82d828

Bousquet, J., Anto, J. M., Czarlewski, W., Haahtela, T., Fonseca, S. C., Iaccarino, G., Akdis, C. A., & Zuberbier, T. (2021). Cabbage and fermented vegetables: From death rate heterogeneity in countries to candidates for mitigation strategies of severe COVID-19. *Allergy, 76*(3), 735–750.

Bridges, D. R., Davidson, R. A., Soule Odegard, P., Maki, I. V., & Tomkowiak, J. (2011). Interprofessional collaboration: Three best practice models of interprofessional education. *Medical Education Online, 16*(1), 6035. https://doi. org/10.3402/meo.v16i0.6035

Carpenter, D. (2012). Is health politics different? *Annual Review of Political Science, 15*, 287–311.

de Leeuw, E. (2009). Evidence for healthy cities: Reflections on practice, method and theory. *Health Promotion International Health Promot Int, 24*(suppl_1), i19–i36. https://doi.org/10.1093/heapro/dap052

de Leeuw, E. (2016). From research to policy and practice in public health. In P. Liamputtong (Ed.), *Public health: Local and global perspectives* (pp. 213–234). Cambridge University Press.

Elazar, D. (1987). *Exploring federalism*. University of Alabama press.

Elgie, R. (2005). From Linz to Tsebelis: Three waves of presidential/parliamentary studies. *Democratization, 12*(1), 106–122. https://doi. org/10.1080/1351034042000317989

Fafard, P., & Cassola, A. (2020). Public health and political science: Challenges and opportunities for a productive partnership. *Public Health, 186*, 107–109.

Fairchild, A. L. (2015). The right to know, the right to be counted, the right to resist: Cancer, AIDS, and the politics of privacy and surveillance in post-war America. *Journal of Medical Law and Ethics, 3*(1–2), 45–64.

Fairchild, A. L., & Bayer, R. (2015). In the name of population well-being: The case for public health surveillance. *Journal of Health Politics, Policy and Law, 3445650.*

Fairchild, A. L., Bayer, R., & Colgrove, J. (2007). *Searching eyes: Privacy, the state, and disease surveillance in America*. University of California Press.

Fearnley, L. (2008a). Redesigning syndromic surveillance for biosecurity. In A. Lakoff & S. J. Collier (Eds.), *Biosecurity interventions: Global health and security in question* (pp. 61–88). Columbia University Press.

Fearnley, L. (2008b). Signals come and go: Syndromic surveillance and styles of biosecurity. *Environment and Planning A, 40*(7), 1615.

Fonseca, S., Rivas, I., Romaguera, D., Quijal, M., Czarlewski, W., Vidal, A., Fonseca, J., Ballester, J., Anto J. M., & Bousquet, J. (2020). Association between consumption of fermented vegetables and COVID-19 mortality at a country level in Europe. *medRxiv*, 2020. https://doi.org/10.1101/2020. 07.06.20147025

Fox, D. M. (2017). Toward a public health politics of consequence: An autobiographical reflection. *American Journal of Public Health, 107*(10), 1604.

Fredette, J. (2014). *Constructing Muslims in France: Discourse, public identity, and the politics of citizenship*. Temple University Press.

Frieden, T. R., & Koplan, J. P. (2010). Stronger national public health institutes for global health. *The Lancet, 376*(9754), 1721–1722.

Gagnon, F., Bergeron, P., Clavier, C., Fafard, P., Martin, E., & Blouin, C. (2017). Why and how political science can contribute to public health? Proposals for collaborative research avenues. *International Journal of Health Policy and Management, 6*(9), 495.

Glazer, N. (1974). The schools of the minor professions. *Minerva, 12*(3), 346–364. https://doi.org/10.1007/bf01102529

Gore, R., & Parker, R. (2019). Analysing power and politics in health policies and systems. *Global Public Health, 14*(4), 481–488. https://doi.org/10.1080/17441692.2019.1575446

Greer, S. L. (2015). John W. Kingdon, agendas, alternatives, and public policy. In S. J. Balla, M. Lodge, & E. C. Page (Eds.), *The Oxford handbook of classics of public policy and administration* (pp. 417–432). Oxford University Press.

Greer, S. L. (2017a). Constituting public health surveillance in twenty-first century Europe. In M. Weimer & A. de Ruijter (Eds.), *Regulating risks in the European Union: The co-production of expert and executive power* (pp. 121–141). Bloomsbury.

Greer, S. L. (2017b). Health policy and territorial politics: Disciplinary misunderstandings and directions for research. In K. Detterbeck & E. Hepburn (Eds.), *Edward Elgar handbook of territorial politics* (pp. 232–245). Edward Elgar. https://deepblue.lib.umich.edu/handle/2027.42/136224.

Greer, S. L. (2019). Comparative federalism as if policy mattered. In S. L. Greer & H. Elliott (Eds.), *Federalism and social policy: Patterns of redistribution in 11 democracies* (pp. 289–309). University of Michigan Press.

Greer, S. L., Elliott, H., & Oliver, R. (2015). Differences that matter: Overcoming methodological nationalism in comparative social policy research. *Journal of Comparative Policy Analysis: Research and Practice, 17*(4), 408–429. https://doi.org/10.1080/13876988.2015.1060713

Greer, S. L., & Jarman, H. (2020). What is EU public health and why? Explaining the scope and organization of public health in the European Union. [8706591]. *Journal of Health Politics, Policy and Law.* https://doi.org/10.1215/03616878-8706591

Greer, S. L., King, E. J., da Fonseca, E. M., & Peralta-Santos, A. (2020). The comparative politics of COVID-19: The need to understand government responses. *Global Public Health, 1*–4. https://doi.org/10.1080/17441692.2020.1783340

Greer, S. L., King, E. J., da Fonseca, E. M., & Peralta-Santos, A. (Eds.). (2021). *Coronavirus politics: The comparative politics and policy of COVID-19.* University of Michigan Press.

Greer, S. L., Rozenblum, S., Falkenbach, M., Löblová, O., Jarman, H., Williams, N., & Wismar, M. (2022). Centralizing and decentralizing governance in the COVID-19 pandemic: The politics of credit and blame. *Health Policy.* https://doi.org/10.1016/j.healthpol.2022.03.004

Greer, S. L., & Kurzer, P. (Eds.). (2013). *European Union public health policies: Regional and global perspectives.* Routledge.

Greer, S. L., & Mätzke, M. (2012). Bacteria without borders: Communicable disease politics in Europe. *Journal of Health Politics, Policy and Law, 37*(6), 887–915.

Hooghe, L., Marks, G., & Schakel, A. (2010). *The rise of regional authority: A comparative study of 42 democracies.* Routledge.

Irwin, R. E. (2020). Misinformation and de-contextualization: International media reporting on Sweden and COVID-19. *Globalization and Health, 16*(1), 62. https://doi.org/10.1186/s12992-020-00588-x

Kingdon, J. W. (2003). *Agendas, alternatives, and public policies.* HarperCollins.

Koivusalo, M. (2015). Health systems and policy space for health in the context of European Union trade policies. In *Services of general interest beyond the single market* (pp. 371–396). Springer.

Laugesen, M. J. (2016). *Fixing medical prices: How physicians are paid.* Harvard University Press.

Lee, L. M., Teutsch, S. M., Thacker, S. M., & St. Louis, M. I. (2010). *Principles and practice of public health surveillance* (3rd ed.). Oxford University Press.

Leider, J. P., Sellers, K., Bogaert, K., Castrucci, B. C., & Erwin, P. C. (2020). Master's-level education in the governmental public health workforce. *Public Health Reports, 135*(5), 650–657. https://doi.org/10.1177/0033354920943519

Lijphart, A. (1984). *Democracies: Patterns of majoritarian and consensus government in twenty-one countries.* Yale University Press.

Lijphart, A. (1999). *Patterns of democracy: Government forms and performance in thirty-six countries.* Yale University Press.

Linz, J. J. (1990). The perils of presidentialism. *Journal of Democracy, 1*, 51–69.

Löblovà, O., Rone, J., & Borbáth, E. (2021). COVID-19 in central and eastern Europe: Focus on Czechia, Hungary, and Bulgaria. In S. L. Greer, E. J. King, E. Massard da Fonseca, & A. Peralta-Santos (pp. 413–435). University of Michigan Press. https://www.press.umich.edu/11927713/coronavirus_politics

Mainwaring, S., & Shugart, M. S. (1997). *Presidentialism and democracy in Latin America.* Cambridge University Press.

Markel, H., Lipman, H. B., Navarro, J., Sloan, A., Michalsen, J. R., Stern, A. M., & Cetron, M. S. (2007). Nonpharmaceutical interventions implemented by us cities during the 1918–1919 influenza pandemic. *JAMA, 298*(6), 644–654. https://doi.org/10.1001/jama.298.6.644

Mätzke, M. (2012). Commentary: The institutional resources for communicable disease control in Europe: Diversity across time and place. *Journal of Health Politics, Policy, and Law, 36*(1), 967–976.

Myhre, S. L., French, S. D., & Bergh, A. (2020). National public health institutes: A scoping review. *Global Public Health, 18*, 1–18.

Park, J. (2021). COVID-19 response in South Korea. In S. L. Greer, E. J. King, E. Massard da Fonseca, & A. Peralta-Santos (Eds.), *Coronavirus politics: The comparative politics and policy of COVID-19* (pp. 105–126). University of Michigan Press. https://www.press.umich.edu/11927713/cor onavirus_politics

Patashnik, E. M., Gerber, A. S., & Dowling, C. M. (2020). *Unhealthy politics: The battle over evidence-based medicine*. Princeton University Press.

Pretti, M. A. M., Galvani, R. G., Vieira, G. F., Bonomo, A., Bonamino, M. H., & Boroni, M. (2020). Class I HLA Allele predicted restricted antigenic coverages for spike and nucleocapsid proteins are associated with deaths related to COVID-19. *Frontiers in Immunology, 11*, 565730. https://doi.org/10.3389/fimmu.2020.565730

Rocco, P., Rich, J. A. J., Klasa, K., Dubin, K. A., & Béland, D. (2021). Who counts where? COVID-19 surveillance in federal countries. *Journal of Health Politics, Policy and Law, 21*, 9349114.

Rojas, F. (2010). *From black power to black studies: How a radical social movement became an academic discipline*. JHU Press.

Rozenblum, S. D. (2021). France's multidimensional COVID-19 response: Ad hoc committees and the sidelining of public health agencies. In S. L. Greer, E. J. King, E. Massard da Fonseca, & A. Peralta-Santos (Eds.), (pp. 264–279). University of Michigan Press. Retrieved from https://www.press.umich.edu/11927713/coronavirus_politics

Rozier, M. D., Willison, C. E., Anspach, R. R., Howell, J. D., Greer, A. L., & Greer, S. L. (2020). Paradoxes of professional autonomy: A qualitative study of US neonatologists from 1978–2017. *Sociology of Health & Illness, 42*(8), 1821–1836.

Shear, M. D., Haberman, M., Weiland, N., LaFraniere, S., & Mazzetti, M. (2021). President's focus in the management of the pandemic: himself. *New York Times*, p. A1.

Skowronek, S. (1982). *Building a New American State: The expansion of national administrative capacities, 1877–1920*. Cambridge University Press.

Timmermans, S., & Berg, M. (2003). *The gold standard: The challenge of evidence-based medicine and standardization in health care*. Temple University Press.

Trump, B. D., Bridges, T. S., Cegan, J. C., Cibulsky, S. M., Greer, S. L., Jarman, H., Lafferty, B. J., Surette, M. A., & Linkov, I. (2020). An analytical perspective on pandemic recovery. *Health Security, 18*(3), 250–256.

Valentine, R., Valentine, D., & Valentine, J. L. (2020). Relationship of George Floyd protests to increases in COVID-19 cases using event study methodology. *Journal of Public Health, 42*(4), 696–697. https://doi.org/10.1093/pubmed/fdaa127

Vinck, D. (2010). *The sociology of scientific work.* Edward Elgar Publishing.

Wagner, M. (1997). Confessions of a dissident. In R. Davis-Floyd & C. F. Sargent (Eds.), *Childbirth and authoritative knowledge: Cross-cultural perspectives* (pp. 366–395). University of California Press.

Zetka, J. R. (2003). *Surgeons and the scope.* Cornell University Press.

Ziemann, A. (2015). *Syndromic surveillance: Made in Europe.* Maastricht University.

CHAPTER 4

Public Health Policymaking, Politics, and Evidence

Anita Kothari and Maxwell J. Smith

1 INTRODUCTION

In this introductory chapter, we discuss the ways in which the public health community tends to understand the intersections of scientific evidence, policymaking, and politics in its pursuit of protecting and promoting the public's health. This is a rather daunting task, not only due to the heterogeneity of perspectives on these matters but also because the work of public health is accomplished by many individuals from several types of organizations. For our purposes, we take 'public health community' to include a range of actors, including public health researchers (e.g., epidemiologists, health promotion scholars, bioethicists, economists, etc.), advocates working in public health-oriented organizations, professional staff (e.g., nurses, nutritionists, community health workers) working in public health agencies, and medical officers of health

A. Kothari (✉) · M. J. Smith
School of Health Studies, Faculty of Health Sciences, Western University, London, ON, Canada
e-mail: akothari@uwo.ca

© The Author(s) 2022
P. Fafard et al. (eds.), *Integrating Science and Politics for Public Health*, Palgrave Studies in Public Health Policy Research,
https://doi.org/10.1007/978-3-030-98985-9_4

affiliated with government and public health agencies. Put another way, public health is an applied field in service of achieving specific outcomes.

Our shared interest in public health is derived from diverse perspectives. Over the last twenty years, Kothari has conducted public health services research in partnerships with public health agencies and decision-makers. She has focused on how these programs are organized in response to legislated mandates; often these arrangements aim to support health equity. Kothari's academic background involved training in health research methodology, population health, and health policy and services. Smith's research is primarily in the area of public health ethics, where he bridges moral and political philosophy and social science methods to examine the pursuit of health equity and social justice in public health, particularly in the context of infectious diseases. Smith's academic background involved training in public health, moral and political philosophy, health law, and bioethics.

Understanding how health is conceptualized and how public health functions is a useful place to start the discussion. It is a common view that health is more than the absence of disease or good physical health for everyday functioning. The elements of health include considerations of physical, social, mental, and spiritual wellness. The public health system tends to work within this holistic framework in its pursuit of protecting and promoting the health of community members. These broad goals are achieved through surveillance and epidemiology; infectious disease detection, outbreak investigation, response, control, and elimination; environmental health; control of risk factors for non-communicable diseases; immunizations; emergency preparedness and response; health promotion and education; and oversight of some clinical services (Bloland et al., 2012). Underlying these functions is a strong mission to promote health equity and limit unjust health disparities. Public health research plays a dominant role in the functions described above through describing the scope of the problem and generating viable solutions.

In the rest of this chapter, we describe how we see the public health view of evidence, policymaking, and the role that research evidence plays in the making of public health policy. We conclude with some reflections on what public health can offer political science and where those fruitful interactions between public health and political science might occur.

2   How Does Public Health
Understand Evidence?

Public health has a complicated relationship with evidence. Like medicine and other health sciences, public health strives and purports to be 'evidence-based' (Water & Doyle, 2002), propped up by epidemiology, the putative 'basic science' of public health (Krieger, 1999). Like other health sciences, an orthodoxy regarding a hierarchy of evidence dominates, privileging evidence generated via randomized controlled trials, systematic reviews, and meta-analyses (Cairney, 2016; Parkhurst & Abeysinghe, 2016). Public health decision-making 'grounded' in the evidence base and its hierarchy of evidence has a veneer of steering clear of value judgements and other forms of evidence prone to bias and error and tends to obscure the political and ethical dimensions of public health decision-making (Goldenberg, 2006). Explicitly grounding decisions in values or other forms of knowledge may be criticized as being overtly 'politicizing' public health decisions, where decisions should instead be 'based on the evidence'.

Yet, by virtue of the nature of public health challenges and the interventions necessary to address them, it is often not possible to conduct randomized controlled trials to make causal inferences or evaluate public health interventions (Frieden, 2017; Kemm, 2006; Raphael, 2000; Victora et al., 2004). Evidence-based decision-making in public health is therefore challenged by the fact that causal interactions often cannot be adequately identified, evidence may not be available, and/or decisions often need to be made early and quickly in order to avoid significant harm to the public's health (Kriebel & Tickner, 2001).

As a partial consequence of these deficits and associated uncertainty, the precautionary principle has enjoyed some prominence in public health decision-making. While there is no consensus definition of the precautionary principle nor agreement about when and how it ought to be applied in public health, the principle generally suggests that a lack of full scientific certainty should not be used as a reason for postponing cost-effective measures to prevent harms when there are threats of serious or irreversible harms to the public's health (Report of the UN Conference on Environment and Development, 1992). For instance, two Canadian judicial inquiries, the Krever Commission of Inquiry on the Blood System in Canada and the Campbell Commission following the outbreak of Severe Acute Respiratory Syndrome (SARS), recommend the use of the precautionary principle to guide Canada's response to public health threats (Campbell, 2004; Krever, 1997). Similar calls were made in relation to the public health response to the Coronavirus 2019 (COVID-19) pandemic (Crosby & Crosby, 2020; Ferrinho et al., 2020). Yet, it is unclear how public health as a field reconciles commitments to evidence-based decision-making with the reality of decision-making that must invariably engage with political and ethical values in contexts of uncertainty.

While evidence-based decision-making and the evidence hierarchy is prominent in public health, some embrace a wide range of disciplinary approaches as constituting public health's 'basic sciences', ranging from political science and sociology to anthropology and economics (Savitz et al., 1999). Others embrace the role of the humanities in public health (Saffran, 2014). And while evidence is still considered important because evidence helps to support justifications for decisions, much like in medicine and other health sciences, the concept of evidence-based decision-making and the evidence hierarchy is problematized from these other disciplinary perspectives (Parkhurst & Abeysinghe, 2016). Given that a number of considerations and outcomes are important to consider in policy debates, a shift has occurred in recent years to acknowledge that evidence is necessary but not sufficient in public health decision-making (Guyatt et al., 2000) and that public health should aim instead to be evidence-informed (Parkhurst & Abeysinghe, 2016).

3   How Does Public Health Understand Policymaking?

Evidence-informed decision-making (EIDM) continues to promote research findings as a major driver of policy by citing the advantage of public accountability and transparency in policymaking. EIDM gained widespread acceptance in the health sciences where proponents suggested that more effective policies and programs, ideally based on systematic reviews of research, would emerge through this approach. This rational approach to policymaking was met with some criticism from both the research supply side and the policymaking demand side. In terms of the former, the way that researchers designed research studies did not lead to findings that answered policymakers' questions about optimal solutions, their local application and implementation; the appropriate research was not available for health systems. In terms of the latter side, multiple influences (e.g., public values) and actors exert pressure on policymaking in the real world.

This view of policymaking intersects with the role of public health—to promote health and prevent disease—and the mechanisms by which to carry out this role. Sometimes public health programs, like a seniors fall prevention program, are introduced locally to address specific community needs. Other times, passive, regional-level strategies that use standardization and legislative enforcement keep communities safe, such as water quality standards or mandatory seatbelt laws. Public health practitioners and researchers intersect with the policymaking process when trying to advocate for this type of legislation, and research findings are the predominant tool used by the public health community in these policy discussions given the strong belief in research evidence as the main justificatory condition for policies. Public health researchers, including epidemiologists and social epidemiologists, can readily establish that a health problem exists and can describe the scope of the problem using research that is timely, accurate, and high-quality. Even complicated issues, like those related to the social determinants of health (e.g., vulnerable circumstances), such as housing or public transportation, can be easily characterized by public health researchers. The challenge comes when trying to 'sell' a public health solution, whether narrow—restricting the availability of alcohol— or broad—implementing a Health in All Policies approach (Crammond & Carey, 2017)—in part because public health researchers may tend to have a simple understanding of the policy process and how to influence it.

This raises the question of why most mainstream public health researchers have limited knowledge of concepts like policy networks, institutions, interests, policy theories, and the like. One possible explanation might be attributed to the policy receptor capacity for public health research. That is, governments might have little time or space to consider the findings from public health research, and thus attempts to determine how to 'break in' to policy discussions might be fruitless. The public health sector competes with resource allocation demands from acute care, long-term care, and community-based health services. Not only is public health typically assigned the smallest portion of the health budget compared to other types of care and services, but it is also a relatively weak lobby group (Vernick, 1999). For example, patients or service recipients can band together to demand more supports for dementia care but recipients of public health services are unlikely to form a pressure group for a condition that was prevented. Similarly, the health professional workforce caring for those with myocardial infarctions will have more clout than their public health counterparts when demanding funding for treatments. Notwithstanding a pandemic or environmental disaster, there are fewer compelling reasons for policymakers to think of public health researchers as anything more than technical experts along with the other technical experts they may wish to consult.

Critical public health scholars, on the other hand, are one of the exceptions to the generalization that mainstream public health researchers have a weak understanding of policymaking. Critical public health scholars focus on and interrogate the structural determinants of health, including the 'political determinants of health', e.g., the effects of neoliberalism, austerity, and income inequality on health (Viens, 2019). Scholarship in the political economy of health, dating back to the 1970's and historically rooted within the Marxian tradition (Harvey, 2020), has examined the relationship between health and, for example, the production and distribution of wealth and issues of capital accumulation and the organization of labor (Raphael & Bryant, 2006). Central to work in the structural determinants of health, political determinants of health, and political economy of health is the examination of political and social forces that create and exacerbate social inequalities, resulting in health inequities (Kittelsen et al., 2019). However, some have argued that political determinants have received less attention in public health scholarship relative to other social determinants (Mishori, 2019), and others still have argued that limited empirical research has sought to study the relationship between political variables and health outcomes (Mackenbach, 2014). In other words, critical public health scholarship acknowledges the political, economic, and social forces that impact the public's health, including the ways in which these forces manifest within the policy process. This has, in turn, led to a greater appetite to understand and interrogate the messy processes of policymaking, in contrast to mainstream approaches that continue to believe in the rational evidence-to-policy model of policymaking. Though, it is important to note that not all critical public health scholarship advances this aim; while critical public health scholarship may engage with the role of politics and power in public health (e.g., the role of neoliberalism, austerity, etc.), this does not necessarily include an understanding and interrogation of the intricacies of the policymaking process itself.

Understanding both the extent of the structural problem and possible ways to alleviate health inequities requires untangling a web of interdependent, multilevel factors with far-reaching and lasting—often intergenerational—effects. These discussions inevitably consider the distribution of power (Harris et al., 2020; Popay et al., 2020), the politics of science and the research evidence (Schrecker, 2017), and, to advance public health action, critical public health scholars may also have established relationships with policymakers. Thus, there is a small sub-population of public health researchers who are entrenched in discussions about health outcomes and policymaking.

4 How Does Public Health Understand Politics?

In characterizing the extent and ways in which public health understands and engages with politics and political science, in the discussion above we identified two poles between which a gradient exists. At one pole, public health is viewed as apolitical and purposefully divorced from thinking about or engaging with politics. At the other pole, public health is viewed *as* politics (Sundin, 2019). Both poles no doubt exist in public health scholarship and practice, though we suspect the majority of public health policymakers, practitioners, and researchers fall somewhere in between.

On one end of the spectrum, public health is viewed as a value-neutral scientific endeavor that is, and perhaps ought to be, divorced from politics and political realities given the view that engagement with politics 'distorts' or in some way 'biases' otherwise 'objective' scientific quests for public health 'truths' (Brown, 2010; Fafard & Cassola, 2020; Krieger, 1999). This corresponds to a long-standing phenomenon in areas of scientific inquiry where research is conducted in a manner that intends to be (and often purports to be) 'unadulterated' by variables considered to be exogenous to science (Proctor and Proctor, 1991). For some, it may be this positivistic view of public health research that is seen as constitutive of what it means for public health to be 'evidence-based'. On this view, the value and extent of political analysis may be limited to evaluation of political interference and the 'political will' to actually do what the evidence suggests as being the proper course of action, as discussed in Chapter 3 (Greer, 2022).

On the other end of the spectrum, public health is viewed as inextricably political; power is exercised over health as part of a wider political, social, and economic system, (Bambra et al., 2005) where health is influenced by different ideological positions, power constellations, and interests (Kickbusch, 2015). Inattention to politics on this critical view would be to ignore that which exerts profound influence on the public's health. This view of public health has a pedigree dating back at least 170 years to Rudolf Virchow and his oft-cited argument that medicine—and here we might include public health as well—is a social science and politics is nothing else but medicine on a large scale (Ashton, 2006; Mackenbach, 2009).

The state's influence on people's lives is deep and pervasive, and the state's role in protecting and promoting public health is no exception. Consequently, precisely how the authority of the state ought to be tamed and justified—a common thread in political science—has been the subject of much scholarship in public health ethics, a sub-field of bioethics. Philosophers and others in this space have drawn upon and generated political theory to answer questions about what justice requires for the public's health (Daniels, 2007), how state intervention for the sake of the public's health can be justified (Jennings, 2003) and even which political theories ought to be used to justify and guide public health activities (Jennings, 2007; Latham, 2016; Powers et al., 2012).

There is wide variation in how public health engages with politics in practice. For instance, academic public health researchers may seek to understand epidemiological trends with the hope that generating this knowledge will be taken up by public health officials in future public health programming or policy. In this role, the academic public health researcher may be more distal from the practice of policymaking and the political dimensions of public health decision-making. This corresponds to a wider phenomenon in science where 'basic' questions in science are studied with little attention paid to whether and how knowledge generated will be taken up in policy or practice (Glasgow et al., 2003; McAteer et al., 2019). With that said, it is common for research funding mechanisms to require researchers to articulate their plans for knowledge translation and exchange and even that they embed 'knowledge users' (e.g., policymakers or decision makers) in research projects. Consequently, it is increasingly likely that public health research is being funded with an explicit, if weakly articulated requirement to focus on whether and how knowledge generated from that research might be used in practice, and in particular, to shape public health policy. This creates pressure on public health scholars to develop at least a cursory understanding and engagement with the policymaking process. Some researchers have observed, however, that traditional knowledge-to-action strategies, which public health scholars will inevitably turn to, are geared to practitioner audiences and may not be directly transferrable as effective knowledge translation strategies for policymakers (Fafard & Hoffman, 2020).

On the other end of the spectrum, public health authorities, such as medical officers of health, are senior officials of governments who often work directly with political leaders. As government officials, while their role may be construed as a voice of science in government, medical officers of health must navigate the political environment in which their expertise and leadership are sought, and therefore often must be politically astute to achieve their goals (Fafard et al., 2018; MacAulay et al., 2021). The upshot is that some working in public health will be far more familiar with, and engaged with, the political dimensions and realities of public health by virtue of their close engagement with decision-makers.

5   How Does Public Health Understand Community in Conceptualizations of Evidence, Politics, and Power?

At the start of this chapter, we noted the applied nature of public health. At its core, the field likes to say that it is driven by community needs. Consequently, the community lens plays a central role in shaping conceptualizations of policymaking and evidence. We talk about 'community' as made up of members of the public to whom a public health agency provides services and have an interest and a duty to understand such that services reflect local values and concerns. This is not to discount residents of the global health community, who also experience health risks and suffer from public health-related conditions, but the discussion in this chapter is particularly applicable to those who live within geographical boundaries associated with legislative mandates for which public health agencies are responsible for fulfilling. This implies that there might be regional or state level agencies who work with specific communities while in parallel a national public health agency will accomplish its work with the larger, country-wide community. The 'community' will benefit, either directly or indirectly, from public health activities.

The intersection of evidence and community plays out in at least two ways. First, those in the public health field who are staunchly evidence-based following the research hierarchy tradition, will seek to understand community health needs to then identify priorities and appropriate solutions or interventions. Classical epidemiological tools will dominate this path. On the other hand, many mainstream public health researchers along with critical public health researchers take up a broader view of evidence. This alternate path requires that epidemiological studies are balanced with local problems and needs *generated from the community*. Essentially, this community lens invites considerations of values and experiential knowledge into how evidence is produced and how evidence is discussed. In this way, health problems and interventions take on their contours in the context of communities. Critical public health researchers may take this even further with attention to power dynamics and the political determinants of health.

Second, not only do local problems and needs derive from the community, but the public health community engages with its constituents in multiple ways. There is a strong tradition in public health practice of 'being political' at the local or regional level through consultation and coalition building, which often includes research activity, as seen through empirical examples discussed in Chapter 6 (Clavier et al., 2022). This makes space for otherwise excluded experiences and perspectives into decision-making structures. There are several examples of grassroots partnerships and advocacy that have forced higher levels of government to act, sometimes on pragmatic grounds, or to achieve consistent standards, e.g., outdoor smoking control policies. While these activities are carried out without formal political science theories or insights in mind, we could discuss at length how these activities emphasize power relations (e.g., working with marginalized sectors of the community); collaborative research (e.g., the democratization of science); group decision-making (e.g., inter-agency collaborations for resources sharing); or other issues related to policy studies.

This brief description touches on the importance of considering the community in the research-to-action cycle. What this means for interdisciplinary scholars is that if you care about public health and the community, then understanding how politics and policy seeps into public health work is vital.

6   Concluding Remarks

The ways and extent to which public health engages with politics and political science may depend, in part, on where one draws the boundaries of 'public health' (Bambra et al., 2005). For some, public health may be characterized narrowly in biomedical terms and individual behaviors and lifestyle choices (Goldberg, 2012). The role or significance of politics and policymaking may be attenuated on this view. For others, public health is viewed as a public matter (Coggon, 2012; Krieger & Birn, 1998) and characterized in a more expansive way to include the contexts in which people are born, live, work, and age, which necessitates the interrogation of social, economic, and political systems and the structures that influence health, including policymaking processes. This has obvious implications for the opportunities for collaboration between public health and political science.

Public health tends to understand and treat the intersections of scientific evidence, policymaking, and politics in a manner similar to other health sciences; that is, with a sometimes unsophisticated, and some might argue naïve, view of evidence-based policymaking. Yet, there are important exceptions. Philosophers of public health, public health ethicists, and critical public health scholars are alive to the social, political, and economic forces that impact the public's health and that exert influence on public health policy and have long-standing engagement with political, ethical, and social theory to understand and interrogate these forces. In many ways, political scientists interested in public health have much to draw from given important work that has been done in public health to understand the nature of a just society, the challenges of understanding and acting on inequality and inequity, the justified use of state coercion for matters of health, and many other big questions of political and social theory.

Yet, if these might be considered 'macro' considerations and issues, public health also offers much insight into what is done at the local, or 'micro', level, e.g., the realities of local government and the power of civil society in shaping public health policy. More specifically, the powerful commitment of public health to engage with and reflect community concerns and building coalitions to advocate for change means that public health practice and scholarship can contribute to our collective understanding of governance at the local level. We have raised the importance of the community as the space from which issues are identified, evidence is generated, and how solutions are context-bound. In particular, issues related to health inequities derive their authority and legitimacy from this 'ground zero' location where partnerships are key. While public health as a multidisciplinary practice had evolved in elaborate partnerships with government, market, and citizens, political science is often still practiced from a monodisciplinary setting. We encourage political science researchers to move away from starting with political science theories, and their accompanying insights, if they want to achieve any practical impact on communities (and the world). Instead, start from where we are at—start with the inequities and community partnerships—and then introduce the relevant policy insights that support sustainable policy action for change.

Perhaps what is most needed, then, is attention to the important work of political science being conducted at the 'meso' level of policymaking—the area where local community interests and needs are navigated alongside (and sometimes in conflict with) political and social forces. We believe that this is perhaps the most fruitful area of potential collaboration between public health and political science.

REFERENCES

Ashton, J. R. (2006). Virchow misquoted, part-quoted, and the real McCoy. *Journal of Epidemiology & Community Health, 60*(8), 671–671.

Bambra, C., Fox, D., & Scott-Samuel, A. (2005). Towards a politics of health. *Health Promotion International, 20*(2), 187–193.

Cairney, P. (2016) *The politics of evidence-based policy making*. Palgrave.

Clavier, C., Gagnon, F., & Poland, B. (2022). Sidestepping the stalemate. The strategies of public health actors for circulating evidence into the policy process. In P. Fafard, A. Cassola, & E. De Leeuw (Eds.), *Integrating science and politics for public health*. Palgrave Springer.

Crammond, B. R., & Carey, G. (2017). Policy change for the social determinants of health: The strange irrelevance of social epidemiology. *Evidence & Policy: A Journal of Research, Debate and Practice, 13*(2), 365–374.

Bloland, P., Simone, P., Burkholder, B., Slutsker, L., & De Cock, K. M. (2012). *The role of public health institutions in global health system strengthening efforts: The US CDC's perspective*. Advance online publication. https://doi.org/10.1371/journal.pmed.1001199

Brown, L. D. (2010). The political face of public health. *Public Health Reviews, 32*(1), 155–173.

Campbell, A. (2004). The SARS commission interim report: SARS and public health in Ontario. *Biosecurity and Bioterrorism: Biodefense Strategy, Practice, and Science, 2*, 118–126.

Coggon, J. (2012). *What makes health public?: A critical evaluation of moral, legal, and political claims in public health*. Cambridge University Press.

Crosby, L., & Crosby, E. (2020). Applying the precautionary principle to personal protective equipment (PPE) guidance during the COVID-19 pandemic: Did we learn the lessons of SARS? *Canadian Journal of Anesthesia/Journal Canadien D'anesthésie, 67*(10), 1327–1332.

Daniels, N. (2007). *Just health: Meeting health needs fairly.* Cambridge University Press. https://doi.org/10.1017/CBO9780511809514

Dawes, D. E. (2020). *The political determinants of health.* Johns Hopkins University Press.

Fafard, P., & Cassola, A. (2020). Public health and political science: Challenges and opportunities for a productive partnership. *Public Health, 186,* 107–109. https://doi.org/10.1016/j.puhe.2020.07.004

Fafard, P., & Hoffman, S. J. (2020). Rethinking knowledge translation for public health policy. *Evidence & Policy: A Journal of Research, Debate and Practice, 16*(1), 165–175.

Fafard, P., McNena, B., Suszek, A., & Hoffman, S. J. (2018). Contested roles of Canada's chief medical officers of health. *Canadian Journal of Public Health, 109,* 585–589. https://doi.org/10.17269/s41997-018-0080-3

Ferrinho, P., Sidat, M., Leiras, G., Cupertino, P., de Barros, F., & Arruda, H. (2020). Principalism in public health decision making in the context of the COVID-19 pandemic. *The International Journal of Health Planning and Management, 35*(5), 997–1000.

Frieden, T. R. (2017). Evidence for health decision making—Beyond randomised, controlled trials. *New England Journal of Medicine, 377*(5), 465–475.

Guyatt, G. H., Haynes, R. B., Jaeschke, R. Z., Cook, D. J., Green, L., Naylor, C. D, Wilson, S. W., & Richardson, M. C. (2000). Users' guides to the medical literature: XXV. Evidence-based medicine: principles for applying the users' guides to patient care. *JAMA, 284*(10), 1290–1296.

Glasgow, R. E., Lichtenstein, E., & Marcus, A. C. (2003). Why don't we see more translation of health promotion research to practice? Rethinking the efficacy-to-effectiveness transition. *American Journal of Public Health, 93*(8), 1261–1267.

Goldberg, D. S. (2012). Social justice, health inequalities and methodological individualism in US health promotion. *Public Health Ethics, 5*(2), 104–115.

Goldenberg, M. J. (2006). On evidence and evidence-based medicine: Lessons from the philosophy of science. *Social Science & Medicine, 62,* 2621–2632.

Greer, S. (2022). Professions, data, and political will. In P. Fafard, A. Cassola, & E. De Leeuw (Eds.), *Integrating science and politics for public health.* Palgrave Springer.

Harris, P., Baum, F., Friel, S., Mackean, T., Schram, A., & Townsend, B. (2020). A glossary of theories for understanding power and policy for health equity. *Journal of Epidemiology & Community Health, 74*(6), 548–552.

Harvey, M. (2020). The political economy of health: Revisiting Its marxian origins to address 21st-century health inequalities. *American Journal of Public Health, 111*(2), 293–300.

Jennings, B. (2003). Frameworks for ethics in public health. *Acta Bioethica, 9*(2), 165–176.

Jennings, B. (2007). Public health and civic republicanism: Toward an alternative framework for public health ethics. *Ethics, Prevention, and Public Health*, 30–58.

Kemm, J. (2006). The limitations of 'evidence-based' public health. *Journal of Evaluation in Clinical Practice, 12*(3), 319–324.

Kickbusch, I. (2015). The political determinants of health—10 years on. *BMJ*. Advance online publication. https://doi.org/10.1136/bmj.h81

Kittelsen, S. K., Fukuda-Parr, S., & Storeng, K. T. (2019). The political determinants of health inequities and universal health coverage. *Global Health*. Advance online publication. https://doi.org/10.1186/s12992-019-0514-6

Krever, H. (1997). *Final report: Commission of Inquiry on the Blood System in Canada*. The Commission.

Kriebel, D., & Tickner, J. (2001). Reenergizing public health through precaution. *American Journal of Public Health, 91*, 1351–1355.

Krieger, N. (1999). Questioning epidemiology: Objectivity, advocacy, and socially responsible science. *American Journal of Public Health, 89*(8), 1151–1153.

Krieger, N., & Birn, A. E. (1998). A vision of social justice as the foundation of public health: Commemorating 150 years of the spirit of 1848. *American Journal of Public Health, 88*(11), 1603–1606.

Latham, S. R. (2016). Political theory, values and public health. *Public Health Ethics, 9*(2), 139–149.

MacAulay, M., Macintyre, A., Yashadana, A., Cassola, A., Harris, P., Woodward, C., et al. (2021). Under the spotlight: Understanding the role of the chief medical officer in a pandemic. *Journal of Epidemiology and Community Health, 0*, 1–5.

Mackenbach, J. P. (2009). Politics is nothing but medicine at a larger scale: Reflections on public health's biggest idea. *Journal of Epidemiology & Community Health, 63*(3), 181–184.

Mackenbach, J. P. (2014). Political determinants of health. *European Journal of Public Health, 24*(1), 2.

McAteer, J., Di Ruggiero, E., Fraser, A., & Frank, J. W. (2019). Bridging the academic and practice/policy gap in public health: Perspectives from Scotland and Canada. *Journal of Public Health, 41*(3), 632–637.

Mishori, R. (2019). The social determinants of health? Time to focus on the political determinants of health! *Medical Care, 57*(7), 491–493.

Parkhurst, J. O., & Abeysinghe, S. (2016). What constitutes "good" evidence for public health and social policy-making? *From Hierarchies to Appropriateness. Social Epistemology, 30*(5–6), 665–679.

Popay, J., Whitehead, M., Ponsford, R., Egan, M., & Mead, R. (2020). Power, control, communities and health inequalities I: Theories, concepts and analytical frameworks. *Health Promotion International.* Advance online publication. https://doi.org/10.1093/heapro/daaa133

Powers, M., Faden, R., & Saghai, Y. (2012). Liberty, mill and the framework of public health ethics. *Public Health Ethics, 5*(1), 6–15.

Proctor, R. N., & Proctor, R. (1991). *Value-free science?: Purity and power in modern knowledge.* Harvard University Press.

Raphael, D. (2000). The question of evidence in health promotion. *Health Promotion International, 15*(4), 355–367.

Raphael, D., & Bryant, T. (2006). Maintaining population health in a period of welfare state decline: Political economy as the missing dimension in health promotion theory and practice. *Promotion & Education, 13*(4), 236–242.

Report of the United Nations conference on environment and development. New York: Department of Economic and Social Affairs, United Nations. (1992 August). [cited 2017 January 30]. Report No.: A/CONF.151/26 (Vol. I)

Saffran, L. (2014). 'Only connect': The case for public health humanities. *Medical Humanities, 40*(2), 105–110.

Savitz, D. A., Poole, C., & Miller, W. C. (1999). Reassessing the role of epidemiology in public health. *American Journal of Public Health, 89*(8), 1158–1161.

Schrecker, T. (2017). "Stop, you're killing us!" An alternative take on populism and public health comment on the rise of post-truth populism in pluralist liberal democracies: Challenges for health policy. *International Journal of Health Policy Management, 6*(11), 673–675.

Sundin, J. (2019). Public health is politics. *Interchange, 50*(2), 129–136.

Vernick, J. S. (1999, September). Lobbying and advocacy for the public's health: What are the limits for nonprofit organizations?. *American Journal of Public Health, 89*(9),1425–1429.

Victora, C. G., Habicht, J. P., & Bryce, J. (2004). Evidence-based public health: Moving beyond randomised trials. *American Journal of Public Health, 94*(3), 400–405.

Viens, A. M. (2019). Neo-liberalism, austerity and the political determinants of health. *Health Care Analysis, 27*, 147–152.

Water, E., & Doyle J. (2002). Evidence based public health practice: Improving the quality and quantity of evidence. *Journal of Public Health Medicine, 24*(1), 227–229.

WHO Commission on Social Determinants of Health & World Health Organization. (2008). *Closing the gap in a generation: Health equity through action on the social determinants of health.* Commission on Social Determinants of Health final report. World Health Organization.

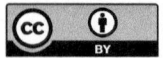

Politics, Evidence, and Policymaking: A Public Health Political Science Approach

CHAPTER 5

How Policy Appetites Shape, and Are Shaped by Evidence Production and Use

"New York is not a City of Alleys", Nick Carr, Location Scout

"I've worked on more films that want to find the imaginary version of New York than the real. The big thing I always get asked to find are dank dilapidated alleys, and New York City has, like, 5 alleys that look like that. Maybe four. You can't film in three of them. So what it comes down to is there's one alley left in New York, Cortlandt Alley, that everybody films in because it's the last place.

I try to stress to these directors in a polite way that New York is not a city of alleys. Boston is a city of alleys. Philadelphia has alleys. I don't know anyone who uses the 'old alleyway shortcut' to go home. It doesn't exist here. But that's the movie you see. Your impression of New York is that it is the city of alleys, and then directors will

K. Oliver (✉)
Faculty of Public Health and Policy, London School of Hygiene and Tropical Medicine, London, UK
e-mail: Kathryn.Oliver@lshtm.ac.uk

© The Author(s) 2022   77
P. Fafard et al. (eds.), _Integrating Science and Politics for Public Health_,
Palgrave Studies in Public Health Policy Research,
https://doi.org/10.1007/978-3-030-98985-9_5

come here, they've seen movies set in New York and they want their movies to have alleys.

And it's this self-perpetuating fictional version of New York that just kills me because movies are so much more interesting when you show a side of New York that actually exists but isn't regularly highlighted".[1]

1   INTRODUCTION

For many years, researchers have advocated for greater research impact on policy. This advocacy has often, in an attempt to be helpful, taken the form of specifying preferred types of evidence (the randomised controlled trial or systematic review, for example) and preferred directions of policy change. A simplistic model, often termed the technocratic or rationalist model, of knowledge uptake is presented: a problem is identified, the most 'robust' research evidence possible is created to solve this problem, the research recommendations are implemented, and the policy problem is solved. Policymakers—who draw on many and varied kinds of evidence—have responded to this advice by funding and supporting particular versions of knowledge (e.g., trials units, systematic review facilities such as the What Works Centres and the National Institute for Health Care and Excellence in the UK).

Yet the production of evidence, and its use are far from simple processes. From discussions about the plurality of evidence (Parkhurst & Abeysinghe, 2016; Petticrew & Roberts, 2003), to the politicisation of research systems and the role research plays in the world, many have argued against the simplistic view of 'best' evidence put forward above, which ignores both values and people. So why does this narrative remain so powerful, even though even many of its proponents would agree that it is an overly simplistic way of understanding how evidence informs policy?

Unfortunately, the dominance of the rationalist model really matters because it affects how policy appetites for evidence, and the actual production of evidence. It narrows the range of evidence available to policymakers in shaping and framing problems and solutions, and consequently there is less support for research which sits outside these framings. This in turn has led to misunderstandings, methodological in-fighting,

---

[1] https://www.citylab.com/design/2011/11/film-location-scout-pet-peeves/521/

misuse of evidence by decision-makers, and vested interests. What might an alternative be?

To better understand how policymakers find and use evidence, we need a broader lens to examine the political economy of knowledge. By understanding what knowledge is, and 'its forms of extraction, points of commodification, how it is refined as intellectual property' (Tilley, 2017), we can better conceptualise its role in decision-making, and begin to imagine the broader evidence-policy system within which knowledge is exchanged. Between 2014 and 2019 in the UK, I conducted 91 interviews with researchers and policymakers in the UK, discussing the challenges of evidence use in policy. I draw on these interviews in this chapter to explore how knowledge production, mobilisation and use shape and are shaped by policy appetites. This offers a new way to begin thinking about how to creatively shape a more helpful environment for both policy and evidence.

2 The Rationalist Model

Researchers and policymakers alike have sought to conquer the challenge of improving health and social outcomes by implementing improved decision-making. Evidence and data use have for decades, if not centuries, been at the heart of this drive. For many, the relationship between these processes is a straightforward, linear one of problem definition, solution creation, and implementation. In this vision, research is there to provide solutions for real-world problems faced by policymakers and practitioners. For their part, policymakers and funders have made investments in applied research tied to explicit policy priorities, with an emphasis on disciplines deemed likely to produce 'economic value' (Bastow et al., 2015). This has broadly meant spending money on solutions-oriented evidence, or to put it another way, research which assists policymakers in selecting options for policy implementation.

From the very beginnings of the evidence-based medicine and evidence-based policy movements (in the UK, usually agreed to be Cochrane's, 1972 'Effectiveness and Efficiency' report (Cochrane, 1972; Oliver & Pearce, 2017), through the growth of evidence-synthesis organisations, to the training of individual researchers to increase their impact, this has come to mean a particular form of evidence and research. Underpinning this is the notion of the hierarchy of evidence, which is a heuristic describing the strength of different methodological designs. Although extensively critiqued, it has also been translated into outcomes-focused decision-making tools such as GRADE (Movsisyan et al., 2018; Shenderovich et al., 2019). This hierarchy affirms and assigns value to different pieces of evidence on the basis of research design; in particular, the randomised controlled trial (RCT), and the systematic review or evidence synthesis. RCTs are valued because this research design minimises the chance that random chance has led to the research finding, meaning that they have high internal validity, and that readers can have confidence that the research finding is reproducible. The systematic review exhaustively brings together evidence on a particular question, assessing the strengths and weaknesses in a body of work. Systematic reviews of RCTs are considered particularly robust—the peak of the evidence hierarchy—but both are prioritised and highly valued (de Souza Leão & Eyal, 2019; Pearce & Raman, 2014; White, 2019). As ably recounted elsewhere, RCTs have been around for almost a century, but in the last 20 years there has been a huge increase in their funding and use (Deaton & Cartwright, 2018; Pearce & Raman, 2014).

The seductively simple process offers an attractive vision of a world where, if only enough research evidence were available, acted on by willing and capable decision-makers, life in general would be better. We could summarise this view as:

- Policy is best made using research evidence.
- RCTs and systematic reviews are the best kind of evidence.
- Researchers should do more, better RCTs and SRs, and maximise their use by policymakers.

This is a very technocratic, rationalised view of policymaking which is still widely held (Wood, 2019). Thus, we find researchers offering aspirational views of their possible impact:

> For our department, [impact] means having certain policies and practices put in place because of our research. (Academic, criminal justice)

> Large national bodies who would then take our research and maybe themselves translate it into guidance, which might be used by non-scientists and non-researchers. (Social scientist)

Well it's good to feel actually that the policy is becoming more evidence based, as long as it doesn't turn into some sort of matrix based thing where you think you measure something and we should change the world to increase that. Everything is matrix based and you can't do anything if you can't find a matrix. But I think that rational view is welcomed. (Social scientist)

I would like our research to ultimately result in some change in the energy system and since we are not in control of the energy system and we do not build energy systems ourselves that means that we will have to have our impact through working with partners. (Engineer)

The version of policy decision-making which these researchers share is quite clear:

It's really important that policy is based on the best evidence that's possible. (Engineer)

Policymaking is seen to be optimised by easy access to high-quality, systematically identified and analysed evidence, which then forms the primary "input" to the policy process (see, e.g., Oxman et al., 2009: 1). The steps within this process are then laid clear for all to see, to enable 'accountability' and revision.

2.1 The Dominance of the Rationalist Model

Given the perceived simplicity of this process, it may be puzzling to its proponents why these improvements often fail to materialise in the real world. Scholars—particularly from the social and political sciences—have problematised the relationship between evidence and policy, recognising its complexity. The policy sciences have demonstrated convincingly that policy operates in a complex, even chaotic fashion. The linear model (positing problems, solutions, evaluations of these solutions, and thus improved policy) bears little resemblance to the multi-level complex adaptive governance that characterises most legislative systems. These days, most policymakers and many (especially social and political researchers) believe that a pluralist, diverse evidence base is the ideal starting point for decisions to be made about public policy and practice (Head, 2008). As a way of achieving this aim, it is now fairly common to see calls for more deliberative, democratic approaches to knowledge production and use (Degeling et al., 2017; Stewart, 2017); see Chapter 13 (Cassola et al., 2022) and Chapter 4 (Kothari & Smith, 2022). This approach recognises that all forms of knowledge are social, in the sense that they are interpreted by humans within social settings, and therefore driven by and subject to societal and political values and interests (Douglas, 2009; Fafard, 2015; Jasanoff & Polsby, 1991). However, despite these efforts, all too frequently the 'problem' is seen as being a 'lack of data', 'lack of evidence', or perhaps 'poor evidence uptake' (where the evidence exists, but is not acted on).

2.2   Why Has This Rationalist Model Held Strong, and Does It Matter?

One reason may be because (ironically) social and political scientists have tended to emphasise the complex nature of policymaking and the intransigent nature of the challenges facing decision-makers. While not wishing to argue with either of these characterisations, a lack of clear, informed lessons for other researchers and decision-makers may have meant that many relied on simplistic, easy-to-understand models of the policy world. So, for many researchers new to this field, their only way of getting a handle on what policy *is*, is to learn from the informal discussions between academics, from funders, or from university-led training courses. These tend to produce generic discourses of a simplified version of how evidence and policy interact, drawing on the misleading advice of unusually successful academics, or otherwise aiming to equip researchers with the idea (and tools to help) of maximising their impact. For example, many universities in the UK and internationally seek to increase their influence in the policy world. To do this, they encourage researchers to engage with government through in-house courses and incentive structures (Fafard & Hoffman, 2020; Hopkins et al., 2021). While well-intentioned, universities tend to rely on the rationalist model of research impact—perhaps because their teaching and examples are often derived from high-status researchers and projects from the faculties of medicine and science, not the political and social sciences. The alternative to the rationalist model is a highly complex evidence-policy ecosystem. For many this is hard to conceptualise, and researchers may feel is too difficult to engage with and influence as a whole. Thus, researchers and policymakers have formed, and are able to continue to promote, an unrealistically simple view of the nature of policy and evidence which is both rationalist and technocratic.

From the political and social sciences, attempts to challenge this over-simplified story have resulted in better conceptualisations of the nature of the problem, but not really in actionable next steps for those wishing to improve the situation. For example, challenges to the evidence hierarchy mostly took the form of methodological debate about the quality of different social research methods (Hammersley, 2005) and the appropriateness of different research designs for use in public policy (Cairney & Oliver, 2017; Head, 2008). These limitations to the RCT are well-documented. RCTs may not be appropriate where complex outcomes may be of interest (such as patient preferences or experiences); policies may operate at a different (e.g., whole-nation) level which is impossible to be randomised; or, as is the case for most public policy interventions, operate within a complex, ever-changing social environment with multiple competing policy interventions influencing individuals at different levels. These limitations to the RCT are of course extremely well-documented and understood by the research and policy community at large. However, this wide understanding of what they can, and cannot tell us has not prevented the even wider uptake of the hierarchy of evidence as a rule of thumb within policy and policy-research circles.

If we look at the three aspects of knowledge production, mobilisation and use together we can see they are a system over and through which we work as individuals and institutions. We operate within a system of funding, institutional roles and activities which incentivises certain activities and behaviours. Any radical approach would need to reimagine this system, but would in doing so challenge deeply held views about how decisions should be made (i.e., based on expertise and/or 'best' evidence) and indeed about the role of science in society.

Yet technocratic and normative polemics are hardly rare. In recent years, there has been a slew of talks and publications in the UK alone calling for more data-driven, technocratic decision-making (Haynes et al., 2012; White, 2019). It is not hard, for instance, to find examples of people advocating for data-driven policymaking with no recognition of the social (and thus non-objective) nature of this data; for the need for more RCTs to inform public policy; and for the importance of strengthening technocratic decision-making structures (Watts, 2019; White, 2019). The COVID-19 pandemic which began in early 2019 is a good example of this cognitive dissonance. It has impacted virtually every population on the planet, with governments adopting a slew of different policy responses to the huge challenge, with different goals (virus transmission suppression, containment, elimination, management), and different strategies to reach these goals (investment in vaccines, additional healthcare resources, public safety announcements, population control measures such as lockdowns, new legislative powers). Yet many in the public health research world continued to insist that evidence needed to be "robust enough" before acting on (meaning, it needed to be RCT evidence). As has been argued, this is simply not an appropriate form of knowledge required to answer the questions raised by the pandemic (Greenhalgh, 2020). Most governments did of course use other forms of evidence, but tended to rely on highly quantitative and—by necessity—reductionist modelling techniques to inform decision-making, rather than on, for example, discussions with anthropologists or sociologists (Cairney, 2021).

The key lesson from the many analyses already written about the covid pandemic, and indeed other disasters, crises, and challenges of more ordinary policymaking, is that multiple forms of knowledge are required (Jasanoff & Polsby, 1991; Sarewitz, 2018; Wynne, 2013). A mixed economy of knowledge and expertise enables a more honest conversation about what implications there are for decision-making. And focusing on how political and social pressures shape our evidence base allows us all to better understand how problems and solutions are framed. How might we do that?

3   AN ALTERNATIVE: THE POLITICAL ECONOMY OF KNOWLEDGE?

Tilley defines the political economy of knowledge as studying 'its forms of extraction, points of commodification, how it is refined as intellectual property' (Tilley, 2017). In short, focusing attention on what is presented and preferred allows us to ask critical questions about who is able to participate in knowledge production and why, what is valued and why, and the impact of these relationships. Using this lens, one can begin to see how misunderstandings, methodological in-fighting, and vested interests shape the evidence available to policymakers, and how this landscape shapes the environment for knowledge production. This offers a new way to begin thinking about how to creatively shape a more helpful environment for both policy and evidence.

Using this lens, I argue how we produce, mobilise, and use evidence has been shaped by the rationalist model, and how this model has shaped policy appetites and continues to influence how we all do our work—even though its failings are so widely understood. I argue that this simple narrative has shaped the evidence-policy environment in three main ways. Firstly, policymakers and researchers *shape the evidence base* through supporting and creating particular forms of evidence. Secondly, it *shapes how evidence is mobilised*, through offering roles and activities for researchers and others to follow. Thirdly, it *shapes how evidence is used* by policymakers, including selective evidence use.

3.1   Shaping the Evidence Base

The rationalist model of evidence-informed policymaking tells us that the main priority for most research funders and researchers is on how to improve the quality of the evidence base. As recounted above, for many this has meant more investment in RCTs. The Education Endowment Foundation (EEF) has, for example, "conducted over 80 randomised controlled trials - often held up as the gold standard in evaluation – and have around 80 more in the field". This is described as "hugely impressive" (Sanders, 2019). The UK government recognised the importance of RCTs in a report written on behalf of the Cabinet Office (Haynes et al., 2012) which argued for more and more RCTs. Alongside, this growth has been a push for more systematic reviews—explicitly, in the case of institutions such as the National Institute for Health and Clinical Excellence (NICE) and the rest of the What Works organisations, which tend to produce systematic reviews to inform policy and practice decisions. As White describes, "more reviews, and more use of reviews" (White, 2019, p. 4) are the explicit aims of these institutions.

In reality, of course, policymakers consume a far more heterogeneous evidence diet than simply RCTs and SRs (Oliver & de Vocht, 2017). Yet for a variety of reasons (including peer pressure, professional standards, and research governance), researchers tend to focus on creating new interventions and evaluations, rather than—for example—analysing local data on behalf of decision-makers. The relative under-investment in social and political research, compared with the vast amounts spent on physical and health sciences, is, I argue, a reflection of the way in which the rationalist model has shaped policymakers' appetites for a particular diet of evidence (Bastow et al., 2015).

Incentive structures within research organisations tend to encourage researchers to do more research (Sarewitz, 2018), of particular design (Oakley, 1990); not to focus on other activities such as 'getting to know policymakers' or mobilising research effectively (Bammer, 2005; Ferlie et al., 2012; Powell et al., 2018). Researchers thus conduct what they consider to be policy-relevant research, which is considered attractive by policymakers, who then ask for more of the same. Public health policy researchers have sometimes referred to this as 'lifestyle drift', where despite understanding the critical role of wider determinants of health like poverty and employment, both researchers and governments focus on policies and programmes which operate at the individual level (Powell et al., 2017; Rutter & Glonti, 2016). RCTs and experimental studies are well-suited to assessing individual-level interventions, such as the 'nudge' techniques which 'encourage' people to make 'better choices' (Thaler & Sunstein, 2008). Today, governments around the world spend billions on R&D, investing in systematic review facilities with explicit remits to inform policy and practice. The What Works model—that is, framing research questions around a solutions-oriented action, answerable by RCT and systematic review, digested with implications for policy and practice—has been exported around the globe (Boaz et al., 2019; Parkhurst, 2017).

One way of disrupting this feedback loop is to make evidence production more democratic and participatory, through co-designing policy-relevant research or interventions, for example, with end-users (see Chapter 13, Cassola et al., 2022). But these are not without their own challenges. How, for instance, could one easily involve a representative sample of all practitioners, officials, politicians, parents, community members, children, professionals who may be affected by a particular policy? How would one identify and reach out to these groups? What about the groups who would be affected by resources being withdrawn from elsewhere to support a new policy? These are extremely challenging steps to take within the confines of a (normal) research project, which risks codesign and coproduction becoming an overly simplified, even tokenistic process which does little to challenge existing social processes and structures through research (Oliver et al., 2019).

How can we reset this conversation between producers and users of evidence? One approach would be to imagine and critically assess the knowledge-policy system in its entirety. One would wish to examine how research funders (including governments) decide on priorities, how these priorities are enacted via funding instruments, committees, and peer review processes, and how researchers respond to these interventions. One could then ask questions about who was involved in these institutions and processes at different levels, and how representative these populations of actors were, compared with those on whom the research may ultimately seek to have impact. There are significant bodies of work which examine research funding allocation (Jones & Wilsdon, 2018; Shepherd et al., 2018), the reliability and replicability of research (Bishop, 2019; Ioannidis, 2005), and the need for transparency and 'openness' in scientific practices (Nosek, 2017). While important, these efforts engage primarily with research practices, not with the political dynamics shaping the evidence base, which lead to what Fricker calls "epistemic injustice" (Fricker, 2007). In essence, if some groups are prevented from having a voice—through lack of participation or representation in research, for example—then they become further disempowered, and policy continues to reinforce existing power imbalances (Holliman, no date). We look towards inclusive research practices (Duncan & Oliver, 2017; Stewart, 2017) to redress this balance, but we need clear, critical perspectives on the roles of sexism, racism, and other biases to explore how our knowledge production systems and outputs could be more representative.

Rather than simply assessing which types of research design were preferred or arguing over which types of research were 'better' for policy, one would wish to assess the broad and catholic appetite for data and evidence of all kinds within policy, and seek to meet and expand this appetite with robust evidence of many types. Perhaps most importantly, one would wish to expand the common understanding of 'evidence production' to include all these social and political processes, rather than to focus merely on what research exists, what is 'best,' and what to do next.

3.2   Shaping Evidence Mobilisation

The simple rationalist, technocratic model of RCT to policy also shapes how researchers and policymakers look for, promote, and engage with evidence. As has been already described, they fund particular organisations and structures which make evidence digestible and accessible, such as systematic reviews or policy briefs. The translation of research into actionable professional/practice guidelines is a key mode of knowledge mobilisation, and the What Works Centres (among others) and the multiple forms of policy lab, unit, or institute attached to universities serve a similar purpose. Yet these activities inevitably focus on the evidence which is there, not the gaps. Many people call for more syntheses (Donnelly et al., 2018), while acknowledging the problems with biased indexing, publication, and dissemination, but producing more academic papers is not going to address the systemic barriers to evidence use. For example, how do researchers and knowledge mobilisers use messaging and communication tools to persuade and engage with decision-makers? If we reject the hierarchy of evidence, how *can* different forms of evidence be assessed and compared? Movements such as *Democratising Evidence*[2] and *Research for All*[3] have begun these conversations, by publishing non-academic outputs and committing to diverse and representative writing teams—but this is still within the context of research production. More thought is required on how this could be operationalised within decision-making contexts.

In addition to the institutional context, the roles of individuals within the rationalist model are clear. Academics and researchers are there not to learn or discuss, but rather as experts there to inform and advise on policy issues:

> I think they'd like to think that their decision-making processes are at least informed by in-house analysis, and then the evidence base" (Health scientist)

> You are advising the chief scientists and they are advising the government on specific policies. (Social scientist)

---

[2] Democratising Evidence is a movement within several disciplines which involves recognising the potential of research as a vehicle for public engagement and equity. See, e.g., Nowotny, H. (2003). Democratising expertise and socially robust knowledge. *Science and Public Policy, 30*(3), 151–156.

[3] *Research for All* is an academic journal focusing on research that involves universities and communities, services or industries working together. Contributors and readers include researchers, policymakers, managers, practitioners, community-based organisations, schools, businesses, and intermediaries. It showcases research done collaboratively and builds a community across academic disciplines, professional sectors, and types of engagement.

Policymakers are there to receive wisdom, by selecting the best evidence available to them. Researchers are encouraged to make their evidence competitive by attending training courses on 'how to increase your impact' to use rhetorical techniques as their opponents, such as appealing to human values and experience, using stories to frame policy debates, and being able to charm and dazzle when networking with policymakers (Oliver et al., 2022; Zardo et al., 2014). Researchers acknowledge that

> You've got to be very careful because the point is, we're not supposed to be marketing our own research and arguing for our own funding. (Social Scientist)

but nevertheless, feel they should advocate for policy positions. Here, a public health clinician/researcher describes how they advised a local commissioner that stroke services should be reorganised towards early intervention in specialist services; despite this not being his specialism:

> One of the most important things I ever did in my medical career was advise a fellow councillor about a new paper that - he's an engineer and couldn't understand it, and I read it to him and said this is good and he went on and he almost single-handedly rearranged stroke management in this country ... I read this thing on stroke for him, and I said, "Yes, the science is fine... What they're saying is what happens, I'm happy with that, no major issues. (Public health clinician)

Many may feel that this is unproblematic, as to compete with other interests within the policy domain, one has to overstate to win any ground. Yet, this overreaching beyond one's expertise, or even beyond the research data can call into question the moral compass of universities and researchers in general:

> the Universities will do anything if you turn to the universities and say well you know I'm really interested in dancing frogs, off they'll nip. They'll be like, where's the grant, where's the money, where's the publication. (Public health researcher)

By extension the credibility of research in general can be questioned, where "scientists as 'strategists' engaged in a struggle for credibility" (Brown, 2015). As described above, by instating that RCT and systematic review evidence forms the only credible basis for action, researchers have opened the door to a relatively easy way for other actors to establish themselves as credible participants in policy debates (see Chapter 9, Hawkins & Oliver, 2022). Much has been written about the ways in which corporations create and curate evidence bases in order to generate lack of certainty, or to attack policy positions which might be detrimental to their growth. One of the starkest examples regards the use of albumin in post-operative patients multiple RCTs were undertaken between 1987 and 2005. A meta-analysis from 2005 showed that albumin killed more critical care patients than saline, and crucially, that this would have been was established by 1989, but for a further 30 years, more RCTs were done mostly funded by albumin producers. The existence of on-going research allowed them to say that it was not yet a settled question, but they were doing their best to establish what was the optimal treatment for patients (Chalmers, 2006). Elsewhere, colleagues have documented the ways in which commercial companies (predominantly pharma, food and alcohol, and tobacco companies) have used this tactic to create uncertainty, establish themselves as credible actors in the policy space, and undermine detrimental policies (Hawkins & Ettelt, 2018; Kickbusch et al., 2016; Knai et al., 2018; McKee & Stuckler, 2018). The existence of a robust evidence base—whether attached to a university, policy, or other entity—thus begins to offer the impression of credibility and security; and its absence, cause for concern (Oreskes & Conway, 2010). If an evidence base can be pointed to or created, the policy or actor is able to present themselves as a disinterested participant in policy debates.

We must acknowledge that appeals to evidence cannot always, and in fact rarely offer clear ways to navigate the political and social challenges of our times (Deeming, 2013). A clearer picture of our values and principles can clarify our aims, what we ask of the evidence base, and the various roles for researchers in this knowledge economy. On the surface, pressures on researchers and funders to increase their 'impact' are, no doubt, well-meaning in their intention to improve outcomes for society through 'improved' decision-making. However, the continued insistence that there is a 'right' form of evidence which should inform decision-making in the 'right' way has several unfortunate effects. As shown, it effectively operates as a counter-argument to those who call for more inclusive and participatory approaches to making and using knowledge. It creates a hierarchy of knowledge which allows research users to assign basically arbitrary values to different pieces of evidence such that some is more 'worthy' than others. This can be taken as a proxy for credibility, which in turn allows policy proposals to be attacked on this basis. And finally, it shapes the behaviours of both research users and producers, in that it creates perverse incentives for researchers to present themselves and their work in particular ways which may undermine their credibility.

3.3 Shaping Evidence Use

Finally, how policymakers use evidence itself is also shaped by the simplistic narrative. By focusing on quality and robustness of research, researchers were naturally enough focusing on those elements in the research-policy environment within their reach; but neglecting to think through either the consequences of these debates, or the broader context within which they were working. For instance, insisting that RCTs are the most, even the only valid form of evidence enables policies to be attacked for *not* being based on RCTs, even where this might be impossible to achieve or inappropriate. RCT evidence is well-suited to establishing effectiveness of individual-level interventions where outcomes are easily quantifiable and measured. Many aspects of public health and social policy and the associated interventions do not fit these criteria. This reality was underscored during the COVID-19 pandemic when debates arose about whether governments should adopt policies with respect to making, physical distancing, or vaccination in the absence of completed RCTs. It is possible that by sidestepping the broader questions of validity to focus on methodological robustness, researchers have enabled policymakers to seize on the RCT as a talisman of quality, making policies harder to challenge and depoliticising, or rather defusing debates about which policies ought to be implemented.

A strong focus on experimental evidence all*ows policymakers to sidestep important questions about systemic problems.* Recent sociological work has pointed to similarities between "randomistas", that is, proponents of RCTs, and philanthro-capitalists in their belief in measurement, mistrust in experts, belief in experimentation as a means to achieve 'leverage, and unstated but present liberal paternalism (de Souza Leão & Eyal, 2019; Deeming, 2013). For example, De Souza Leão et al. describe the case of a deworming RCT in Africa which showed increased educational attainment for both treated and untreated children, although this later proved to be unreplicable. Millions of dollars were invested in deworming, rather than in improving school access, teacher training, or the many other elements which combine to influence educational attainment. De Souza

Leão et al. show that the presence of the RCT allowed donors and decision-makers to sidestep complex, moral questions about resource allocation and systems change, focus on what could be measured, and evaluate only what was easily available. This is important, as these evidence bases then become the justification for further political action.

Another example concerns the UK Department of Health refusing to fund an RCT of the Sure Start programme (thus ensuring no negative results could be found (Melhuish et al., 2008, 2010). The preference for certain methods and epistemologies allows policymakers to use legitimate concerns about methods or generalisability to undermine and dismiss evidence which may be inconvenient. This could enable the politicisation of research activities, where researchers are unable to test hypotheses effectively, nor able to discuss their findings openly or honestly (Hartley et al., 2017).

Thus, by insisting on the primacy of certain forms of knowledge, researchers may be opening the door to a policy focus on interventions for which experimental data is available and proliferating. Researchers and funders thus interpreted policy as being rationalist and technocratic, and responded with an increased focus on individual-level interventions, in a feedback loop, leading to an overall lack of attention to gaps in the evidence base, possible alternative policies, systems-level thinking, and non-incremental change (Baum & Fisher, 2014).

The rationalist model also enables poor evidence use behaviours among policymakers. For example, cherry-picking data. The classic example is the youth recidivism intervention, Scared Straight, in which 'at-risk' youths were exposed to the prison environment, in an attempt to demonstrate its awfulness and prevent further crime. Proponents of Scared Straight prefer an evaluation which demonstrates raised awareness of prison immediately following the visit (Finckenauer & Finckenauer, 1999; Petrosino et al., 2003), which they argue demonstrated effectiveness, but a systematic review of long-term evaluations shows increased offending in the intervention arm (Petrosino et al., 2013). Similarly, the UK government's flagship Troubled Families policy has shown no effect on its target outcomes "despite persistent claims by politicians that it had 'turned around' the lives of tens of thousands of families and saved over a billion pounds" (Butler, 2016). Sure Start is talked about both as a success (Glass, 1999; Melhuish et al., 2010) and a failure (Clarke, 2006; Melhuish et al., 2008), according to whether one measures social exclusion/participation, or educational attainment.

Evidence is 'used' when it enables a decision to be made. Yet we know that decisions are rarely clear-cut, and where they are, evidence rarely allows decision-makers to choose between options (Cairney et al., 2016). To better understand how evidence is used in decision-making, we must move past diagnosing 'correct' types of evidence or 'correct' types of use, towards understanding the knowledge ecosystem within which the policy problems are framed and discussed.

4   Conclusions

Evidence is shaped by those who create it (as funders, as participants, or as researchers), those who curate and promote it (as writers, disseminators, or synthesisers), and by those who use it. As Weiss argued in 1977, improving evidence 'use' means, fundamentally, improving decision-making. Her primary concern, as an evaluator and scholar of public policy, was on how to improve the quality of public decision-making; and for her, as for many of us, improving use of research evidence played an important role in that process. Yet almost from its inception, the evidence-based policy and practice movement has somehow conflated these goals. Parsing them out allows us to ask what 'quality' evidence or decisions look like, and who should participate in them. But too often, the assumption has been made that good evidence will automatically lead to better decisions.

Despite a good understanding of how evidence and policy interact developed in the social and political sciences, many researchers continue to misunderstand policy. Even when acknowledging its complexity and arbitrariness, they offer rationalist conceptualisations, and technocratic preferences regarding decision-making. In this world, policymakers seek (and are offered) clear answers to defined problems, or arbitration between clear policy options. The researcher becomes an individualist entrepreneur, attempting to maximise their own influence, often without considering the moral, ethical, or political dimensions of their claims or actions.

The technocratic vision has real dangers for democratic decision-making, and for the credibility of evidence more generally. Either the technocrats are simply unaware of the strength of the arguments made by the democratisers, or they disagree with their stance. Is any reconciliation possible?

Framing the relationships between research and evidence production, mobilisation, and use as a social construction shaped by power dynamics and social interactions allows us to interrogate how these forces determine behaviours and outcomes, and we can start to see the knowledge economy as an interrelated, mutually shaping dynamic system. Bringing critical perspectives into this systemic approach to the study of knowledge production, mobilisation, and use, we can illuminate the social pressures which influence these processes.

This offers a new way to begin thinking about how to creatively shape a more helpful environment for both policy and evidence. To return to Nick Carr's quote at the start of this article, we all know that New York is not a city of alleys—that there is an evidence base beyond the hierarchy of evidence, and that use is not always instrumental—but somehow this realisation does not translate into more complete depictions. We can ask why not. We can also ask what to do about it.

While useful for illuminating social dynamics which reinforce power imbalances, this may not be a perfect lens for exploring evidence-based policymaking. We do need to ask where responsibility and power lie; how consensus about policy preferences is generated, and what are the various roles of researchers and policymakers, and the importance of agency within this system.

Finally, merely describing a problem is not a means to deal with it. Yet by arming researchers and policymakers with critical perspectives on how evidence and policy shape one another, we can start to have more informed conversations about what a healthy system might look like. At the very least, we need to start asking serious questions about the roles of researchers and policymakers in sustaining the current system. Is it our job as researchers to monitor and assess how well policymakers used evidence? Is transparency enough? And how do the broader societal and cultural aspects of the knowledge production system influence our practice as researchers?

References

Bammer, G. (2005). Integration and implementation sciences: Building a new specialization. *Ecology and Society, 10*(2), 6.

Bastow, S., Dunleavy, P., & Tinkler, J. (2015). *The impact of the social sciences: How academics and their research make a difference.* How Academics and Their Research Make a Difference. Sage. https://doi.org/10.4135/978147 3921511

Baum, F., & Fisher, M. (2014). Why behavioural health promotion endures despite its failure to reduce health inequities. *Sociology of Health and Illness, 36*(2), 213–225. https://doi.org/10.1111/1467-9566.12112

Bishop, D. (2019). Rein in the four horsemen of irreproducibility. *Nature.* https://doi.org/10.1038/d41586-019-01307-2

Boaz, A. et al. (2019) *What works now? Evidence-informed policy and practice revisited.* Policy Press. Available at: https://policy.bristoluniversitypress.co.uk/what-works-now. Accessed 17 July 2018.

Brown, M. B. (2015). 'Politicizing science: Conceptions of politics in science and technology studies. *Social Studies of Science. SAGE PublicationsSage UK: London, England, 45*(1), 3–30. https://doi.org/10.1177/030631271455 6694

Butler, P. (2016). More than £1bn for troubled families "has had little impact". *The Guardian.* Available at: https://www.theguardian.com/society/2016/oct/17/governments-448m-troubled-families-scheme-has-had-little-impact-thinktank. Accessed 4 June 2019.

Cairney, P. (2021). The UK government's COVID-19 policy: What does "guided by the science" mean in practice?, *Frontiers in Political Science. Frontiers Media SA, 3.* https://doi.org/10.3389/FPOS.2021.624068/FULL

Cairney, P., & Oliver, K. (2017). Evidence-based policymaking is not like evidence-based medicine, so how far should you go to bridge the divide between evidence and policy? *Health Research Policy and Systems, 15*(1).https://doi.org/10.1186/s12961-017-0192-x.

Cairney, P., Oliver, K., & Wellstead, A. (2016). To bridge the divide between evidence and policy: Reduce ambiguity as much as uncertainty. *Public Administration Review, 76*(3), 399–402. https://doi.org/10.1111/puar.12555

Cassola, A., Fafard, P., Palkovits, M., & Hoffman, S J. (2022). Mechanisms to bridge the gap between science and politics in evidence-Informed policymaking: Mapping the landscape. In P. Fafard, A. Cassola, & E. De Leeuw (Eds.), *Integrating science and politics for public health.* Palgrave Springer.

Chalmers, I. (2006). Meeting the research information needs of patients and clinicians more effectively. In *Equator Network, 1st Annual Lecture.*

Clarke, K. (2006). Childhood, parenting and early intervention: A critical examination of the Sure Start national programme. *Critical Social Policy. 26*(4), 699–721. Sage. https://doi.org/10.1177/0261018306068470

Cochrane, A. L. (1972). Effectiveness and efficiency: Random reflections on health services. *BMJ.* https://doi.org/10.1136/bmj.328.7438.529

Deaton, A., & Cartwright, N. (2018). Understanding and misunderstanding randomised controlled trials. *Social Science & Medicine. Pergamon, 210,* 2–21. https://doi.org/10.1016/J.SOCSCIMED.2017.12.005

Deeming, C. (2013). Trials and tribulations: The "use" (and "misuse") of evidence in public policy. *Social Policy & Administration. Wiley-Blackwell, 47*(4), 359. https://doi.org/10.1111/SPOL.12024

Degeling, C., et al. (2017). Influencing health policy through public deliberation: Lessons learned from two decades of Citizens'/community juries. *Social Science and Medicine, 179*, 166–171. https://doi.org/10.1016/j.socscimed.2017.03.003

Donnelly, C. A., et al. (2018). Four principles to make evidence synthesis more useful for policy. *Nature. Nature Publishing Group, 558*(7710), 361–364. https://doi.org/10.1038/d41586-018-05414-4

Douglas, H. (2009). *Science, policy, and the value-free ideal.* University of Pittsburgh Press.

Duncan, S., & Oliver, S. (2017). Editorial. *Research for All, 1*(1), 1–5. https://doi.org/10.18546/RFA.01.1.01

Fafard, P. (2015). Beyond the usual suspects: Using political science to enhance public health policy making. *Journal of Epidemiology and Community Health, 1129*, 1–4. https://doi.org/10.1136/jech-2014-204608

Fafard, P., & Hoffman, S. J. (2020). Rethinking knowledge translation for public health policy. *Evidence and Policy, 16*(1), 165–175. Policy Press. https://doi.org/10.1332/174426418X15212871808802

Ferlie, E. et al. (2012). Knowledge mobilisation in healthcare: A critical review of health sector and generic management literature. *Social Science & Medicine, 74*(8), 1297–1304. The Boulevard Langford Lane Kidlington, Oxford OX5 1GB UK: Pergamon/Elsevier Science Ltd. https://doi.org/10.1016/j.socscimed.2011.11.042.

Finckenauer, J. O., & Finckenauer, J. O. (1999) *Scared straight!: The panacea phenomenon revisited.* Waveland Press. Available at: https://www.ncjrs.gov/App/Publications/abstract.aspx?ID=178617. Accessed 31 January 2018.

Fricker, M. (2007). *Epistemic injustice: Power and the ethics of knowing.* Oxford University Press. https://doi.org/10.1093/acprof:oso/9780198237907.001.0001

Glass, N. (1999). Sure Start: The development of an early intervention programme for young children in the United Kingdom. *Children & Society, 13*(4), 257–264. Blackwell. https://doi.org/10.1002/CHI569

Greenhalgh, T. (2020). Will COVID-19 be evidence-based medicine's nemesis? *PLOS Medicine. Public Library of Science, 17*(6). https://doi.org/10.1371/JOURNAL.PMED.1003266

Hammersley, M. (2005). Is the evidence-based practice movement doing more good than harm? *Reflections on Iain Chalmers' Case for Research-Based Policy Making and Practice', Evidence & Policy: A Journal of Research, Debate and Practice.* https://doi.org/10.1332/1744264052703203

Hartley, S., Pearce, W., & Taylor, A. (2017). Against the tide of depoliticisation: The politics of research governance. *Policy & Politics, 45*(3), 361–377. https://doi.org/10.1332/030557316X14681503832036

Hawkins, B., & Ettelt, S. (2018). The strategic uses of evidence in UK e-cigarettes policy debates. *Evidence & Policy: A Journal of Research, Debate and Practice.* https://doi.org/10.1332/174426418X15212872451438

Hawkins, B., & Oliver, K. (2022). Select committee governance and the production of evidence: The case of UK E-cigarettes policy. In P. Fafard, A. Cassola, & E. De Leeuw (Eds.), *Integrating science and politics for public health.* Palgrave Springer.

Haynes, L., et al. (2012). *Test. Developing public policy with randomised controlled trials,* SSRN. https://doi.org/10.2139/ssrn.2131581

Head, B. W. (2008). Three lenses of evidence-based policy. *Australian Journal of Public Administration, 67*(1), 1–11. https://doi.org/10.1111/j.1467-8500.2007.00564.x

Holliman, R. (n.d.). Fairness in knowing: How should we engage with the sciences? *Engaging Research.* Available at: http://www.open.ac.uk/blogs/per/?p=8197 (Accessed: 17 May 2019).

Hopkins, A. et al. (2021). Are research-policy engagement activities informed by policy theory and evidence? 7 challenges to the UK impact agenda. *Policy, Design and Practice.*

Ioannidis, J. P. A. (2005). Why most published research findings are false. *PLoS Medicine, 2*(8). https://doi.org/10.1371/journal.pmed.0020124

Jasanoff, S., & Polsby, N. W. (1991). The fifth branch: Science advisers as policymakers. *Contemporary Sociology, 20*(5), 727. https://doi.org/10.2307/2072218.

Jones, R., & Wilsdon, J. (2018) *The biomedical bubble.* Available at: www.nesta.org.uk. Accessed 17 May 2019.

Kickbusch, I., Allen, L., & Franz, C. (2016). The commercial determinants of health. *The Lancet Global Health.* https://doi.org/10.1016/S2214-109X(16)30217-0

Knai, C., et al. (2018). Systems thinking as a framework for analyzing commercial determinants of health. *Milbank Quarterly, 96*(3), 472–498. https://doi.org/10.1111/1468-0009.12339

Kothari, A., & Smith, M. J. (2022). Public health policymaking, politics, and evidence. In P. Fafard, A. Cassola, & E. De Leeuw (Eds.), *Integrating science and politics for public health.* Palgrave Springer.

McKee, M., & Stuckler, D. (2018). Revisiting the corporate and commercial determinants of health. *American Journal of Public Health.* https://doi.org/10.2105/AJPH.2018.304510

Melhuish, E., Belsky, J., & Barnes, J. (2010). Evaluation and value of sure start. *Archives of disease in childhood, 95*(3), 159–161. BMJ. https://doi.org/10.1136/adc.2009.161018.

Melhuish, E., Belsky, J., & Leyland, A. (2008). *The impact of sure start local programmes on three-year-olds and their families.* Available at: http://eprints.bbk.ac.uk/7579/. Accessed 31 January 2018.

Movsisyan, A., et al. (2018). Rating the quality of a body of evidence on the effectiveness of health and social interventions: A systematic review and mapping of evidence domains. *Research Synthesis Methods.* https://doi.org/10.1002/jrsm.1290

Nosek, B. (2017). Opening science. In *Open: The philosophy and practices that are revolutionizing education and science.* https://doi.org/10.5334/bbc.g.

Oakley, A. (1990). Who's afraid of the randomised controlled trial? *Women & Health.* https://doi.org/10.1300/j013v15n04_02

Oliver, K. A., & de Vocht, F. (2017). Defining 'evidence' in public health: A survey of policymakers' uses and preferences. *European Journal of Public Health, 27*(suppl_2), 112–117.

Oliver, K. A. et al. (2022.). What works in academic-policy engagement? *Evidence and Policy.* https://doi.org/10.1332/174426421X16420918447616

Oliver, K., Kothari, A., & Mays, N. (2019). The dark side of coproduction: Do the costs outweigh the benefits for health research? *Health Research Policy and Systems, 17*(1). https://doi.org/10.1186/s12961-019-0432-3.

Oliver, K., & Pearce, W. (2017). Three lessons from evidence-based medicine and policy: Increase transparency, balance inputs and understand power. *Palgrave Communications, 3*(1), 43. https://doi.org/10.1057/s41599-017-0045-9

Oreskes, N., & Conway, E. M. (2010). *Merchants of doubt: How a handful of scientists obscured the truth on issues from tobacco smoke to global warming* (p. 355). Bloomsbury Press.

Oxman, A. D. et al. (2009). SUPPORT tools for evidence-informed health policymaking (STP) 16: Using research evidence in balancing the pros and cons of policies. *Health Research Policy and Systems, 7*(1). CAMPUS, 4 CRINAN ST, LONDON N1 9XW, ENGLAND: BMC. https://doi.org/10.1186/1478-4505-7-S1-S16.

Parkhurst, J. (2017). *The politics of evidence: From evidence-based policy to the good governance of evidence.* Routledge Studies in Governance and Public Policy. https://doi.org/doi:10.4324/9781315675008

Parkhurst, J. O., & Abeysinghe, S. (2016). What constitutes "good" evidence for public health and social policy-making? From hierarchies to appropriateness. *Social Epistemology, 30*(5–6), 665–679. https://doi.org/10.1080/02691728.2016.1172365

Pearce, W., & Raman, S. (2014). The new randomised controlled trials (RCT) movement in public policy: Challenges of epistemic governance.

Policy Sciences,47(4), 387–402. Springe. https://doi.org/10.1007/s11077-014-9208-3

Petrosino, A. et al. (2013). "Scared straight" and other juvenile awareness programs for preventing juvenile delinquency. *Cochrane Database of Systematic Reviews* (3). https://doi.org/10.1002/14651858.CD002796.pub2.

Petrosino, A., Turpin-Petrosino, C., & Buehler, J. (2003). Scared straight and other Juvenile awareness programs for preventing Juvenile delinquency: A systematic review of the randomised experimental evidence. *The ANNALS of the American Academy of Political and Social Science, 589*(1), 41–62. Sage. https://doi.org/10.1177/0002716203254693

Petticrew, M., & Roberts, H. (2003). Evidence, hierarchies, and typologies: Horses for courses. *Journal of Epidemiology and Community Health.* https://doi.org/10.1136/jech.57.7.527

Powell, A., Davies, H. T. O., & Nutley, S. M. (2018). Facing the challenges of research-informed knowledge mobilisation: 'Practising what we preach?', *public Administration, 96*(1), 36–52. WIley. 111 RIVER ST, HOBOKEN 07030–5774. https://doi.org/10.1111/padm.12365.

Powell, K. et al. (2017). Theorising lifestyle drift in health promotion: Explaining community and voluntary sector engagement practices in disadvantaged areas. *Taylor & Francis. Routledge, 27*(5), 554–565. https://doi.org/10.1080/095 81596.2017.1356909

Rutter, H., & Glonti, K. (2016). Towards a new model of evidence for public health. *The Lancet, 388,* S7. https://doi.org/10.1016/S0140-6736(16)322 43-7

Sanders, M. (2019). *We owe a debt to Kevan Collins.* KCL News Centre. Available at: https://www.kcl.ac.uk/news/we-owe-a-debt-to-kevan-collins. Accessed 17 May 2019.

Sarewitz, D. (2018). Of cold mice and isotopes or should we do less science? In *Science and politics: Exploring relations between academic research, higher education, and science policy summer school in higher education research and science studies.* Bonn. Available at: https://sfis.asu.edu/sites/default/files/sho uld_we_do_less_science-revised_distrib.pdf.

Shenderovich, Y., Sutherland, A., & Grant, S. (2019) *Assessing confidence in "what works" in social policy.* RAND blog.

Shepherd, J. et al. (2018). Peer review of health research funding proposals: A systematic map and systematic review of innovations for effectiveness and efficiency. *PloS One, 13*(5), e0196914 (Ed., G. E. Derrick). Public Library of Science. https://doi.org/10.1371/journal.pone.0196914.

Souza Leão, D. L. & Eyal, G. (2019). The rise of randomised controlled trials (RCTs) in international development in historical perspective. *Theory and Society* (pp. 1–36). Springer. https://doi.org/10.1007/s11186-019-093 52-6.

Stewart, R. (2017). Terminology and tensions within evidence-informed decision-making in South Africa over a 15-year period. *Research for All.* https://doi.org/10.18546/RFA.01.2.03

Thaler, R., & Sunstein, C. (2008). *Nudge: Improving desicions abouth health, wealth and happiness, Nudge: Improving decisions about health, wealth, and happiness.* https://doi.org/10.1007/s10602-008-9056-2.

Tilley, L. (2017). Resisting piratic method by doing research otherwise. *Sociology, 51*(1), 27–42. https://doi.org/10.1177/0038038516656992. Sage. https://doi.org/10.1177/0038038516656992.

Watts, C. (2019). *Using RCTS to evaluate social interventions: Have we got it right? | LSHTM.* CEDIL and Centre for Evaluation Lecture Series. Available at: https://www.lshtm.ac.uk/newsevents/events/using-rcts-evaluate-social-interventions-have-we-got-it-right. Accessed 20 May 2019.

Webel, A. R. et al. (2010). A systematic review of the effectiveness of peer-based interventions on health-related behaviors in adults. *American journal of public health, 100*(2), 247–253. American Public Health Association. https://doi.org/10.2105/AJPH.2008.149419.

White, H. (2019). *The twenty-first century experimenting society: The four waves of the evidence revolution, 5*(1). https://doi.org/10.1057/s41599-019-0253-6.

Wood, M. (2019). *Hyper-active governance: How governments manage the politics of expertise.* How governments manage the politics of expertise. Cambridge University Press. https://doi.org/10.1017/9781108592437

Wynne, B. (2013). Social identities and public uptake of science: Chernobyl, Sellafield, and environmental radioactivity sciences. *Radioactivity in the environment, 19,* 283–309. https://doi.org/10.1016/B978-0-08-045015-5.00016-2

Zardo, P., Collie, A., & Livingstone, C. (2014). External factors affecting decision-making and use of evidence in an Australian public health policy environment. *Social Science & Medicine, 108*(SI), 120–127. Elsevier Science Ltd., The Boulevard Langford Lane Kidlington Oxford OX5 1GB UK. https://doi.org/10.1016/j.socscimed.2014.02.046.

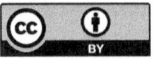

CHAPTER 6

Sidestepping the Stalemate: The Strategies of Public Health Actors for Circulating Evidence into the Policy Process

Carole Clavier, France Gagnon, and Blake Poland

1 Introduction

We have argued elsewhere that public health actors often display a certain naiveté when it comes to the policy process. They tend to believe that

C. Clavier (✉)
Department of Political Science, Université du Québec à Montréal, Montréal, QC, Canada
e-mail: clavier.carole@uqam.ca

F. Gagnon
School of Administration Sciences, Université TÉLUQ, Quebec City, QC, Canada

Quebec Population Health Research Network, Quebec City, QC, Canada

B. Poland
Dalla Lana School of Public Health, University of Toronto, Toronto, ON, Canada

© The Author(s) 2022
P. Fafard et al. (eds.), *Integrating Science and Politics for Public Health*,
Palgrave Studies in Public Health Policy Research,
https://doi.org/10.1007/978-3-030-98985-9_6

presenting evidence to policy-makers should be sufficient to change policies. They also tend to ignore the inherently political nature of public health, the characteristics of the policy process or the competing priorities and factors that guide public policymaking (Bernier & Clavier, 2011; de Leeuw et al., 2014). As de Leeuw succinctly puts it: "The moral high ground that many if not most health professionals and scholars occupy may also stand in the way of a realistic appraisal of the complex and competitive nature of integration efforts. There is significant naiveté when it comes to the politics and power games and the role that the health sector can or should play" (de Leeuw, 2017, p. 344). This is consistent with the premise of this book that public health policymaking is locked in a stalemate between the evidence-based and the politics-driven policy-making perspectives. Public health actors are thought to rely solely or primarily on scientific evidence to guide their influence strategies over the policy-making process, thus setting their efforts apart from and above politics. By contrast, elected officials, their political advisors and senior civil servants take the broader view that party politics, public opinion, interests, past decisions and other political factors influence policymaking, thus resisting the sole influence of scientific evidence. Overcoming the stalemate would require more overlap between the two worlds of scientific evidence and politics.

By contrast, in this chapter, we take a nuanced perspective on the stalemate between evidence and politics by revisiting our earlier claim that public health actors are naive about the policy process. What prompted us to do so are the results from a recent comparative study of active transportation policies in Montréal and Toronto. We have found that local public health actors (professionals and senior officials from local public health agencies) are very involved in official policy processes (e.g. public consultations, committees). They have developed sustained interactions with other local actors interested in active transportation policy (from elected officials to NGOs) with the explicit aim of influencing the emergence and implementation of active transportation policies (Clavier et al., 2019). Evidence is central to the arguments that they put forward, but what public health actors do to circulate evidence suggests that they engage strategically with the policy process. These findings lead us to question the extent of the political naiveté or, to the contrary, political savviness of local public health actors.

The central question we address in this chapter is: what do the strategies that local public health actors used to circulate evidence suggest about their conception of the policy process and about the role of evidence in the policy process?

The next two sections present the active transportation policy study, including the methods used for data collection and analysis, as well as insights from theories on policy coalitions, actor interactions and the reception of policy transfer that will be useful to examine the insertion of evidence into the policy process. The results are organized into two main sections, (1) the strategies that public health actors used to circulate evidence into the policy process and (2) how local public health actors conceive of the policy process.

2   Theory and Methods—Considering Strategies for Evidence Circulation in Local Policy Subsystem

2.1   Evidence and the Policy Process

The debate juxtaposing evidence-based policymaking and politics is an enduring feature of the literature (Newman, 2017; Standring, 2017), as is the quest for methods to produce the "right kind of evidence" for use by policy-makers and understanding how policy-makers use evidence (for instance: Hunter, 2009; Ouimet et al., 2010; Pawson, 2002; Whitehead et al., 2004). Policy studies are also concerned with how theories of the policy process conceptualize evidence and the realities of introducing evidence into the political process of policymaking (Béland & Katapally, 2018; Cairney, 2016; Fafard, 2008; Parkhurst, 2017; Smith, 2013). This latter stream of research has highlighted the competing ideas, social values, interests and issues that characterize the policy process; the challenges to democratic legitimacy posed by evidence and expert knowledge, and the limitations of experts' understanding of the policy process. Among theories of the policy process, the Advocacy Coalition Framework (ACF) (Sabatier & Weible, 2007) considers that technical information contributes to policy learning, i.e. it contributes to transforming how policy actors view a public problem and its solutions. Policy learning is one way to bring about public policy change. More generally, the ACF maps interactions between actors involved in one policy and seeks to identify coalitions among these actors, based on their sustained interactions and shared beliefs about the policy. It explains policy change through the opposition between policy coalitions, when the dominant coalition may be replaced by a contestant, or through changes in the beliefs of the dominant coalition.

Our primary interest is not how actors in the dominant coalition come to include new evidence (new technical information) into their policy beliefs. It is, rather, how actors from opposing coalitions (or from the fringes of the dominant coalition) circulate new evidence so that it comes to the attention of the dominant coalition. Considering actor interactions on the basis of their shared belief systems brings attention to two issues relevant to the strategies of evidence circulation, namely the processes of actor inclusion and actor exclusion from the policy process and the ideas that bring coalitions together (Clavier & O'Neill, 2017). If some actors are not in a position to cooperate closely with decision makers from the dominant coalition, how else do they circulate their knowledge? Do they seek cooperation with actors sharing similar, or at least compatible, ideas about the policy? Do they try and introduce their evidence into other narratives about active transportation so as to influence policy? Based on these questions, this chapter focuses specifically on our research about what public health actors do for circulating evidence in the policy process and towards the dominant coalition in the case of active transportation policies in Montréal and Toronto (Clavier et al., 2019). Going back to the starting point for this chapter, we will then reflect on what these strategies tell about how public health actors conceive of the policy process.

2.2   The Active Transportation Policy Study

Empirically, this chapter draws on data gathered in a comparative research study on the processes underlying the implementation of active trans-portation policies in Montréal (Québec, Canada) and Toronto (Ontario, Canada). This was a funded study with human subjects review.[1] We studied active transportation policies as potential healthy public policies. As such, one of the research objectives was to question the role of public health actors and knowledge in the emergence and implementation of active transportation policies.

---

[1] The research project was funded by the Heart and Stroke Foundation as part of the CIHR competition for Population Health Intervention Research (2014–2018). It was approved by the Ethics Committees of the Université du Québec à Montréal (# S-703818–66), of the University of Toronto (# 31,140) and of Toronto Public Health (# 2015–06).

To achieve our objectives, we used the ACF as a template to identify the contours of the active transportation policy subsystem. We identified policy actors involved in the emergence and implementation stages of the policy process, while recognizing that these stages do not logically follow one another (DeLeon, 1999), their belief systems as well as their interactions. We collected data through document analysis (official plans and reports) and semi-structured interviews with key policy subsystem actors (20 in Montréal and 20 in Toronto) conducted between 2015 and 2017. In this chapter, we rely on interviews with public health actors in both cities (two in Toronto, three in Montréal). Although the sample is small, interviews with other actors from their respective active transportation policy subsystem confirm their practices for the circulation of evidence. The public health actors under study here are professionals and senior officials in local public health agencies, that is Montréal Public Health and Toronto Public Health. Their job descriptions entail programme and policy development, programme implementation—in conjunction with local partners from different institutions or community organizations—and research. This means that they not only circulate evidence but also produce evidence, either on their own or through collaborations with academics and NGOs. We use the term "evidence" in a broad sense here to refer to conclusions of research projects carried out by local public health actors, reports based on literature reviews and original data, and experiences from active transportation policies in other cities and countries.

We conducted thematic data analysis (Braun & Clarke, 2006) of the verbatim transcripts of interviews using an online data analysis platform (Dedoose). We established a list of themes related to the conceptual categories of the ACF (actors, interactions, belief systems, relatively stable parameters and external events) and added to that list inductively during data analysis. The research yielded data on the role of public health actors and public health knowledge in the processes of active transportation policy emergence and implementation (Clavier et al., 2019). This chapter builds on the data presented in the 2019 article to identify strategies that public health actors used to circulate evidence. However, the arguments we make here about how public health actors conceive of the policy process go beyond the scope of the original comparative research on active transportation policy. Besides, we do not consider how municipal decision makers weigh evidence from public health actors as compared to evidence from other sources (private consultants, industry lobbies and so on): focusing on public health actors only may overstate the coherence and influence of their narrative about active transportation.

3   STRATEGIES OF PUBLIC HEALTH ACTORS TO CIRCULATE EVIDENCE INTO THE POLICY PROCESS

The strategies that local public health actors used to circulate evidence address different dimensions of the policy process, namely ideas, the existence of competing interests, the formal instruments of public participation/consultation, the interactions of policy and politics as well as the interactions of actors. As these dimensions are closely related, we have organized the presentation of these strategies into two categories: those that address ideas and framing and those that address actor interactions.

3.1   Framing Active Transportation and Health Through Evidence

In both Montréal and Toronto, local public health actors have become involved in the development of active transportation policies by building evidence about the links between air pollution, transportation and health and about the links between the built environment, physical activity, collisions and health. Toronto Public Health has published a series of reports on the built environment and health titled *Healthy Toronto by Design* as well as a series on walking, cycling and the built environment (Toronto Public Health, 2011, 2012, 2013, 2014). "*Le transport urbain, une question de santé*" is a key publication by Montréal Public Health on the links between transportation, health and the built environment, including suggestions for action (Direction de santé publique, 2006). In addition, public health employees with a research role have published reports that local actors promoting active transportation policies often reference. Among these, two reports analyze what makes neighbourhoods walkable (Paquin & Pelletier, 2012) and the numbers of pedestrians and cyclists injured in collisions at intersections in Montréal (Morency et al., 2013).

In building this evidence base, local public health actors reference the influence of public health actors in other jurisdictions as an incentive to address the subject of active transportation, as well as the importance of research and academic publication. Working with other public health institutions in an intervention research partnership broadens the scope of issues that the local public health units work with. Involvement in academic research and publication also lends legitimacy to their involvement in active transportation:

> Then by 2011, came this concept of Healthy Toronto by Design, and again broadening our focus. So you get a healthy city because of many spheres, but, of course, transportation is one. Then things like Walkable City. And here, what I want to say is I think a key influencer is Dr. David Mowat from Peel. And he was the one who encouraged a number of health units including Toronto Public Health to be joined on a grant from CPAC (Canadian Partnership Against Cancer). (Public health actor, Toronto)

> This is what allowed me to survive, so to speak: producing academic research is a way to gain legitimacy, so that I could give talks for citizens, NGOs, the public. Academia has been an ally. (Public health actor, Montréal)

If building an evidence base was a necessary first step, local public health actors have also sought ways to communicate this evidence effectively. Data visualization is one of them. In Montréal, several local public health actors—including a researcher employed in the provincial public health agency—have mentioned the importance of maps in their efforts at building evidence:

> Maps [displaying the number of pedestrians injured at each intersection in the city] raised profile because they were accessible to the public and citizens brought them up at city council or borough council meetings saying, 'People get injured on my street.' (Public health actor, Montréal)

Visualizing data about injuries at intersections proved a powerful tool for communicating the data and for promoting its uptake by citizens, NGOs and other actors. In the case of pedestrian injuries at intersections, it also provided another angle to raise awareness about active transportation. As another public health actor put it, transportation safety provided a more compelling agenda for citizens and policy-makers than arguments about the effects of active transportation on the reduction of greenhouse gas emissions. It contributed to the introduction of security measures such as reduced speed limits in residential neighbourhoods in the City's transportation plan.

In their efforts to frame evidence so that it makes sense for other policy actors, local public health actors have also mentioned the need to consider how others perceive the problem, based on their own professional norms and objectives. For instance, one public health actor in Montréal says that while his professional experience leads him to consider the influence of the built environment on collisions involving pedestrians and cyclists, the police look at the situation from another standpoint as they are responsible for implementing regulations about individual behaviour. Another public health actor recounts efforts to understand the values and opinions of local politicians before presenting them with policies from other jurisdictions. This, he said, was part of the strategy to construct health, transportation and the built environment as a public problem in the late 1990s in Montréal:

> Before you start tackling a problem, it is important to understand how people perceive this problem, what they know about it, what are their values, their attitudes. … If you want to change behaviours and paradigms, you have to find out what they think first. (Local public health actor, Montréal)

Local public health actors have used a number of strategies to make the case for the health benefits of promoting active transportation. They have built evidence, presented and framed that evidence so as to create interest in active transportation and changes to the built environment. This denotes an understanding of the processes of framing and the construction of public problems, as well as an understanding that changing policy paradigms will not result from merely framing evidence in a compelling way. It is also necessary to recognize and work with the competing paradigms, values and professional norms of the different actors involved.

3.2   Circulating Evidence Within the Local Policy Subsystem

Complementary to their strategies for building an evidence base and for framing policy problems, local public health actors have developed several strategies to circulate evidence among other actors in the local policy subsystem.

First, we consider how local public health actors share evidence with municipal politicians and civil servants who are in a position to make decisions about active transportation policy. Practices in the two cities differ slightly in this respect given that Montréal Public Health is a local unit of the provincial health and social services administration, whereas Toronto Public Health is part of the municipal administration.

In Montréal, local public health actors take advantage of formal policy mechanisms such as public consultations and membership of municipal committees on active transportation and related issues. They regularly write briefs as part of official consultation processes on a range of issues related to transportation. Past briefs dealt with the revision of the city's road classification (which has implications for speed limits, the volume of traffic and which administration gets responsibility for pedestrian and cyclist infrastructure), major road works such as the renovation of the Turcot Interchange, pedestrian street designations and so on. Montréal Public Health is also a member of the municipal Cycling committee, although the role of this committee has fluctuated over time, from being rarely convened to holding regular meetings.

In Toronto, some public health actors that we interviewed mentioned that they shared their evidence with other public health professionals within their own organizations and that they worked with service delivery programmes such as diabetes and obesity. Primarily, local public health actors describe how they cooperate with managers and professionals from other municipal services over significant periods of time to bring about changes to the built environment. For instance, the report *Air Pollution Burden of Illness from Traffic in Toronto* (2007) was prepared in collaboration with Transportation Services and its publication was announced in a joint press conference. Public health actors also mention that municipal services tasked with implementing changes to the built environment used evidence from public health community consultations about how to increase walking, cycling and health in several neighbourhoods of the City:

> For instance, they're [Transportation Services] getting some opposition out in the east end of the city to sidewalks being put in on a particular street, because it's a higher income street, they don't want to lose their front lawn. So they're now going back to the demonstration project that was in that area to say the community identified sidewalks as being very important in this area. So they're going back and referencing some of the reports that we've done. So it's a good use of how Public Health can have an influence. (Public health actor, Toronto)

Local public health actors also mention other opportunities that they use to establish collaborations with other municipal services, for instance, helping with the cost of buying documentation on active transportation, creating information packages for local transportation coordinators and including their own reports on health, the built environment and transportation in the packages. Overall, they describe long-term efforts to build alliances and frame policy issues. They explained that building trust and collaboration with managers and professionals from other services was an ongoing process, influenced by the formal responsibilities of each policy sector; the hierarchical accountability structure within the organization and the individual managers and professionals perceptions of their own role within the formal municipal organization.

Second, local public health actors in both cities have developed collaborations with NGOs interested in active transportation, urban planning and the environment to promote active transportation. These collaborations are opportunities to circulate evidence among a broader audience. Montréal public health actors, who are not part of the municipal administration, claim this strategy more forcefully than their counterparts in Toronto. Nevertheless, in Toronto, NGOs and local public health actors view their partnerships positively, the latter sharing evidence that the former use in their advocacy efforts.

In Montréal, public health actors have developed long-term collaborations with NGOs advocating for active transportation and for changes to urban planning and the built environment. These collaborations include cultivating relationships with NGO representatives and journalists in all their areas of expertise (notably smog, air quality and the built environment); jointly developing research on shared areas of interest (for instance, the health impact of smog among populations living along urban highways); organizing and participating in meetings with NGO representatives and politicians to advocate for policy changes (for instance, inviting prominent speakers such as architect Jan Gehl to present examples from other countries); sharing evidence. Montréal Public Health also supports specific NGO interventions related to active transportation and related topics through regular funding programmes under its control.

These long-standing collaborations appear to help build the credibility of novel ideas: sustained interactions between local public health actors, NGOs and professionals from municipal services through professional training, conferences and accounts of policies in other cities and countries help frame the agenda around active transportation. In that sense, public health actors embed their production and sharing of evidence in those interactions with other actors concerned with active transportation. This public health actor even considers that his mandate is to build evidence and share it with NGOs so that they can use it into their advocacy efforts:

> Our service is to do research and share the results, namely to transfer the results to NGOs. They are the ones that set the policy agenda, much more than I can do. (Public health actor, Montréal)

As mentioned above, local public health actors in Montréal work in a local unit of the provincial health and social services administration. They are civil servants in a different order of government than municipalities. Although Montréal Public Health has historically enjoyed some latitude in sharing public health concerns about municipal and provincial policies, they have no formal status within municipal administrations. Therefore, collaborations with NGOs and municipal services such as described above are a valuable way to circulate evidence among the local policy subsystem to indirectly influence municipal officials. This was what happened with the data displaying the number of injured and deceased pedestrians at each intersection across the city of Montréal. The report also formulated several recommendations to increase safety at intersections, such as building sidewalk bump outs and changing pedestrian and cyclist crossing signs (timers, dedicated lights). Although municipal councillors and employees appeared initially reluctant to acknowledge the data, its distribution among NGOs and citizens provided an alternate way to share and discuss the evidence with municipal actors. It appears to have swayed the discussion on this topic as the city has been redesigning intersections to make them safer for pedestrians (e.g. building bump outs to reduce the width of intersections) for the past few years.

In sum, public health actors in Montréal and Toronto focus their work around evidence of the links between health, transportation, the built environment and the environment (air quality, climate change). They have developed a series of strategies to facilitate the uptake of evidence by local actors and to change how they frame policy issues. Joining health and urban planning, for instance, provides a different way of considering the effects of transportation on health and the possibilities for public action. Collaborations with other actors, whether municipal services or NGOs, provide ways of circulating evidence but also of strengthening advocacy efforts. These strategies suggest that, although evidence is the core of their work, public health actors conceive of municipal policymaking as a political process that requires changing how policy issues are framed and requires building alliances with like-minded actors. In the next section, we question this perception of the policy process in greater detail.

4   How Local Public Health Actors Conceive of the Policy Process

The conception of the policy process that emerges from interviews with local public health actors as part of the active transportation policy study is ambiguous. It certainly contains traces of the "moral high ground" (de Leeuw, 2017, p. 344) but it also denotes an awareness of how politics and policymaking affect their work and should shape their strategies for circulating evidence. This ambiguity is noticeable in how politicians perceive the role of public health actors.

4.1   Traces of the Moral High Ground in How They Engage with Other Policy Sectors

Taking the moral high ground translates into claims about the superior value of health and health-related evidence. Public health research and public health actors are then legitimate to make suggestions about other sector policies, so that they become healthier. In our exploration of the strategies that public health actors use to share evidence with other actors, we have noted their awareness of the different paradigms and interests of other policy sectors. This awareness, however, appears a little ambiguous as a conception of health as a superior value may come in the way of engaging those other sectors:

> [Our data] is always perceived as a criticism of their practices. But no [it is not a criticism], it is a problem. People get hit, they get injured, that's how it is in large cities. [...] But the initial reaction is always defensive: 'Is that true? We do our job, we do what's best, we conform to the guidelines.' (Local public health actor, Montréal)

> Our MOH [medical officer of health] met relatively recently, I don't know, a few months ago, with the chair, the councillor chair of the Public Works and Infrastructure Committee [...] And she kind of felt that the MOH was encroaching on other people's mandates and was working well beyond

the health mandate. So not understanding and not accepting the health mandate, our health mandate comes from the WHO, where health is not just absence of disease, it's wellness, mental health, you know, physical health, the whole thing. So we got a little bit more work to do to bring people into that understanding. (Public health actors, Toronto)

This last excerpt does not mean that local public health actors are unaware that the formal mandate of public health units in the province of Ontario is legislated. Rather, it speaks to their conception of health as encompassing all areas of life and, therefore, government activity.

Considering health as a superior value has consequences for how local public health actors engage with other sector actors. Is the benefit to public health an argument compelling enough that other sector actors should accept policy recommendations that come in conflict with their own norms and practices? Despite these traces of the moral high ground, local public health actors recognize that understanding the legitimacy of other policy ideas is a necessary first step to changing them through training and education:

"But I also learned to be very respectful of, they're all trying to protect people, they're trying to build good safe roads and to challenge their beliefs is not something that we're trying to do; what we were trying to do is to say that we also have our mandate, so how can we work together and still build safe transportation structures, but do it in a way that helps people to be more active? [...] ['Somebody that teaches road design "] did not know what a Complete Street was. So yeah. And if these are the people that are teaching the new students that are actually doing the road design, the surveyors, the engineers, then we're going to have to make sure that we sort of go down that stream" (Local public health actors, Toronto).

4.2 Attention to Politics

Alongside this moral position, local public health actors—especially senior civil servants—are also attentive to the politics of active transportation policymaking. Interviews with local public health actors indicate that they understand the confrontation of interests and the varied political benefits of different types of policy instruments. For instance, in the early days of raising awareness for a policy that would reduce air pollution in Montréal, one interviewee mentioned that it was easier for local decision makers to limit emissions from wood-burning stoves than from motor vehicles.

Although the logic of the argument was not fully explicit in the interview, interests were stronger and better organized in the transportation sector than in the domestic heating subsector. Besides, municipalities may regulate the maximum amount of emissions allowed from wood-burning stoves in their constituency (wood-burning stoves are static, identified in building and renovation permits, subject to inspection) whereas a similar measure concerning cars or trucks would be outside the remit of their constitutional responsibilities and political influence.

Senior local public health actors in Montréal are also aware of the implications of the current governance of transportation and planning at the local level. The governance of transportation spreads across the province, the metropolitan area of Montréal, the city of Montréal and the adjacent municipalities. Responsibilities are also segmented by modes of transportation, which is detrimental to a general policy of sustainable transportation that plans for how best to move people around, rather than how to develop separate transit, roads and bicycle lane networks:

> What we would like is an integrated governance for planning and for transportation systems, road transportation as well as transit and bicycle lanes, with actual political and spending powers. (Local public health actor, Montréal)

Similarly, another actor reflects upon the applicability of different strategies to increase active transportation, showing an understanding of the limits of certain types of policy instruments, of the multi-level governance of planning and how certain instruments may be more amenable to municipal intervention than others.

Local public health actors are also aware of electoral cycles and of sectoral politics—in the sense that politicians and senior administrative officials are keen to protect, even extend, the contours of their policy sectors, just like the public health sector does. Some describe pragmatic attitudes towards electoral cycles and government changes. For instance, if a mayor and municipal council dropped policy changes that public health actors and NGOs advocated for, the latter would take up their advocacy efforts again with the new administration. In Toronto, city politics has had a strong influence on active transportation policy under the populist mayorship of Rob Ford, known, among other things, for his vocal criticisms of the "war on cars." As a consequence, professionals in Transportation Services had limited abilities to invest major time and resources in active transportation because of the tense political climate around this issue. According to local public health actors, this led to postponing an update of the city's cycling plan.

Local public health actors are also mindful of the political capital of senior public health officials, that is of the potential political consequences of the evidence and proposals to change active transportation policy that they put forward:

> P1: I think really the most important role for both [P2] and myself is to be able to provide good evidence and good information and good strategic advice to the MOH. He really cares about these issues. He is our spokesperson and does it very well. And so the rest of us work to create a good package, and sometimes we have to bring him along because he's dealing with... I don't know, about 200 different health issues. And we all have to be careful with reputation management. Like how much political capital did he lose on the speed limit, you know, fiasco. He got a lot of very positive emails, he became like a local hero for getting beat up by the mayor at the time, but then again on some level, everyone's a bit careful. Like we don't want repeats of that. That's not a winning strategy. (Local public health actor, Toronto)

The very public controversy that followed a proposal to impose a 30 km/h speed limit in residential neighbourhoods sheds light on how local politicians view public health's proposals about active transportation policy and ambition to introduce more health into non-health policies. Following Toronto Public Health's work on the *Road to Health* report, the City's Chief Medical Officer put forward one of the report's proposals to limit maximum speed limits in residential neighbourhoods to 30 km/h. Although the proposal received positive support from City Planning, it caused a controversy with Transportation Services and, primarily, with the Chair of Public Works Committee and with the Mayor. Consistent with his earlier positions, Mayor Ford called the proposal, "nuts, nuts, nuts." He went so far as to ask, "why does he [the Chief Medical Officer of Health] still have a job?", before he had to apologize a few months later (Dale, 2012). The politician who chaired the city's Public Works committee took a similar stance, claiming that the Chief Medical Officer of Health had no legitimacy to make transport-related recommendations: "If he wants to lower speed limits, maybe he should apply for the general manager's job in the transportation department" (Dale, 2012). The Chief Medical Officer of Health stood behind the maximum speed limit proposal citing that scientific evidence proved its effectiveness in reducing the number and seriousness of injuries to pedestrians and cyclists resulting from collisions with cars. He further stated the limits of his role by saying that politicians then had to weigh the different interests and make decisions (Rider, 2012). This whole episode was widely reported in the media both as a fiasco for public health and as a heroic stance against the Mayor. More to the point, it establishes a distinction between political decision-making and expert advice, with public health actors in the role of experts that politicians may trust and value (or not) but may also ignore. This local politician expects public health actors—who are city staff—to provide the City with the best possible evidence-based advice, regardless of local politics:

> That's why you pay these guys [public health staff] the big bucks, speaking truth to power. And so another sub-issue in this, and this thing here is the integrity and autonomy of the public service. They don't work for the politicians individually, they work for council, they don't work with the grassroots community organizations … they don't work for them, they're not their mouthpieces, they have an integrity and autonomy and professionalism and that's what we want them to do. […] I go back to that line that I said to [the Chief Medical Officer of Health] all the time is, 'I'm grateful to you because you have the temerity to tell me what I need to hear, not what I want to hear.' And that doesn't mean that on the political side, that I'm going to vote the way you recommend. That's my prerogative. In this world of ours, democracy gives the generalists, i.e. the politicians, the final say on public policy. And I might for totally different reasons vote another way. That's my right. But it's not my right to tell you what advice you should be giving me. (City Councillor, Toronto)

Local public health actors concerned with active transportation in Montréal similarly consider that their responsibility is to build and share evidence about the public health impacts of policies that relate to transportation and the built environment. As we have mentioned above, they have also sustained long-term interactions with NGOs sharing similar objectives to influence public policies. Just as in Toronto, this perceived mandate of public health has spurred criticisms from some politicians. In the period leading to public consultations on the refection of the largest highway interchange in Montréal, public health actors organized a conference and a bus tour of the area with journalists and politicians, including the deputy minister of Transportation, to share evidence about transportation and health and discuss policy options. Widely covered in the media, the event caused angry exchanges between the provincial Ministry of Transportation, the provincial Ministry of Health and Social Services and the local public health unit. Just like Toronto's Chief Medical Officer of Health was "invited" to apply for a job in Transportation services, public health actors in Montréal were "invited" to become candidates in the next election since they wanted to meddle with politics:

> The Transportation minister told the Health minister that 'if the Montréal Public Health gang wants to do politics, they should stick their faces on telephone poles and become candidates.' [...] He said we were doing politics. No, we don't do politics: we share evidence. (Local public health actor, Montréal)

We could interpret this last sentence as yet another trace of the moral high ground. We could also read it as an acknowledgement that public health actors should frame health-related evidence and share it with other actors in the policy subsystem so that it becomes part of the decision-making process. Whether such practices overstep the administrative duties of public health actors employed in public administrations is not a topic that can be settled here (Fafard & Forest, 2016).

5   Discussion

We started this chapter with the following question: what do the strategies that local public health actors used to circulate evidence reveal about their conception of the policy process and about the standing of evidence in the policy process? The short answer is that local public health actors place evidence at the core of their practice, but that they handle evidence in the local policy subsystem based on their expertise and political knowledge. They frame evidence in ways that showcase how health is intertwined with other areas of municipal responsibility, in that case especially with transportation and the built environment. They work together with municipal civil servants from other policy sectors, advocacy groups and NGOs to make sure evidence is part of policy discussions. Interviews indicate that local public health actors have a certain expectation of being right about the importance of health, but a pragmatic view of how to convince others. This pragmatic view draws on their understanding of competing policy

objectives, framing policy issues, influence of electoral cycles and politics on policymaking, governance arrangements and their implications for
policy.

The worlds of politics and evidence appear to overlap at local level. In
that sense, we could say that local public health actors sidestep the stalemate between evidence and politics by developing politically savvy ways
of circulating evidence among other actors in the local policy subsystem.

How does this relate to the challenges of improving collaboration
between public health and political science? To a certain extent, it stands
in contrast to Fafard and Cassola's (2020) claim that the lack of a
common language between political science and public health, especially
as regards the conception of evidence, impedes collaboration. Indeed,
political interests are not only obstacles to the strategies of public health
actors to influence policy: some become opportunities to share evidence
with other actors and to build narratives to increase the legitimacy of their
preferred policy. However, the conclusions from this chapter agree with
these authors' second challenge, embracing complexity, which calls for
political scientists and public health researchers to consider several ways
of knowing about public health policy, including "public health actors'
frontline knowledge of policy implementation from both a clinical and
community perspective" (Fafard & Cassola, 2020, p. 108).

Within public health, there appears to be a fault line between public
health researchers—whose conception of evidence presumably ignores the
complexities of the policy process—and public health practitioners, whom
we have shown to have a more pragmatic understanding of politics, interests and how to influence policy through the circulation of evidence. Our
results suggest that the stalemate is less at the frontlines of public health
practice and more among (academic) analysts of healthy public policymaking, who come from different academic departments and intellectual
traditions. However, this chapter builds upon a small sample of interviews
with public health actors, all of them involved in the same policy area,
given that this was not the original focus of the research. It also describes
the situation in two of Canada's larger cities, each with long histories of
healthy public policy advocacy. To what extent might these findings hold
in smaller centres without such a history of accumulated experience and
expertise? Further research could help build a more complex portrait of
how public health actors conceive of the policy process. Does it, as we
assume based on our interviews, vary according to their position in the
hierarchy of their institutions, with senior public health actors (managers)

having a more politically informed view of the policy process than professional or junior public health actors? Do their views of the policy process vary depending on their policy area or public health problem of expertise? To what extent do public health researchers and senior public health practitioners have different conceptions of the policy process? In turn, this knowledge would provide a stronger basis for collaborations between public health and political science that make better use of the diversity of expert and experiential knowledge while recognizing their respective scope and aim (Gagnon et al., 2017).

Our results also echo findings from other studies that consider "strategic public health advocacy" (Smith & Weishaar, 2018) crucial for networks to influence policymaking. According to Smith, network theories, such as the ACF, tend to overestimate the influence of values in the formation and success of policy coalitions. Communication between network members, collectively engaging in political trade-offs, leadership by policy brokers and a supportive context are crucial to networks developing a coherent, cohesive and timely strategy to influence policy (Smith & Weishaar, 2018). ACF scholarship also points to the importance of social interactions among coalition members, of the support that coalitions derive from related networks to explain coalition behaviour and of the influence and of their ability to rely on political institutions (Kübler, 2001).

What are the implications for resolving the stalemate between science and policy in public health policymaking? Taking inspiration from our earlier proposals for research collaborations between political science and public health and from Cairney's "theory-led academic-practitioner discussions" (Cairney, 2014), we suggest that part of the way forward to overcome the stalemate between public health and political science is to go beyond the circulation of evidence from researchers to practitioners, or from public health practitioners to other sector practitioners. It is important to consider also how institutions and governance practices across levels of government and across policy sectors frame and influence the ability to make policies for health (Clavier & Gagnon, 2013). Political science researchers, public health researchers and practitioners, practitioners from other policy sectors who work within and outside public administration each have different understandings of politics and policymaking, and of the role of evidence in the policy process. Collaborations between all these actors could be a starting point for conversations about how to build policies for health using theoretical and practical knowledge of the complexities of the policy process.

For these actors to more fully engage with each other, we suggest three related tips: (1) better connecting public health evidence with practical policy solutions, in their social, political and institutional context; (2) developing sustained interactions with non-public health actors working with or advocating for these policy solutions and (3) to accomplish this, getting the help of boundary actors skilled in connecting problems and solutions across policy sectors. Indeed, public health policy problems—in particular those concerned with influencing the more distal determinants of health—relate to several policy areas (see how health, transportation and urban planning are closely intertwined in our active transportation policy study). Actors working as boundary spanners or policy brokers (Nay & Smith, 2002; Stern & Green, 2005; Williams, 2002) have the resources and skills to create links between a variety of policy actors and problems, within a coalition and between coalitions. De Leeuw et al. (2018) suggest overlaying the analysis of networks with the analysis of policy frames defended by actors in the network to identify boundary actors that could bring together actors and their conception of the policy problem.

References

Béland, D., & Katapally, T. R. (2018). Shaping policy change in population health: Policy entrepreneurs, ideas, and institutions. *International Journal of Health Policy and Management, 7*(5), 369–373. http://www.ijhpm.com/art icle_3451_b32faa0e01cc2a181c3b89245b9749d0.pdf

Bernier, N. F., & Clavier, C. (2011). Public health policy research: Making the case for a political science approach. *Health Promotion International, 26*(1), 109–116.

Braun, V., & Clarke, V. (2006). Using thematic analysis in psychology. *Qualitative Research in Psychology, 3*(2), 77–101. https://doi.org/10.1191/147808 8706qp063oa

Cairney, P. (2014). How can policy theory have an impact on policy making? The role of theory-led academic–practitioner discussions. *Teaching Public Administration, 33*(1), 22–39. https://doi.org/10.1177/0144739414532284

Cairney, P. (2016). *The politics of evidence-based policy making*. Palgrave Macmillan.

Clavier, C., & Gagnon, F. (2013). L'action intersectorielle en santé publique ou lorsque les institutions, les intérêts et les idées entrent en jeu. *La Revue de l'innovation : La Revue de l'innovation dans le secteur public, 18*(2), article 2.

Clavier, C., Gagnon, F., Paquin, S., Hayes, K., Poland, B., Savan, B., et al. (2019, mai). La santé publique, un acteur majeur des politiques urbaines de transport actif? *Revue Francophone sur la Santé et les Territoires*, 1–13. https://rfst.hypotheses.org/clavier-carolegagnon-france-paquin-sophie-hayes-katie-poland-blake-savan-beth-escoute-nina

Clavier, C., & O'Neill, M. (2017). The role of policy coalitions in understanding community participation in healthy cities projects. In E. de Leeuw & J. Simos (Eds.), *Healthy Cities* (pp. 359–373). Springer.

Dale, D. (2012, April 24, 2012). Lower Toronto speed limits by 10 to 20 km/h to protect pedestrians, chief medical o!cer says. *The Toronto Star*. Retrieved from https://www.thestar.com/news/city_hall/2012/04/24/lower_toronto_speed...y_10_to_20_kmh_to_protect_pedestrians_chief_medical_officer_says.html

de Leeuw, E. (2017). Engagement of sectors other than health in integrated health governance, policy, and action. *Annual Review of Public Health, 38*(1), 329–349. https://doi.org/10.1146/annurev-publhealth-031816-044309

de Leeuw, E., Browne, J., & Gleeson, D. (2018). Overlaying structure and frames in policy networks to enable effective boundary spanning. *Evidence & Policy: A Journal of Research, Debate and Practice, 14*(3), 537–547. https://doi.org/10.1332/174426418X15299595767891

de Leeuw, E., Clavier, C., & Breton, E. (2014). Health policy—Why research it and how: Health political science. *Health Research Policy and Systems, 12*(1), 55. http://www.health-policy-systems.com/content/12/1/55.

DeLeon, P. (1999). The stages approach to the policy process: What has it done? Where is it going? In P. A. Sabatier (Ed.), *Theories of the policy process*. Westview.

Direction de santé publique. (2006). *Le transport urbain, une question de santé*. Montréal: Agence de la santé et des services sociaux de Montréal.

Fafard, P. (2008). *Données probantes et politiques publiques favorables à la santé: Pistes fournies par les sciences de la santé et la science politique*. Centre de collaboration nationale sur les politiques publiques et la santé.

Fafard, P., & Cassola, A. (2020). Public health and political science: Challenges and opportunities for a productive partnership. *Public Health, 186*, 107–109. https://doi.org/10.1016/j.puhe.2020.07.004

Fafard, P., & Forest, P.-G. (2016). The loss of that which never was: Evaluating changes to the senior management of the Public Health Agency of Canada (https://doi.org/10.1111/capa.12174). *Canadian Public Administration, 59*(3), 448–466. https://doi.org/10.1111/capa.12174.

Gagnon, F., Bergeron, P., Clavier, C., Fafard, P., Martin, E., & Blouin, C. (2017). Why and how political science can contribute to public health? Proposals for collaborative research avenues. *International Journal of Health Policy and Management, 6*(9), 495–499. https://doi.org/10.15171/ijhpm. 2017.38

Hunter, D. J. (2009). Relationship between evidence and policy: A case of evidence-based policy or policy-based evidence? *Public Health, 123*(9), 583–586.

Kübler, D. (2001). Understanding policy change with the advocacy coalition framework: An application to Swiss drug policy. *Journal of European Public Policy, 8*(4), 623–641. https://doi.org/10.1080/13501760110064429

Morency, P., Archambault, J., Cloutier, M.-S., Tremblay, M., Plante, C., & Dubé, A. S. (2013). *Sécurité des piétons en milieu urbain: enquête sur les aménagements routiers aux intersections*. Direction de la santé publique de l'Agence de la santé et des services sociaux.

Nay, O., & Smith, A. (2002). Les intermédiaires en politique. Médiation et jeux d'institutions. In O. Nay, & A. Smith (Eds.), *Le gouvernement du compromis. Courtiers et généralistes dans l'action politique* (pp. 1–21). Economica.

Newman, J. (2017). Deconstructing the debate over evidence-based policy. *Critical Policy Studies, 11*(2), 211–226. https://doi.org/10.1080/19460171. 2016.1224724

Ouimet, M., Bédard, P.-O., Turgeon, J., Lavis, J. N., Gélineau, F., Gagnon, F., et al. (2010). Correlates of consulting research evidence among policy analysts in government ministries: A cross-sectional survey. *Evidence & Policy, 6*(4), 433–460.

Paquin, S., & Pelletier, A. (2012). *L'audit de Potentiel Piétonnier Actif et Sécuritaire du quartier Centre-Sud. Pour un quartier qui marche*. Montréal: Direction de la santé publique   Agence de la santé et des services sociaux de Montréal.

Parkhurst, J. (2017). *The politics of evidence: From evidence-based policy to the good governance of evidence*. Routledge.

Pawson, R. (2002). Evidence-based policy: The promise of 'realist synthesis'. *Evaluation, 8*(3), 340–358. https://doi.org/10.1177/135638902401 462448

Rider, D. (2012, May 2). Toronto's medical officer unfazed by Ford brothers' criticism. *Toronto Star*. Retrieved from https://www.thestar.com/news/city_hall/2012/05/02/torontos_medical_officer_unfazed_by_ford_brothers_criticism.html

Sabatier, P. A., & Weible, C. M. (2007). The advocacy coalition framework: Innovations and clarifications. In P. A. Sabatier (Ed.), *Theories of the policy process* (2nd ed., pp. 189–220). Westview Press.

Smith, K. E. (2013). *Beyond evidence-based policy in public health: The interplay of ideas*. Palgrave Macmmillan.

Smith, K. E., & Weishaar, H. (2018). Networks, advocacy and evidence in public health policymaking: Insights from case studies of European Union smoke-free and English health inequalities policy debates. *Evidence & Policy: A Journal of Research, Debate and Practice, 14*(3), 403–430. https://doi. org/10.1332/174426418X15299596208647

Standring, A. (2017). Evidence-based policymaking and the politics of neoliberal reason: A response to Newman. *Critical Policy Studies, 1–8*. https://doi.org/ 10.1080/19460171.2017.1304226

Stern, R., & Green, J. (2005). Boundary workers and the management of frustration: A case study of two Healthy City partnership. *Health Promotion International, 20*(3), 269–276.

Toronto Public Health. (2007). *Air pollution burden of illness from traffic in Toronto—Problems and solutions*.

Toronto Public Health. (2011). *Healthy Toronto by design*.

Toronto Public Health. (2012). *Road to health: Improving walking and cycling in Toronto*. Toronto Public Health, Healthy Public Policy Directorate.

Toronto Public Health. (2013). *Next stop health: Transit access and health inequities in Toronto*. Toronto Public Health.

Toronto Public Health. (2014). *Active city: Designing for health*. Toronto Public Health.

Whitehead, M., Petticrew, M., Graham, H., Macintyre, S. J., Bambra, C., & Egan, M. (2004). Evidence for public health policy on inequalities: 2. Assembling the evidence jigsaw. *Journal of Epidemiology and Community Health, 58*, 817–821.

Williams, P. (2002). The competent boundary spanner. *Public Administration, 80*(1), 103–124.

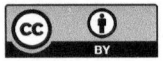

CHAPTER 7

Beyond the Public Health/Political Science Stalemate in Health Inequalities: Can Deliberative Forums Help?

Katherine E. Smith, Anna Macintyre, and Sarah Weakley

1 INTRODUCTION: MINI-PUBLICS AND DELIBERATIVE FORA AS A SOLUTION TO THE STALEMATE?

As this book explores, we have recently witnessed multiple efforts to counter some of the shortcomings of the evidence-based policy ideal, many of which include strategies for democratising the production and utilisation of evidence. A 2020 special issue of *Evidence & Policy* suggests such strategies are much needed, given the 'uneasy tension' that exists between EBP and public participation (Stewart et al., 2020). Deliberative forums involving a small number of lay citizens ('mini publics') appear

K. E. Smith (✉) · A. Macintyre
School of Social Work and Social Policy, University of Strathclyde, Glasgow, UK
e-mail: katherine.smith.100@strath.ac.uk

S. Weakley
College of Social Sciences, University of Glasgow, Glasgow, UK

© The Author(s) 2022   127
P. Fafard et al. (eds.), *Integrating Science and Politics for Public Health*,
Palgrave Studies in Public Health Policy Research,
https://doi.org/10.1007/978-3-030-98985-9_7

to be one of the most popular innovations for engaging publics in policy discussions (Jacquet & van der Does, 2020). This chapter explores one specific type of mini-public known as 'citizens' juries' (see Box 1).

Box 1: What Are Citizens' Juries?

Citizens' juries are a method of deliberation, originally developed by the Jefferson Center in the USA. They involve a group of 12–24 individuals, selected to represent the demographics of the area or population of interest, being brought together to deliberate on a policy issue (generally clearly framed as a question), over the period of between two and seven days. 'Jury' reflects the design inspiration, taken from juries used within legal court cases: the 'jurors' are 12–24 demographically diverse participants, while the 'witnesses' are individuals invited to 'give evidence' to the citizens' jury based on their expertise (e.g. in available evidence, personal or professional experiences, or a combination). The topics on which citizens' juries deliberate tend to be complex policy issues (Wakeford, 2002), often involving normative/ethical dimensions. Over the period in which the jury meets, facilitators schedule structured encounters, which routinely involve the delivery of pre-conceived activities designed to help participants consider evidence and debate potentially desirable policy approaches (hence, these are spaces in which publics, evidence, and policy are all considered). Juries are intended to facilitate public engagement in democratic processes and so, ideally, ought to also involve commitments from decision-makers to engage with the results (Carney & Harris, 2013). There are multiple examples in which this has been the case, including several in Australia over the past decade (Victorian Local Government Association, Undated). However, in many cases, citizens' juries are used for research purposes, albeit with some effort to bring findings to the attention of policy audiences (Street et al., 2014).

This chapter begins by outlining the case for citizens' juries (and similar mini-publics) as a means of overcoming the 'uneasy tension' that Stewart et al. (2020) describe between efforts to promote evidence-informed policymaking and efforts to support democratically engaged policymaking. Next, it introduces the topic of health inequalities in the UK as a case study, explaining how efforts to achieve policy ambitions to reduce health differences between social groups achieved only limited success, despite a strong commitment to evidence-based policymaking from 1997 onwards. It notes that many of the key actors (in research and policy) have attributed this to a presumed lack of public support for research-informed policy proposals to address health inequalities via redistributive, macro-level policies. It then challenges this presumption via a range of evidence, including qualitative studies, a national representative survey and a series of three citizens' juries, reflecting on the potential for citizens' juries to help overcome the apparent tensions that exist between evidence, policy and publics when it comes to tackling health inequalities in the UK. In the concluding discussion, this chapter returns to the broader literature on mini-publics to argue that deliberative spaces do appear to offer constructive discursive spaces in which it is possible to overcome potential tensions between evidence, policy and publics. However, it also argues there are reasons to be cautious about the potential role of deliberative forums, given the limited political engagement to date, concerns about potential tensions between representative and deliberative democracy, the high resources required, and challenges around ethically representing minority groups.

2   THE CASE FOR MINI-PUBLICS IN PUBLIC HEALTH POLICY

A 2014 systematic review of the use of citizens' juries in health policy research identified 37 studies that, between them, reported results from 66 juries (Street et al., 2014). One particularly high profile example has been in Ireland, where a citizens' assembly (similar to citizens' juries but slightly larger in format) informed a referendum on the topic, which subsequently led to a change in the law (Carolan, 2020). Yet, despite being widely used in health policy, there are only a small number of examples of published accounts of citizens' juries engaging in discussions about public (population) health, such as health inequalities, obesity, smoking or alcohol, with a view to influencing national health policy. This is despite the fact that a high-level review of the evidence on the social determinants of health specifically identified citizens' juries as a promising mechanism for those seeking to address the social determinants of health (Marmot, 2013).

Where deliberative methods have been used to explore citizen perspectives on tackling health differences, it has most often been at local, community level (Subica & Brown, 2020), which tends to restrict the potential policy options that can be discussed to those which are controlled by local decision-makers. However, there have been some interesting deliberative experiments on the topic of tackling obesity in

Australia (Anaf et al., 2018; Moretto et al., 2014; Street et al., 2017). For example, one of these citizens' juries 'unanimously called for government regulation to ensure that transnational fast food corporations pay taxes on profits in the country of income' (Anaf et al., 2018). A two-thirds majority of jury members 'also recommended government regulation to reduce fast food advertising, and improve standards of consumer information including a star-ratings system' (Anaf et al., 2018). In a separate citizens' jury, in South Australia, jury members agreed that obesity prevention requires multifaceted government intervention and made recommendations around health promotion and education, regulation of food marketing, taxation/subsidies and called for a parliamentary enquiry (Street et al., 2017). These two examples suggest, as did the Irish abortion example, that public views can sometimes be more sympathetic to the need for policy change than policymakers may presume.

3   THE CASE STUDY: TACKLING HEALTH INEQUALITIES IN SCOTLAND AND ENGLAND

This chapter builds on the conclusions of an earlier study that the lead author undertook of the relationship between evidence and policy relating to health inequalities in Scotland and England (Smith, 2013). The study, based on documentary analysis and a series of interviews with researchers and policymakers, found that a key issue was that most researchers and policy actors believed there was a lack of public support for the kinds of more egalitarian, macro-level policy changes research suggested was required to substantially reduce health inequalities. For example:

> Policy advisor (interviewed 2011): *"Even if all the evidence said we must do this, but then again if there's a whole opinion, national public opinion saying, well actually, no, we disagree with this approach, as an MP you would have to, obviously you have to weigh that in."*

> Senior academic (interviewed 2005): *"We're not willing to live in societies where there's equality in other domains, other than health. [...] In virtually every other domain of life, we don't want equality; we actually worship inequality."*

Overall, only 8 out of the 112 interviewees I interviewed in two linked studies (my PhD research 2004–2007 and a post-doctoral study that ran

2011–2012) claimed there was any public appetite for more egalitarian policies in the UK and no one claimed there was much media or political interest in such policies. This, then, was a powerful belief which worked to undermine and 'filter out' the research-informed ideas that pointed to the need for more egalitarian policy responses to inequalities in wealth, housing, education, etc. In effect, 'the public' were repeatedly implicated across interviews as political actors resistant to the kinds of policy proposals supported by the health inequalities research community. Yet, it was unclear how interviewees had reached this conclusion. When asked about the basis of these claims, interviewees' accounts were often vague but commonly referred to media coverage, voting in general elections and general social attitudes surveys/polls. There were no references to empirical evidence relating to public understandings of health inequalities or specific views about responses to health inequalities. This is perhaps unsurprising given there has actually been very little research to explore public understandings of health inequalities and even less about public views on potential policy responses to health inequalities. Reflecting all this, suggests that the way in which interviewees referred to public preferences and beliefs is akin to Walker et al.'s (2010, p. 932) account of 'the public' as 'imaginaries' who were invoked in policy discussions, given agency and sometimes employed for strategic reasons (often in accounting for the failure of policy action to reflect prominent research-informed ideas, even though these ideas often featured in policy documents).

4   Empirical Evidence Demonstrating Greater Than Perceived Alignment Between Public Views of, and Research on, Health Inequalities

Informed by the above work, the lead author began asking questions about research on precisely this topic: what do members of the public in the UK think about health inequalities and potential policy responses, how has this been explored to date and are there any gaps in our knowledge. After considering multiple different options, it was decided to use a threefold approach involving: (i) a review of existing academic literature on this topic; (ii) a new national survey (which would follow up and expand some earlier survey work so allow some exploration of changes over time); and (iii) a series of deliberative citizens' juries in three UK cities that had been widely studied in the health inequalities literature

(Glasgow, Manchester and Liverpool). The following sections provide a brief overview of the results of these three ways of trying study what members of the public think about health inequalities and potential policy responses.

4.1   What Does Existing Qualitative Research Tell Us About Public Understandings of Health Inequalities and Potential Policy Responses to These Inequalities in the UK?

As a first step, the project tried to identify all published academic literature exploring public understandings of health inequalities and of potential policy responses (see Smith & Anderson, 2018). Despite a comprehensive search strategy, we identified only 17 relevant studies, most of which were qualitative, which we brought together as a meta-ethnography (informed by Noblit & Hare's [1988] approach to synthesising qualitative research). The findings of this synthesis (Smith & Anderson, 2018) suggest that people have sophisticated understandings of the underlying causes of socioeconomic health inequalities that closely mirror popular, research-informed theories about health inequalities (Bartley, 2004; Marmot, 2010). As Bolam et al. (2006) conclude, people's accounts tend to highlight the importance of both material-structural factors and social constructions of individual and collective experiences (i.e. of the deeply intertwined nature of materialist and psychosocial explanations of health inequalities). In particular, the emphasis that people place on experiences of employment, poor quality jobs and worklessness as health determinants, reflects extensive epidemiological evidence (Bambra, 2011). Indeed, while the complex and dynamic relationships linking people's experiences of socioeconomic deprivation to poor health make singular policy solutions unlikely, the findings add weight to calls for macro-level policy responses to health inequalities and suggest supportive employment policies are one of the most promising areas to focus on.

Likewise, the importance participants attached to experiencing fear, stress and social isolation, and their concern (and sometimes anger) at feeling judged or disrespected, all reflect research evidence concerning psychosocial pathways and relative social status and equality (Marmot, 2015). A recently published ethnographic and interview-based study of lay perspectives on health inequalities in north east England (not included in our meta-ethnography as it was published subsequently to our searches) also emphasised the importance of psychosocial pathways, identifying 'fatalism' (linked to low sense of control) as a key psychosocial pathway linking disadvantage to poor health (Garthwaite & Bambra, 2017). This dimension of the findings underlines the importance of the ways in which public servants (from teachers to Job Centre staff and social workers) interact with the communities they serve. Indeed, in several cases, single experiences of disrespect, coercion or discrimination appeared to have had long-term consequences for participants. This suggests that the increased conditionality of welfare support (combined with cuts in public spending), in which those seeking benefits are required to provide an array of information to demonstrate their commitment to finding work (or to support their claim to be unable to work) is impacting negatively on health in Britain's poorer communities, further exacerbating health inequalities.

Finally, participants consistently described proximal, behavioural contributors to poor health, such as high alcohol consumption, drug use, unhealthy diets and smoking, as 'coping' mechanisms or forms of escapism (i.e. as understandable responses to the multiple other factors impacting on wellbeing). This reinforces research claims that policy interventions aimed only at this level are unlikely to be effective in reducing health inequalities (Scott et al., 2013; Whitehead, 2007).

In sum, the lay explanations for the drivers of health inequalities in the UK appear to be sophisticated, multidimensional and in line with academic accounts (Marmot, 2010; Smith et al., 2016). Yet, seemingly paradoxically, the findings also suggest that people experiencing socioeconomic deprivation are often unwilling to acknowledge the logical consequence of the impacts of the pathways linking structural disadvantage to poor health, i.e. the existence of health inequalities. We argue in the published paper (Smith & Anderson, 2018), following several authors of included studies, that this reflects an attempt to resist some of the stigma and shame associated with poverty (Walker et al., 2013), poor health (Scambler, 2008) and place (Wacquant et al., 2014) and to, instead, exert a sense of individual agency in the face of adversity. As Elliot and colleagues note, this presents a dilemma for researchers since, 'acknowledging the impact of deprivation, disadvantage and exclusion is potentially to reinforce an identity that people may be trying to resist' (Elliot et al., 2016, p. 229).

This paper made three suggestions as to how researchers might engage in public discussions that both avoid contributing to the stigmatisation of particular places and communities (labels that, Pearce [2012] notes, can be both enduring and highly mobile) and begin enabling people to 'imagine transformation' (Elliot et al., 2016). First, we emphasised the importance of taking care with the choice of language used to discuss health inequalities, especially when focusing on particular places or communities. Second, we argued that researchers could do more to challenge binary oppositions (e.g. 'poor' versus 'rich', 'healthy' versus 'unhealthy') and instead explore the consequences of inequality for everyone. Hence, rather than yet more research focusing on disadvantaged communities, we made a case for studying how people across the social gradient (Marmot, 2010) understand health inequalities. Third, we argued that the focus of future health inequalities research should move beyond analysing the problem of health inequalities to better understanding potential proposals for their amelioration. As part of this, we called for more experimentation with deliberative democratic forms of engagement (Blacksher, 2013) and/or with participatory practices specifically intended to overcome alienation (Blencowe et al., 2015). These findings directly informed the development of a subsequent study that combined a representative sample survey with citizens' juries to explore public views on potential policy responses to health inequalities in the UK.

4.2   What Do Surveys Tell Us About Public Understandings of Health Inequalities and Potential Policy Responses to These Inequalities in the UK?

We designed a national cross-sectional survey that was administered online by Opinium Research in August 2016 and involved 1,717 nationally (UK) representative respondents (for full methodological details, please see Smith et al., 2021). The survey asked questions on: perceptions of health inequalities; perceptions of 12 potential policy responses, selected on the basis that an earlier survey found they attracted significant support among researchers (Smith & Kandlik Eltanani, 2014); the role of government in tackling health inequalities; perceptions of income inequalities in the UK; sense of fairness; factors affecting participants' health and key sociodemographic characteristics. For the purposes of this chapter, we are going to highlight three key findings.

First, the results suggest that ~70% of respondents were aware richer people live longer but most people did not seem to think poorer people were more likely to experience key NCDs (heart disease and cancer), mental ill health or accidents. In other words, while people are aware of overarching inequalities in life expectancy, they seem less aware of the morbidity and mortality patterns underlying this overarching pattern. In this respect, the results were surprisingly similar to a survey undertaken almost two decades earlier, in 1997, described by Macintyre et al. (2006). This suggests public recognition of health inequalities and the patterns of ill health underlying health inequalities has not increased since 1997. Given the amount of policy attention that has been invested in health inequalities in the UK in the intervening period (Mackenbach, 2011; Marmot, 2010; Smith, 2013), this was surprising.

The second and third key findings draw on survey responses to a series of questions that used a Likert scale to ask respondents how likely they felt particular policy responses were to reduce health inequalities in the UK, with 5 signalling strongly agree and 1 strongly disagree. Table 1 presents an overview of the mean scores and standard deviation for each policy proposal included in the survey and uses colour shading to distinguish distinctive types of policy response.

The second key finding is that, when it comes to public views about proposals for tackling health inequalities, support seems particularly strong for the notion that the National Health Service (NHS) can and should play a key role in responding to health inequalities (the top two proposals focus on the NHS—a general investment in the NHS and a specific investment in GP services). The popularity of these two policy proposals is unsurprising in the context of research undertaken by The Health Foundation around the same time demonstrating that the NHS is held in very high regard by members of the UK public (Gershlick et al., 2015). However, this finding is important because it is out of line with the views of many health inequalities researchers, who tend to believe that the NHS (a service primarily designed to treat—rather than prevent—ill health) can play only a limited role in tackling health inequalities (Smith, 2013; Smith & Kandlik Eltanani, 2014).

The third key finding is that, contrast to the beliefs of the interviewees in my earlier research (see Sect. 3 of this chapter), most respondents supported most of the macro-level policy proposals included in the survey as likely to be effective responses to health inequalities. This included two economic proposals focusing on wealth, increasing the minimum wage and introducing higher taxes for richer people, as well as a range of proposals to provide various forms of social support, broadly with a view to improving living and working conditions. The three proposals

Table 1 Average public support for policy proposals for tackling health inequalities according to the national sample survey (from most to least popular)

Specific policy proposal	Broader policy approach (colour coded)	Average public support within national survey (n=1717)		Ranking (most support = 1, least support = 12)
		Mean (SD)	% agree /strongly agree	
Spend more money on the National Health Service (NHS)	Health Services	4.33 (0.93)	79%	1.
Spend more money on General Practitioner (GP) services	Health Services	4.12 (0.95)	73%	2.
Provide more support for unemployed people to find jobs	Social support	3.91 (0.98)	65%	3.
Spend more money on support services	Social support	3.90 (1.02)	65%	4.
Limit advertising of unhealthy products	Regulatory driven behavioural change	3.86 (1.17)	62%	5.
Increase the Minimum Wage	Economy-wealth	3.86 (1.12)	61%	6.
Spend more money on social housing	Social support	3.75 (1.12)	58%	7.
Provide the public with more health information	Health promotion	3.59 (1.08)	50%	8.
Introduce higher taxes for richer people	Economy-wealth	3.54 (1.30)	53%	9.
Plain packaging for cigarettes	Regulatory driven behavioural change	3.36 (1.37)	43%	10.
Increase the price of unhealthy products	Fiscally driven behavioural change	3.32 (1.32)	45%	11.
Spend more on smoking cessation services	Health promotion	3.20 (1.17)	37%	12.

that performed least well in the survey, the only three to achieve less than 50% of respondents agreeing/strongly agreeing they were likely to reduce health inequalities, were all targeted at trying to achieve behavioural change (two focused on smoking). Here, the findings suggest public views are more in line with researchers' own views about the kinds of policy responses that are likely to be effective in reducing health inequalities (Smith, 2013; Smith & Kandlik Eltanani, 2014).

A survey like this is limited in the insights it can provide. It tells us only how the sample of participants responded at a given point in time, and it asked people to respond 'off the top of their heads', providing no additional information or opportunity for discussion. We therefore know very little about why participants answered as they did or whether, had they had an opportunity to engage with evidence and to deliberate with others, their views might have shifted. The data from the citizens' juries are much more informative in this regard.

4.3 What Do Citizens' Juries Tell Us About Public Understandings of Health Inequalities and Potential Policy Responses to These Inequalities in the UK?

Three two-day citizens' juries were undertaken in July 2016 in Glasgow ($n = 20$), Liverpool ($n = 20$) and Manchester ($n = 17$) (total $n = 57$)[1] (again, for full methodological details, please see Smith et al., 2021). These cities were purposively sampled, as they all have large health gaps within their populations and share a similar socio-political context, including experience of post-industrial decline; all of which have led to previous comparative studies of health inequalities across the three cities (Walsh et al., 2010). Table 2 summarises the sociodemographic characteristics of the final sample.

The profile of recruits was broadly in line with the quota targets, notwithstanding a slight overrepresentation of Scottish National Party voters in Glasgow, and Green party voters in Manchester (compared to the voting profiles of those cities at the time of recruitment). To compensate individuals for the significant time commitment and to cover any travel, subsistence and caring related costs, jurors received £220 for participating.

---

[1] One participant was excluded from the quantitative analysis since they provided no demographic information so, for the quantitative data, $n = 56$.

Table 2 Citizen juries sample description ($n = 56$)

		Frequency	Percentage (%)
Gender	Male	28	50.00
	Female	27	48.21
	Neither	1	1.79
Age	18–34	27	48.21
	35–54	14	25.00
	55+	15	26.79
Income	Low	13	24.07
	Middle	30	55.56
	High	11	20.37
Political Party 2015	Conservatives	9	16.07
	Labour	19	33.00
	Liberal Democrats	1	93.00
	Scottish National Party	12	21.43
	Green Party	6	10.71
	Did not vote	9	16.07

Across the two days, we collected data in four ways: individually, via (i) questionnaires (which mirrored the national survey) completed at the beginning (t1), mid-point (t2) and end (t3) of the juries; collectively, via (ii) ethnographic notes throughout (including during social breaks); (iii) audio recordings of all full and small group discussions and (iv) photos and notes of 'sticky wall' exercises, including two full group exercises where participants were asked to vote for their top policy choices. The main task given to the juries was to address the following question:

> Some people think that in a fair society, the government should work to try to limit health differences between richer and poorer groups. Others think that in a fair society, it is up to individuals. Other people have opinions somewhere in between. What should the government do about these health differences, and why?

During each jury, participants undertook a range of exercises to get to know each other, to develop 'rules of engagement' and to find out more about health inequalities research and potential policy solutions. This included hearing from two 'witnesses' in person and four via pre-recorded, specially-commissioned videos (four researchers, one public health practitioner and advocate and a General Practitioner doctor [GP]).

Each provided a different perspective, with the intention of reflecting research and policy debates in the UK. Jurors were given an opportunity to develop questions in small group discussions and then to reconvene as a full group, at which time they could put their questions directly to the 'witness' or (for the videos) facilitators with health inequalities research expertise. Each jury culminated in a collective voting and ranking exercise over two rounds (with a discussion in between), focusing on potential policy responses to health inequalities.

Table 3 summarises the quantifiable findings from the citizens' juries. The results demonstrate that responses between jury members and the national survey sample were similar, though not identical (compare Tables 1 and 3). It also shows that some jury members amended their

Table 3 Average public support for policy proposals for national survey and average public support and group voting for citizens' juries

Broader policy approach[a]	Average public support within Citizen Juries T1 (n=56)		Average public support within Citizen Juries T3 (n=56)		Change in individual support following deliberation	Rank position at T1 & T3 in individual responses (1=most popular)	Rank position of original proposals in group voting (1=most popular)[b]		
	Mean (SD)	% agree /strongly agree	Mean (SD)	% agree /strongly agree			Glasgow	Liverpool	Manchester
Spend more money on the NHS	4.75 (0.51)	96%	4.43 (0.87)	88%	-0.32	T1: 1 T3: 1	7	1	2
Spend more money on GP services	4.50 (0.75)	89%	4.41 (0.71)	91%	-0.09	T1: 4 T3: 2	6	4	8
Provide more support for unemployed people to find jobs	4.56 (0.71)	87%	4.32 (0.75)	87%	-0.24	T1: 2 T3: 3	5	3	11 tied
Spend more money on support services	4.53 (0.77)	87%	4.29 (0.71)	86%	-0.24	T1: 3 T3: 4	10	11 tied	11 tied
Spend more money on social housing	4.12 (0.92)	72%	4.16 (0.78)	80%	+0.04	T1: 7 T3: 5	9	8	5
Increase the Minimum Wage	4.43 (0.85)	87%	4.14 (0.98)	70%	-0.29	T1: 5 T3: 6	2 tied	2	3
Provide the public with more health information	4.28 (0.98)	80%	4.00 (0.97)	69%	-0.28	T1: 6 T3: 7	12	11 tied	13
Limit advertising of unhealthy products	3.84 (1.14)	62%	3.96 (1.11)	69%	+0.12	T1: 8 T3: 8	8	10	10
Introduce higher taxes for richer people	3.62 (1.20)	54%	3.62 (1.39)	54%	+/- 0	T1: 9 T3: 9	2 tied	14	1
Increase the price of unhealthy products	3.39 (1.22)	44%	3.61 (1.17)	56%	+0.22	T1: 11 T3: 10	11	6	9
Spend more on smoking cessation services	3.48 (1.19)	50%	3.31 (1.07)	44%	-0.17	T1: 10 T3: 11	15	17	15 tied
Plain packaging for cigarettes	3.25 (1.43)	37%	3.04 (1.31)	33%	-0.21	T1: 12 T3: 12	14	16	15 tied

[a] The colour coding of proposals mirrors that of Table 1, indicating the broad type of proposal.
[b] The colour coding of the rank position provides a quick visual sense of which proposals were ranked highest (green signifies top 5, orange signifies ranked 6-10, red signifies proposals were ranked outside the top 10). Some rank positions are missing because some juries included their own proposals but these are not included in Table 3 (see Table 4 & Smith et al, 2021).

views following exposure to research evidence, expert opinion and jury discussions (i.e. that the results from the questionnaire responses of individual jury members are different between time-point 1 and time-point 3, albeit often only marginally). More noticeable, however, is the fact that jury members responded differently when reporting their individual views and when voting collectively. It is particularly striking that the two economic proposals, one focusing on increasing the wealth of poorer groups by increasing the minimum wage and another focusing on more egalitarian distribution of wealth via tax increases for richer people, both performed much better in group voting (with the exception of tax increases in Liverpool). This suggests that, when groups are working collectively, they are more supportive of these kinds of policies (see also Table 4). Each jury was also encouraged to suggest additional proposals, some of which they decided to consider in the group voting (see in Table 4). These proposals also suggest a clear interest in more 'upstream' policy proposals, focusing on improving living and working conditions or on economic policy reform.

The qualitative data (transcriptions of group discussions and ethnographic notes) provide further insights and, in some cases, led us to reach rather different conclusions about the quantitative data than we might have otherwise done. For the purposes of this chapter, we will highlight six aspects that we I feel stand out, before taking a step back to reflect

Table 4   The top ranked proposals in each jury in final group voting round

Glasgow	Liverpool	Manchester
1 Close the tax loopholes*	1 Spend more money on the NHS	1 = Introduce higher taxes for rich people
	2 Increase the national minimum wage	
2 = Increase national minimum wage		1 = Spend more on the NHS
2 = Introduce higher taxes for (*very) rich people	3 Provide more support for people seeking jobs	2 = Close corporate tax loopholes*
3. Reduce the price of healthy products*	4 = Spend more on GP services	2 = Increase the national minimum wage
4. Provide more support for people seeking jobs	4 = Ban zero hour contracts*	3. Invest more money in social housing

*Signifies participants' own addition/suggestions

on what the combined findings (Sects. 4.1–4.3) suggest about the potential of deliberative spaces to overcome the 'stalemate' on which this book focuses.

First, as was the case with some participants featured in the meta-ethnography (see Sect. 4.1), some participants were resistant to the idea of health inequalities:

> We don't necessarily agree a hundred percent with the fact that if you're wealthy you're healthy and if you're unwealthy you're unhealthy. (Male participant, Glasgow)

> It seemed like [...] it was like everyone was saying you're a stereotype that if you're there you're that and if you're there you're that. [...] It's stereotyping the actual character isn't it? That poor people are like this, and the rich people are like this. It's wrong. (Female participant, Manchester)

These responses can be understood as resisting a message experienced as disempowering and, at times, stigmatising (Smith & Anderson, 2018). This concern was so great in the Liverpool discussions that one member proposed an additional policy response of tackling 'stereotyping of people in poverty'. This perspective, which was often linked to a sense of poor health being down to serendipity, potentially undermined the value of the whole exercise since, if participants did not believe that anything other than luck explained health differences, it implied there was no issue for policy to address. However, despite evidence of this perspective in all three juries, it was far from dominant, and everyone continued to engage in discussions. Moreover, the space that the juries provided to discuss health inequalities in depth seemed to increase participants' willingness to explicitly acknowledge their existence (there were far fewer references to this view on day two of each jury compared to day one). Reflecting this, the idea that nothing should be done to tackle health inequalities was unpopular in group voting (no one voted for it in Glasgow or Liverpool and only one person voted for this option in Manchester). This suggests that providing spaces to explore health inequalities in depth may increase people's willingness to explicitly acknowledge the issue (a necessary foundation of meaningful discussions about potential policy responses).

Second, mirroring the results of the national sample survey, Table 3 shows that health service based responses remain the most popular but that, beyond this, public views on the kinds of policy responses likely to reduce health inequalities are relatively well-aligned with those of researchers (Smith & Kandlik Eltanani, 2014), with a clear focus on improving living and working conditions and (especially in group voting) improving the material and economic circumstances of poorer groups.

Third, the qualitative data did not always appear well aligned with the quantitative data or, at least, provided a rather different perspective on the quantitative findings. Two examples illustrate this. First, although health service (NHS and GP) focused policy proposals were among the most popular proposals in individual group voting across time-points 1 and 3 (as they had been in the national survey), the qualitative data suggest these kinds of investments were nonetheless contested, usually on the basis of concerns about efficiency and management:

> We could probably do it more [invest in the NHS] but I think there's more than enough there, or there's nearly enough there I should say. But we're constantly mopping a bath that's flooding instead of turning the tap off. (Male participant, Liverpool)

> I think the NHS thing with GP services, I agree with that. I think it's a case of restructuring them rather than actually throwing more money at it.... (Female participant, Glasgow)

> But it's because everybody's so hung up about the NHS has got to have more money, but is it being managed correctly? (Manchester participant, female)

Hence, although these proposals were popular (and it was also clear from discussions that health service staff, especially doctors, were held in high regard), they were accompanied by some consistent reservations (in contrast to many of the other proposals).

The second example of the varying insights provided by different elements of the data relates to an archetypal health promotion proposal; to provide the public with more health information. In jury discussions, participants often referred to this as 'health education'. However, in using this language we noticed there appeared to be some quite different perspectives on what this proposal involved:

I think a wee bit more education for some people to, instead of taking their kids to McDonald's and spending £10 or £15 on that, they could buy a bag of shopping, buy fresh fruit, fresh veg, go somewhere. [...] So if they actually had that bit of background on how to make all these things, it would maybe help them. (Glasgow participant, female)

Thank you very much. Anyone who has something that is more or less related? (Facilitator)

I agree with that because it talks about education which I think is the fundamental. It's the level that you educate people. It allows them to make the right choice with whatever resources they've got. The more money that's thrown at education across the board, and the earlier it starts. [...] Education, it underpins everything else, it underpins everything we do. It informs our choices, it explains your actions, it does everything. Unless you have it, you don't really have much. (Glasgow Jury, male participants)

The female participant quoted above framed health education as health promotion (teaching people about healthier eating), which was how we (the research team) also interpreted this proposal. In contrast, the male participant appeared to be envisioning a much broader policy, involving an investment in education 'across the board' (which we would have categorised as a rather different kind of policy response). This is important because it highlights that respondents' understandings of the proposals put forward varied, sometimes fundamentally. Hence, this was a proposal that, while not especially popular according to the quantitative data, nonetheless appeared to garner consensus within discussions and this appeared to be, at least in part, because there were varying interpretations about what this proposal would involve.

The fourth aspect of the data worth highlighting is that proposals involving tax increases (whether via income tax increases for richer people or increased taxes on unhealthy products) were relatively popular in individual responses and in group voting but generated considerable controversy in group discussions. For example:

I do think the more you earn, the more income you earn the more tax you should pay, I just think that's how it should be. Not like extortionate amounts but people can. (Female participant, Liverpool)

Yeah, well we think if you've worked hard to get to the top, why take your wages off you and bring you down? I don't think that's right. (Female participant, Liverpool)

As we see above, whether increased taxation was supported appeared to relate partly to participants' individual perceptions of fairness. Other aspects of the qualitative data suggest views changed, depending on the tax rate and income threshold being proposed, perhaps because this affected who, within the juries, would have to pay more tax, as one participant in Glasgow suggested.

The juries in Glasgow and Manchester both discussed the threshold for being 'rich' in detail, with varying views about who increased taxation would (and should) impact. The Glasgow jury agreed the threshold for increased taxation should be £200,000+ (a threshold advocated by a vocal male participant and formally agreed by the group, though quietly criticised by three female participants who felt it should be around £50,000), whereas the Manchester jury agreed it should be £100,000+. Overall, although the proposal to require richer people to make more tax achieved significant support, these variations and discussions underline the contested nature of this proposal. Discussions around the proposal to increase taxes on unhealthy products fared similarly, though with this proposal, the transcripts capture more examples of participants trying to persuade others to support the proposal on the basis of efficacy in reducing consumption and a 'polluter pays' type principle, as well as the potential to raise public revenue.

Fifth, beyond the discussions around specific policy proposals, the data suggest that at least three factors intersected to reduce (the relatively high) support for macro-level policy proposals. As Table 5 illustrates, this included a lack of trust in (local and national government) and discourses of individualism and fatalism.

The three factors outlined in Table 5 sometimes coalesced to challenge support for macro-level policy proposals, though not consistently. For example, while the lack of trust in government consistently undermined support for proposals involving taxation (whether via income tax changes or unhealthy product taxes), discourses around individual responsibility were sometimes used to reinforce arguments against tax-based proposals but, at other times, were used to support tax increases on unhealthy commodities since these were positioned by some jurors as maintaining choice, while reducing consumption.

Table 5 Three intersecting factors that appeared to reduce (the relatively high) support for macro-level policy responses to health inequalities

Factor	Illustrative data extract
Lack of trust in local and national governments	'I don't really think politicians know what they're doing. [...] The politicians, they can't do anything about it [health inequalities], they can't even run the country for god's sake, so you know. We're lost really aren't we?' (Female participant, Liverpool) 'Councils steal money' (Male participant, Glasgow)
A prevalent discourse around individual responsibility	'I get that the Government plays a part, no one's denying that, on advertising and marketing and things. But when it comes down to it, it is individual responsibility, you're responsible for your own health. You're responsible for your own life' (Female participant, Glasgow) 'it's all up to the individual how they conduct and live their lives. If they want to eat healthy fine, if you don't, fine' (Female participant, Liverpool)
Fatalistic discourses about human nature	'People have smoked and drank for god knows how long. It's down to their personal choice. And people who are under large stress in society use alcohol and whatever as a form of escapism, to get away from their troubles and the worries. [...] You can lead the horse to water but you can't make it drink' (Female participant, Liverpool) 'So some people find happiness in comfort food, smoking, alcohol, all these different things [...] even if they know they're unhealthy, they know the health risks, they've been educated but they don't care. They actually just enjoy it and want to do it. Should they be convinced or should they just be allowed to do what they want?' (Male participant, Manchester)

Sixth, at least some jury members adjusted their responses following exposure to evidence, expert views and discussions with one another (Table 3). All three sources were also drawn on in the discussions around the group voting exercises. This suggests that allowing people to find out about an issue via research and expert testimony, and to discuss and deliberate on the issue with a view to making policy recommendations, does result in a rather different 'public view' than opinion polling. Here, the qualitative data suggest that expert testimony from trusted sources (academic researchers, policy advisors, a health advocate and a GP) had a greater impact on jury members than quantified evidence (e.g. graphs and statistics that they were shown in presentations and also had in individual participant packs). The most persuasive evidence, however, appeared to be jury members' accounts of their own personal experiences, perhaps because this was the most uncomfortable to openly challenge in a group setting, especially one in which respect for fellow participants had been strongly emphasised.

5   Concluding Discussion

The data presented in this chapter suggest that policy and researcher perceptions of public opinions about health inequalities in the UK are not especially well-aligned with actual public opinions. We employed multiple ways of exploring public views about potential policy responses to health inequalities and all of these methods suggested that, in contrast to policymakers' and researchers' perceptions (Smith, 2013), public views are relatively well-aligned with researcher perspectives on health inequalities. Both the meta-ethnography and the qualitative data generated in the citizen jury discussions suggest that people generally (but especially those with personal experience of disadvantage) have a good understanding of the ways in which social determinants shape health and of how the unequal distribution of these determinants underlies health inequalities.

The survey and citizen jury data further demonstrate that public views on potential policy responses to health inequalities are, with the exception of the consistently high public support for health service led responses, remarkably similar to the views of researchers, with evident support for more upstream policy responses that aim to improve living and working conditions and to tackle poverty and the unequal distribution of wealth. This suggests that perceived tensions between evidence, policy and publics around the issue of health inequalities are not as great as many policy-makers and researchers appear to believe. Moreover, the citizens' juries provided a space in which members of the public became, via exposure to evidence, expert testimony and discussions with fellow jury members, more willing to acknowledge the existence of health inequalities. The jury data also demonstrate that at least some participants adjusted their policy preferences following this exposure, which suggests that the responses of this kind of informed 'mini-public' are distinct from the more spur-of-the-moment responses that opinion polls generate. It is perhaps also worth noting that the jury discussions seemed very well-received by participants, according to their exit questionnaires and the comments made to us, as organisers, as they left. This feedback suggested most participants enjoyed the experience, with several noting they felt this kind of approach should be taken more often. All of this suggests that deliberative spaces such as citizens' juries may well provide a means of helping to overcome (actual or perceived) stalemates between evidence and politics.

However, there are also three reasons to remain cautious about the potential role that deliberative forums might play in overcoming such stalemates. First, this is a much more expensive way of assessing public opinion than polling and the final results of the individual responses of the informed jury members were not radically different from the uninformed national sample (comparing Tables 1 and 3), which raises questions about the relative return on investment for policy audiences interested in public perspectives (though the group ranking results of the three juries were substantially different). Second, it proved hard to attract policy interest in the juries so, while the juries provided a very useful means of bringing researcher and professional perspectives into dialogue with members of the public, the juries lacked the kind of political-policy engagement that the original architects of citizens' juries intended (Fishkin, 1995). This may reflect the wider, much discussed tension between representative and deliberative democracy (e.g. Pickard, 1998). Finally, the small nature of the juries meant that diversity was inevitably limited; a common criticism of citizens' juries (Smith & Wales, 2006). Although we were able to include a good range of participants for some demographic characteristics (notably gender, age groups, socioeconomic position and political preferences), there are a host of potentially relevant demographic characteristics for which key groups were either not present or not well-represented (e.g. people with particular disabilities and long-term health conditions and people from specific minority ethnic groups). In sum, the small scale of mini-publics means it is impossible to capture the diversity of the wider public in a meaningful way. This means the perspectives and experiences of some groups are inevitably under-represented; a particular concern where the issue in question relates to intersecting societal inequalities, as is the case with health inequalities in the UK.

Reflecting on the work presented in this chapter, our own conclusion is that deliberative mini-publics can be extremely insightful for research in ways that may well contribute to overcoming the stalemate between evidence and publics (i.e. key component of politics in democracies). The highly positive feedback from most participants about their jury experiences, combined with the multifaceted nature of the data they generated, left us convinced that these kinds of deliberative spaces can serve a very useful purpose as spaces of research-informed public dialogue. Moreover, for the most part, the focus on policy solutions did appear effective in reducing the potential for discussions about health inequalities to feel disempowering for those bearing the greatest burden of these inequalities. Hence, as a mechanism for bringing researchers and publics into conversation about persistent societal challenges, we feel these kinds of deliberative forums have huge potential, especially if combined with methods to address some of the significant limitations (e.g. methods to capture a wider diversity of views, such as surveys, and efforts to ensure a wide range of social groups are informing the overall data).

Viewed from a policymakers' perspective, deliberative mini-publics certainly have limitations that may reduce their capacity to overcome the stalemate between evidence and politics, not least the cost involved and some concern that these forms represent a challenge to representative democracy. However, if the idea is simply that these are useful tools to inform policy discussions within representative democracies, the case for further experimentation with mini-publics seems convincing. Indeed, since these juries were conducted, multiple policy-led deliberative forums have been undertaken with further commitments recently arising across the UK, notably in Scotland (Lacelle-Webster & Warren, 2021; Wells et al., 2021). Deliberative forums are certainly no panacea for overcoming the stalemate with which this book is concerned, and more work is needed to develop ways of ensuring minority groups are better represented, but they may be a promising means of identifying potential routes to get beyond a stalemate situation for issues in which there is a perceived gap between research-informed policy proposals and public preferences.

Acknowledgements and Funding The initial scoping review work for the meta-ethnography was supported by The Samaritans. The national sample survey and the citizens' juries were funded by a Leverhulme Prize (Sociology & Social Policy) that the lead author was awarded in 2014. Thanks are due to all of the research respondents as well as to: Opinium for undertaking the national sample survey; Ipsos MORI for recruiting participants to the juries; Rosie Anderson for conducting secondary reviews for the meta-ethnography and helping to organise and run the citizens' juries; Oliver Escobar for helping design the citizens' juries and acting as the facilitator; Alexandra Wright, Gillian Fergie and Rebecca Hewer for data collection and organisational support with the juries; Rebecca Hewer for assistance coding the qualitative data; Linda Bates, Jeff Collin, Sarah Hill, Kate Pickett, David Walsh, Graham Watt and Richard Wilkinson for expert witness contributions; and the editorial team involved in this book for constructive reviewer feedback.

REFERENCES

Anaf, J., Baum, F., & Fisher, M. (2018). A citizens' jury on regulation of McDonald's products and operations in Australia in response to a corporate health impact assessment. *Australian and New Zealand Journal of Public Health, 42*(2), 133–139.

Bambra, C. (2011). *Work, worklessness, and the political economy of health.* Oxford University Press.

Bartley, M. (2004). *Health inequality: An introduction to theories, concepts and methods.* Polity Press in Association with Blackwell Publishing Ltd.

Blacksher, E. (2013). Participatory and deliberative practices in health: Meanings, distinctions, and implications for health equity. *Journal of Public Deliberation, 9*(1): Article 6 (unpaginated).

Blencowe, C., Brigstocke, J., & Noorani, T. (2015). Theorising participatory practice and alienation in health research: A materialist approach. *Social Theory & Health, 13*(3), 397–417.

Bolam, B., Murphy, S., & Gleeson, K. (2006). Place-identity and geographical inequalities in health: A qualitative study. *Psychology & Health, 21*(3), 399–420.

Carney, G., & Harris, C. (2013). Citizens' voices: Experiments in democratic renewal and reform. *Political Studies Association of Ireland.*

Carolan, E. (2020). Constitutional change outside the courts: Citizen deliberation and constitutional narrative(s) in Ireland's abortion referendum. *Federal Law Review, 48*(4), 497–510.

Elliot, E., Popay, J., & Williams, G. (2016). Knowledge of the everyday: Confronting the causes of health inequalities. In K. E. Smith, C. Bambra & S.

E. Hill (Eds.), *Health inequalities: Critical perspectives* (pp. 223–237). Oxford University Press.

Fishkin, J. (1995). *The voice of the people: Public opinion and democracy*. Yale University Press.

Garthwaite, K., & Bambra, C. (2017). "How the other half live": Lay perspectives on health inequalities in an age of austerity. *Social Science & Medicine, 187*, 268–275.

Gershlick, B., Charlesworth, A., & Taylor, E. (2015). *Public attitudes to the NHS: An analysis of responses to questions in the British Social Attitudes Survey.* The Health Foundation. https://www.health.org.uk/publications/public-att itudes-to-the-nhs

Jacquet, V., & van der Does, R. (2020). Deliberation and policy-making: Three ways to think about minipublics' consequences. *Administration & Society.* 0095399720964511.

Lacelle-Webster, A., & Warren, M. E. (2021). *Citizens' assemblies and democracy.* Oxford University Press.

Macintyre, S., McKay, L., & Ellaway, A. (2006). Lay concepts of the relative importance of different influences on health; are there major sociodemographic variations? *Health Education Research, 21*(5), 731–739.

Mackenbach, J. P. (2011). Can we reduce health inequalities? An analysis of the English strategy (1997–2010). *Journal of Epidemiology and Community Health.*

Marmot, M. (2010). *Strategic review of health inequalities in England post-2010* (Marmot review final report). University College London.

Marmot, M. (2013). *Review of social determinants and the health divide in the WHO European Region: final report*. World Health Organization Regional Office for Europe. https://apps.who.int/iris/bitstream/handle/10665/108 636/9789289000307 eng.pdf. Accessed 20 November 2020.

Marmot, M. (2015). *Status syndrome: How your place on the social gradient directly affects your health*. Bloomsbury.

Moretto, N., Kendall, E., Whitty, J., Byrnes, J., Hills, A., Gordon, L., Turkstra, E., Scuffham, P., & Comans, T. (2014). Yes, the government should tax soft drinks: Findings from a citizens' jury in Australia. *International Journal of Environmental Research and Public Health, 11*, 2456–2471.

Noblit, G. W., & Hare, R. D. (1988). *Meta-ethnography: Synthesizing qualitative studies*. Sage Publications Inc.

Pearce, J. (2012). The 'blemish of place': Stigma, geography and health inequalities. A commentary on Tabuchi, Fukuhara & Iso. *Social Science & Medicine, 75*(11), 1921–1924.

Pickard, S. (1998). Citizenship and consumerism in health care: A critique of citizens' juries. *Social Policy & Administration, 32*(3), 226–244.

Scambler, G. (2008). Deviance, sick role and stigma (Chapter 13). In *Sociology as applied to medicine* (6th ed., pp. 205–216). Saunders (Elsevier).

Scott, S., Curnock, E., Mitchell, R., Robinson, M., Taulbut, M., Tod, E., & McCartney, G. (2013). *What would it take to eradicate health inequalities? Testing the fundamental causes theory of health inequalities in Scotland*. NHS Health Scotland.

Smith, G., & Wales, C. (2006). *Citizens' juries and deliberative democracy*. Democracy as Public Deliberation.

Smith, K. E. (2013). *Beyond evidence-based policy in public health: The interplay of ideas*. Palgrave Macmillan.

Smith, K. E., & Anderson, R. (2018). Understanding lay perspectives on socioeconomic health inequalities in Britain: A meta-ethnography. *Sociology of Health & Illness, 40*(1), 146–170.

Smith, K. E., Bambra, C., & Hill, S. E. (Eds.). (2016). *Health inequalities: Critical perspectives*. Oxford University Press.

Smith, K. E., & Kandlik Eltanani, M. (2014). What kinds of policies to reduce health inequalities in the UK do researchers support? *Journal of Public Health, 37*(1), 6–17.

Smith, K. E., Macintyre, A. K., Weakley, S., Hill, S. E., Escobar, O., & Fergie, G. (2021). Public understandings of potential policy responses to health inequalities: Evidence from a UK national survey and citizens' juries in three UK cities. *Social Science & Medicine, 291*, 114458.

Stewart, E., Smith-Merry, J., Geddes, M., & Bandola-Gill, J. (2020). Opening up evidence-based policy: Exploring citizen and service user expertise. *Evidence & Policy: A Journal of Research, Debate and Practice, 16*(2), 199–208.

Street, J., Duszynski, K., Krawczyk, S., & Braunack-Mayer, A. (2014). The use of citizens' juries in health policy decision-making: A systematic review. *Social Science & Medicine, 109*, 1–9.

Street, J. M., Sisnowski, J., Tooher, R., Farrell, L. C., & Braunack-Mayer, A. J. (2017). Community perspectives on the use of regulation and law for obesity prevention in children: A citizens' jury. *Health Policy, 121*(5), 566–573.

Subica, A. M., & Brown, B. J. (2020). Addressing health disparities through deliberative methods: Citizens' panels for health equity. *American Journal of Public Health, 110*(2), 166–173.

Victorian Local Government Association. (Undated). *Citizen juries—An overview*. Victorian Local Government Association. https://www.vlga.org.au/sites/default/files/v4-Citizen-Juries-an-overview.pdf. Accessed 30 November 2020.

Wacquant, L., Slater, T., & Pereira, V. B. (2014). Territorial stigmatization in action. *Environment and Planning A, 46*(6), 1270–1280.

Wakeford, T. (2002). Citizens juries: A radical alternative for social research. *Social Research Update, 37*. University of Surrey. https://www.sru.soc.surrey.ac.uk/SRU37.PDF. Accessed 6 April 2022.

Walker, G., Cass, N., Burningham, K., & Barnett, J. (2010). Renewable energy and sociotechnical change: Imagined subjectivities of 'the public' and their implications. *Environment and Planning A, 42*(4), 931–947.

Walker, R., Kyomuhendo, G. B., Chase, E., Choudhry, S., Gubrium, E. K., Nicola, J. Y., LØDemel, I., Mathew, L., Mwiine, A., Pellissery, S., & Ming, Y. A. N. (2013). Poverty in global perspective: Is shame a common denominator? *Journal of Social Policy, 42*(2), 215–233.

Walsh, D., Bendel, N., Jones, R., & Hanlon, P. (2010). It's not 'just deprivation': Why do equally deprived UK cities experience different health outcomes? *Public Health, 124*(9), 487–495.

Wells, R., Howarth, C., & Brand-Correa, L. I. (2021). Are citizen juries and assemblies on climate change driving democratic climate policymaking? An exploration of two case studies in the United Kingdom. *Climatic Change* Pre-print (online first).

Whitehead, M. (2007). A typology of actions to tackle social inequalities in health. *Journal of Epidemiology and Community Health, 61*(6), 473–478.

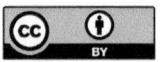

CHAPTER 8

Is Local Better? Evolving Hybrid Theorising for Local Health Policies

Evelyne de Leeuw

The birth of modern public health is the flip-side of the coin of rapid urbanisation in the nineteenth century. Public health, urban governance and politics go together. More recently, the realisation that health is not created by the medical care delivery system and its associated industries has been rediscovered since Thomas McKeown (1976) showed that sewers, not drugs, improved population health. Public health adepts knew this since the German princely states' Gesundheitspolizey (Gaißert, 1909), the occupational health equity analyses in France by Villermé (1840), Virchow's aphorisms about politics being medicine writ large and of course British advances around removal of pump handles and early forms of Geographic Information Systems (Snow, 1855). Over the last half century, this call to cast the net wider, or even in different directions, has not relented.

E. de Leeuw (✉)
University of New South Wales, Sydney, NSW, Australia
e-mail: e.deleeuw@unsw.edu.au

© The Author(s) 2022   153
P. Fafard et al. (eds.), *Integrating Science and Politics for Public Health*,
Palgrave Studies in Public Health Policy Research,
https://doi.org/10.1007/978-3-030-98985-9_8

Roughly since McKeown's analysis, the health field has called for making health policy development the responsibility of all sectors, not just the health care systems. Such calls include the Alma Ata Declaration (World Health Organization [WHO], 1978), the Ottawa Charter for Health Promotion (WHO, Health Canada, and Canadian Public Health Association, 1986) and United Nations (UN) high-level ministerial statements on the control and management of chronic disease (e.g., by UN, WHO, cf. Glasgow & Schrecker, 2016). Interestingly, global governance parameters dictated that most of these statements and compacts aimed at the nations-state, with the exception of the Ottawa Charter—which embraced a 'settings' approach as it recognised that health is made not in the capital, but in the streets, corridors, schools and marketplaces of localities. The urgency to integrate echoes calls from administrative and political science, also first voiced in the 1970s, to join up policy systems. There is a range of monikers for either, from *Healthy Public Policy* and *Health in All Policy* to *Whole-of-Government* and *Integrated Governance*. Whatever it is called, it remains what Peters has called 'the holy grail of public administration'. Wholesome integration is a good thing, and the WHO has enthusiastically been compiling vast series of case studies around successful intersectoral action (de Leeuw, 2021a).

But systematic appraisals of integrated health policy—and the processes that brought them about—are few and far between. The integration rhetoric seems strong, and the evidence appears light. The practical reality that a sewer line is not within the policy or operational remit of a medically qualified professional is immutable, but also of such an esoteric nature that its cognitive consequences are not successfully moved into other realms. The clinic does not run sewerage infrastructure. When Nancy Milio exhaustively documented how virtually every government sector impacted on health (1981a), the implication of a necessity to join up public policy for health was equally irrefutable. However, the practical demonstrations of such integrated policies were limited and deemed too unique to their contexts to be of replicable global relevance. The North Karelia project (Puska, 2002), the Norwegian Farm-Food-Nutrition approach (Milio, 1981b) and Heartbeat Wales (Nutbeam & Catford, 1987) were heralded as great successes of integrated approaches for health. But political science, administrative science and policy studies scholars have rarely applied a rigorous (theory-based) lens to explain these professed triumphs. Health promotion and public health policy appear to remain adrift on a sea of case studies.

Considering the place of 'the local' in the context of 'the global' is similarly challenging. Barber (2013) argues in a popular meme that cities collect the garbage, and that mayors should rule the world. The systematically compiled evidence that this makes sense, particularly in the health realm, continues to emerge.

Chapter Navigation

The nature of this chapter is part scholarly, part personal journey. In my reflections on the use of political science in understanding social choice (i.e., policy) for health, my occasionally ill-informed career choices have led me to a place where I am convinced that, most of the time, local is better. Acuto and Leffel (2020) and Acuto et al. (2021), in fact share my views and add a strong conceptual call that local must also become global. This is my gaze: I hope to cast a political science look at local health processes—not with an ambition to be comprehensive but to illustrate that this yields superior insight. First, I illustrate the rise of local perspectives in health policymaking through a case study that describes agenda setting for health policy (also known as Healthy Public Policy, or—more recently—Health in All Policy). This research demonstrates that local health policy developments are delivering better processes and outcomes. From this, the argument progresses to look at policy analyses of the European WHO Healthy Cities network and contrasts some of its premises to other global urban health efforts. The key lesson seems to be that value-based (i.e., community inspired and supported, solidarity and equity driven, ecological and sustainability targeting) local health engagement seems better than a more traditional neo-liberal (i.e., new public management) Key Performance Indicator hinged approach. The question then becomes how successful local health policy in one spatial context may lead to policy learning and transfer elsewhere. The first stage in answering this question is found in a critique of mechanistic 'knowledge translation approaches'. The second is a demonstration of the more switched-on political nature of political science approaches to policy learning. Here, I argue—based on our research in local health policy—that the very nature of local government and community allows for easier and more transparent policy inspiration. I make a case for policy development processes through mapping networks of policy language and policy actors and I argue that this would be easier at local level than elsewhere. Thirdly, there is a normative dimension. With over 15,000 'Healthy Cities' (de Leeuw &

Simos, 2017) and probably thousands more that are willingly struggling with the nature of health in their governance remits, there is simply a need to address the determinants of health (be they social, commercial, or political) with clearer guidance for political leadership at the local and global levels. Finally, with the reader joining my journey, you will also experience the increasingly complex nature of my theoretical choices and applications between 1986 and 2021... I have landed in a health political science space where an eclectic amalgamate of theoretical insights makes perfect sense. I am in good company, I feel: Paul Cairney (2013) suggests that there is added value to be found in added theories.

1   The Rise of Local

Based on pronouncements by Milio and Hancock, the Ottawa Charter for Health Promotion called for the 'Building of Healthy Public Policy' (Milio, 1981a). A natural sceptic, in 1986 I found this an intriguing message: would it really be possible for a nation-state to embrace the evidence—and then formulate and implement policy—that health and health equity can only be developed and boosted through truly integrated approaches? The Netherlands' government had published its intentions in a discussion document—accompanied by an exhaustive series of sectoral background briefings—called 'Nota 2000'. It took the Lalonde Report (Laframboise, 1990) one step further: all Ministries and public sectors were identified as having a role and responsibility in the promotion and maintenance of health. In 1989, my study of this Nota 2000 concluded that the development of 'Healthy Public Policy' *at the level of the nation-state* is virtually impossible (de Leeuw, 1989; de Leeuw & Polman, 1995). I arrived at this conclusion based on two core lines of reasoning.

First, I used Cobb and Elder's agenda setting theory (Cobb & Elder, 1971, 1983). The two American political scientists, in the spirit of the day, had formulated a relatively straightforward and functional 'strong theory' (see Sabatier's initial casting, 1999, for his views what such a theory ought to do). My inquiry concluded that 'health policy' (aka 'Healthy Public Policy') was not going to be endorsed and implemented at the national level in the country. Yet there was great enthusiasm for its potential at regional and local jurisdictional levels. In Table 1, the key propositions and predictive capabilities of the theory are presented (left column) as are some key inferences about how nation-state policy processes are

Table 1 Cobb & Elder agenda-setting parameters against their operations at local level

Cobb and Elder's theoretical dimensions	Implications for national versus local policy
There is a distinction between the social (aka 'systemic') and the political (aka 'institutional') agenda, and 'issues' (contentious matters) need to penetrate the barrier between the two to arrive at the level of political discourse and (parliamentary) decision-making	At national levels, operators in either agenda can pretend to be and act separate. At the local level, it is undeniable that they have a presence in both: a Councillor at the local butcher's is instantly held accountable. A national Minister at a capital supermarket will likely remain anonymous
Three models are applying this 'barrier penetration' idea: the outside initiative (classic romantic democratic ideas of social activism); the mobilisation model (certain actors launch an issue onto the social agenda and manipulate it towards and within the political agenda) and the inside initiative model (bureaucrats and technocrats with direct connection to policy and politics shape political discourse)	Communications operations to advance any of these three are sometimes more easily identified and debunked at the local level, in particular for the mobilisation model. The local level creates a 'forced transparency' and at the same time interesting wheeling-and-dealing. (In these days of glocal virtual connectedness and WikiLeaks, 'alternative facts' and bots and trolls, this may not hold true any more)
Pushing issues from one on the other agenda requires 'issue expansion' from small—often tiny—interest groups to the public at large. Various denotations of these 'publics' are given. Directly affected small interest groups should mobilise their embracing larger publics—the broadest is the 'general public' which isn't necessarily deemed driven by credible sources of information	At the local level, members of the various publics are not abstract 'actors' or 'stakeholders' but real people in real environments. At national levels, they are 'faceless' and/or 'hollowmen'. Yet, current social movement insights show simultaneous memberships across different 'publics'. (again, the advance of social media, 'alternative facts' and distrust of the public sector may have changed this)
Key to this 'issue expansion' across concentric circles of publics to secure issues entering the political agenda hinges on representations of the issue: It is defined and perceived ambiguously/equivocally; the social relevance is perceived as high; the issue relates to the long term; it is represented as not technical or technocratic; and it has few historical precedents	At the local level, issue expansion dimensions are more 'in your face' and directly observable Cobb and Elder were strong proponents of the view that, in politics, perception is reality. For local conversations, there may be more and better opportunity to test and apply the issue expansion rhetoric, and gauge whether the agenda is in fact being advanced. Nationally, publics and authorities may need to resort to more distant tools like polls and focus groups

qualitatively different from those lower jurisdictions (right column). I investigated the issue at the jurisdictional level of the nation-state. Surprisingly, and un-prompted, most interview respondents volunteered an opinion that Healthy Public Policy had more promise at the local government level (in the Netherlands, one of then ~700 municipalities) than nationally.

Second, my analysis why the Netherlands' national government was unable to develop, accept and implement a national Healthy Public Policy hinged on issues associated with power and, in particular, theories like the power-distance-reduction theory (Mulder, 1977; see also Harris et al., 2020). For Mulder, at the individual level:

1. More privileged individuals tend to try to preserve or to broaden their power distance from subordinates.
2. The larger their power distance is from a subordinate, the more the power holder would try to increase that distance.
3. Less powerful individuals try to decrease the power distance between themselves and their superiors.
4. The smaller the power distance, the more likely is the occurrence of less powerful individuals trying to reduce that distance.

When applied to institutional actors, the national level of policymaking was a far more stable (or rather, stale) environment than the local level where perceptions of power difference between the actors in the policy game were more easily overcome.[1] In terms of the punctuated equilibrium types of theories of the policy process (e.g., True et al., 2019), local policy processes seemed more punctuated and less balanced than national ones. At the local level, therefore, we could find faster responsiveness to (health) policy challenges. Local, in policy terms, is certainly quicker and may indeed be better.

Practical knowledge and procedural knowledge are at least as insightful as scholarly knowledge—and often more so. The 'discovery' that 'health policy' at the nation-state level was hard to accomplish was already foreshadowed by the visionaries behind the Ottawa Charter. In parallel to

---

[1] As an aside, organisational psychologist Geert Hofstede has applied this idea of 'power distance' to typify national—organisational—cultures and found that this approach may work well in more egalitarian societies such as The Netherlands, Sweden and Costa Rica, but not necessarily in authoritarian places like the Soviet Union or Chile under Pinochet.

its development, they had accumulated a critical mass for a demonstration project at the local level (de Leeuw, 2017; Hancock, 2017). The World Health Organization in Europe, followed by (networks of) cities in North America, Australia and New Zealand, was exploding with enthusiasm for 'Healthy Cities', originally cast by Duhl (1963), formally posited by Hancock in 1984, substantiated by Hancock and Duhl in 1986, and boosted by Kickbusch and Tsouros into an urban social movement in the second half of the 1980s. These cities were to pursue eleven qualities (Table 2). Individually and as a network, they actively

Table 2 Hancock and Duhl (1986) evidence-based recommendations for the values of a healthy city

A Healthy City should strive to provide	
1.	A clean, safe, high quality physical environment (including housing quality)
2.	An ecosystem which is stable now and sustainable in the long term
3.	A strong, mutually supportive and non-exploitative community;
4.	A high degree of public participation in and control over the decisions affecting one's life, health and well-being
5.	The meeting of basic needs (food, water, shelter, income, safety, work) for all the city's people
6.	Access to a wide variety of experiences and resources with the possibility of multiple contacts, interaction and communication;
7.	A diverse, vital and innovative city economy
8.	Encouragement of connectedness with the past, with the cultural and biological heritage and with other groups and individuals
9.	A city form that is compatible with and enhances the above parameters and behaviour
10.	An optimum level of appropriate public health and sick care services accessible to all
11.	High health status (both high positive health status and low disease status)

endeavoured to move from temporally and substantively limited projects into larger programmes and long-term policies for health (de Leeuw & Simos, 2017), even when their national governments failed to do so. The collateral by-catch of the national-level investigation revealed a much more exciting local opportunity.

De Leeuw et al. (2020) show that 'Healthy Cities' was the first transnational and global network of local governments and their communities pursuing a joint goal (before the mid-1980s international collaboration between local governments usually took the shape of more symbolic 'twin city' arrangements, e.g., Jayne et al., 2011, who also note that the context for city engagement in global affairs continues to change). Healthy Cities were followed by Sustainable Cities, a network formed in the lead-up to the Rio Earth Summit Conference (1992) and formalised in 1994 through commitments to an 'Aalborg Charter' and later a 'Basque Declaration' (cf Pinto et al., 2015). de Leeuw et al. (2020) analyse some of these 'Theme City Networks' against their stated impacts on health equity. They list in their review, among many others, Just Cities, Green Towns and Cities, Transition Towns and Ecodistricts, Winter Cities, Resilient Cities, Creative Cities, Knowledge Cities, Safe Cities and Communities, Festive Cities, Slow Cities as well as Happy Cities, Smart Cities, Child-friendly Cities, Age-friendly Cities, Conscious Cities and Inclusive Cities....

2   'Healthy Cities' as Policy Code, and 'Health Cities' as a Rhetoric

In the—notably European—assessments of Healthy Cities, one thing becomes abundantly clear. Although 'Healthy Cities' adopt and build on an ambitious value system (including the pursuit of equity, solidarity, sustainability, empowerment, etc.), each locality follows its own path. These over 15,000 different paths are determined by history, culture, geopolitical connection, spatial dimension, growth and access to services, industrial and economic bases, etc. The maxim *'If you've seen one Healthy City, you've seen one Healthy City'* is clear. In their essence, 'Healthy Cities' are localised health aspirations. The smallest self-declared 'Healthy City' is l'Isle-aux-Grues (a community on an island in the St. Lawrence River in Québec with around 200 inhabitants). The largest is the conurbation of Shanghai with over 16 million people. Brenner's multi-scalar perspective on urbanity seems to be of particular relevance in understanding these thousands of diverse local health ambitions (e.g., Brenner, 2019).

In particular where there are strong and codified networks of Healthy Cities, there is coherence between the approaches and paradigms that they apply to their activities (de Leeuw, 2015). Beginning in 1986, the designated cities within the WHO/EURO Network had to formally commit to a clearly defined set of values, including the above Eleven Qualities. For each (approximately) 5-year 'Phase', European cities must commit to a collection of policy priorities set in connection with WHO's global and regional (in this case European) work plans. For the current Seventh Phase of the European designated Healthy Cities network, these priorities are captured in the Six Ps (Fig. 1).

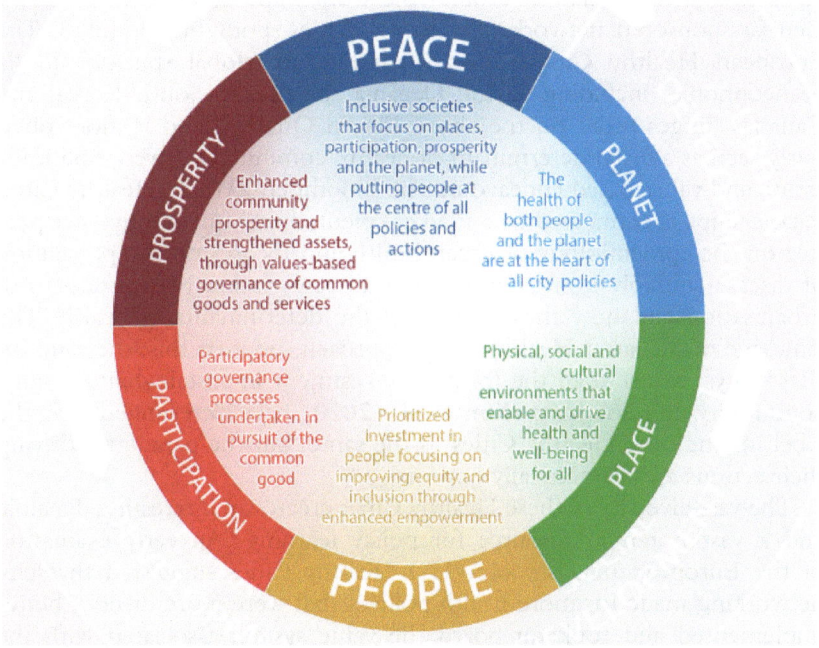

Fig. 1 Current WHO/EURO Healthy City priorities (cf http://www.euro.who.int/en/health-topics/environment-and-health/urban-health/who-european-healthy-cities-network/healthy-cities-vision)

Such a systematic and comprehensive approach to making Healthy Cities work is not universal for all the 15,000 self-identified Healthy Cities around the world. Currently, the Eastern Mediterranean Region of WHO is implementing a designation scheme focusing on the role of local government in Universal Health Coverage, and the Pan American Health Organization encourages local governments to achieve health equity through the systematic application of consultancy findings by Sir Michael Marmot (Rodríguez et al., 2019).

It is clear that different and relatively separate epistemic communities put their stamps on different 'Healthy Cities' networks (e.g., Goumans & Springett, 1997). This has in fact resulted in unproductive disconnects and often a focus on the development of policies and interventions that cannot necessarily be deemed the best or most appropriate ones. One of the most blatant disconnects is the one between European Healthy Cities (and its epistemic relatives around the world) and a Bloomberg/WHO Geneva sponsored network (see https://cities-spotlight.who.int/). The European Healthy Cities vision (including its global spin-offs in 'la Francophonie' including Africa, Oceania, Japan and South Korea, and Canada) hinges more on the above Eleven Qualities and is more obviously seen as a distal determinant of health, community driven, politically astute and value-based endeavour. The Bloomberg/WHO Healthy Cities Partnerships is connected to a market-oriented and quantitative perspective on the epidemiology of urban health and focuses on the prevention of disease (notably non-communicable disease) rather than processes of urbanisation and how they impact on the determinants of health. The language of the latter Healthy Cities approach supports this: they aim for 'Best Buys' rather than the former's investment in sustainability, equity, community and solidarity. Kim et al. (2020) have determined that the label for the two 'Healthy Cities' is the same, but the paradigms driving their actions are diametrically opposed.

The vast diversity of these Healthy Cities creates an interesting dynamic and a vast potential resource for policy learning. An early evaluation of the European network of WHO Healthy Cities suggested that city networking made for more health policies that were more diverse, better implemented and took on board the value system associated with the social determinants of health, health justice and health equity (Camagni & Capello, 2004). Nation-state health policy diffusion has not been documented with rigour, as far as I know, although there is emergent research in tobacco control (e.g., Studlar, 2015). Locally, cities themselves claimed to have learned from each other and WHO how to integrate 'upstream public health' considerations in their policy repertoire (Farrington et al., 2015). The political science literature frames this phenomenon as policy learning or policy transfer. Hawkins et al. (2020) provide a concise overview of the pertinent literature. They frame effective policy learning and transfer as a multi-level governance challenge.

In the context of the premise of this chapter, it is important to make this point: policy learning and transfer (whether horizontal [from city to city] or vertical [from city to region, country and beyond]) are conditional on prevailing socio-cultural and political paradigms and associated epistemic communities. I will continue the exploration of the premise that local may be better by first looking at the nexus between research, policy and practice, and then consider a more socially dynamic understanding of policy transfer.

3   TRANSLATING KNOWLEDGE OR MOVING IT THROUGH THE SYSTEM?

In a more romantic world view—and many public health professionals espouse this as they believe that 'health' is an unchallenged aspiration of all humanity—there is an assumption that good evidence must automatically lead to good policy and its implementation. The underlying idea is borrowed from clinical research. It has led to what is commonly known as 'implementation science'—not to be confused with policy implementation parameters... (Nilsen et al., 2013). New treatments and diagnostics need to diffuse and permeate into healthcare delivery systems. Individual and organisational behaviour change—often protocolised—are the tools of this trade. It uses language from the areas of diffusion of innovation and psychological behaviour change realms. Public health has similarly embraced this mantra of evidence-based policy and practice. But all too often solid evidence does not find an unobstructed way from research into practice, and practice is not adequately reflected in the scientific endeavour. This remains a frustration for the public health community which tends to operate, pragmatically, at the nexus between policy, research and practice. The gap between effectiveness on evidence, policy development, and practical intervention design and fidelity (implementing what was designed) has achieved increasing systematic attention in, for instance, Cochrane and Campbell Collaboration reviews.

The embrace of systematically generated evidence as a sine qua non for clinical practice has been powerful and pervasive. It has led to mechanistic clinical accountabilities, and some medical practitioners maintain that individual creative response to complex morbidities should transcend the results of Randomised Controlled Trials (Richter et al., 2020). Yet, the idea of 'Knowledge Translation' (KT) has become a major industry in the health field, essentially driven by a core logic of linear rational reasoning. Critics of the concept view it as a bad metaphor (Greenhalgh & Wieringa, 2011) that may have done the field more bad than good. 'Translation' as a metaphor would relate either to linguistics or to mathematics. Either one language (Clinician) is turned into another (Policy-ese), or in Euclidean geometry, a geometric transformation moves every point of a figure or a space by the same distance in a given direction, or as shifting the origin of the coordinate system. Neither of these is the perspective in health system implementation science, and its uncritical application to policy development may be considered fraught. The naïve view is also referred to as the 'two communities' hypothesis, an idea that has been rejected as mechanistic and stagnant (Lin & Gibson, 2003).

There are also conceptual and substantive problems with the KT suite of approaches (defined as a 'dynamic and iterative process that includes synthesis, dissemination, exchange and ethically-sound application of knowledge to improve health' (Straus et al., 2009, p. 165)). First, it is grounded in a presumed value-free Cartesian world view where facts are facts, and only facts matter. I and others have argued that facts, particularly in policy development and politics, are always subject to framing, morphing and negotiation. Facts are thoughts, thoughts are perceptions, perceptions are emotions, and we do not tend to think of emotions as facts. Cairney and Oliver (2020) build on this haiku and generate some evidence-based (but warranty-free) suggestions for engagement at the interface between scholarship, policy and practice.

I have called this interface *the nexus*. What happens at the nexus, and connects or separates the three domains of policy, research and practice can and should be studied. Understanding processes and structures that determine overlaps and gaps would enable us to generate better ways of generating knowledge for practice and policy. A systematic narrative review elicited two things about this arena (de Leeuw et al., 2007, 2008): (a) what tried-and-tested theoretical and conceptual models for work at the research-policy-practice nexus have been reported in the international peer-reviewed scholarly literature, and (b) are there organisations

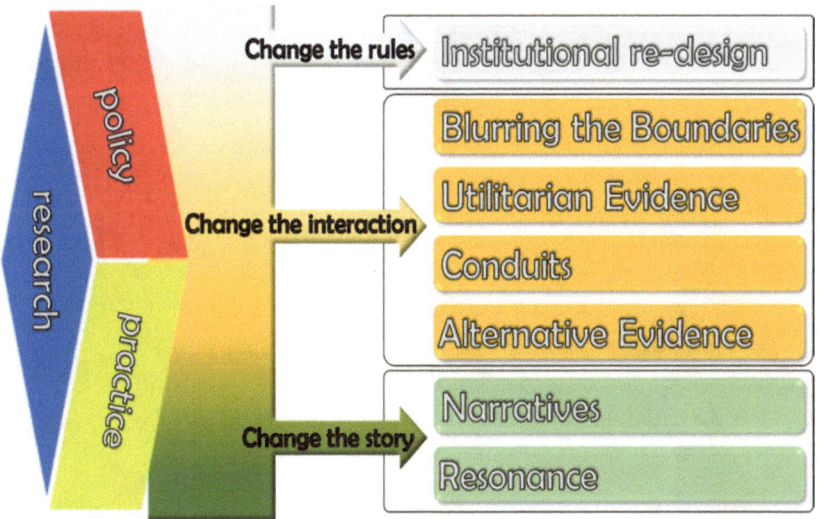

Fig. 2 Seven categories of theories and conceptual frameworks that explain what happens between research, policy and practice for health

or groups that have a reputation for success in acting at the nexus, and do they follow the processes and parameters identified theoretically and conceptually?

Nearly thirty different theoretical frameworks specifically dealing with actions at the nexus were reported to have been applied. For analytical purposes, we grouped them into seven categories, which could then be put into three groups (Figs. 2 and 3).

The categories of practice-affirmed and tested conceptual models and theory-based evaluation build on and reinforce each other.

The *Institutional Re-Design* category of theories finds that to bridge the gap between research, policy and practice, you can set and enforce rules and other institutional arrangements. For instance, one could imagine that research is only financed once applied in practice (this would require a fundamentally different world view where base funding for research is guaranteed, and applied research rewarded[2]) to secure

---

[2] There is an interesting hypothetical healthcare funding parallel: what if, instead of paying fee-for-service, or by case load, health services and their professionals would be

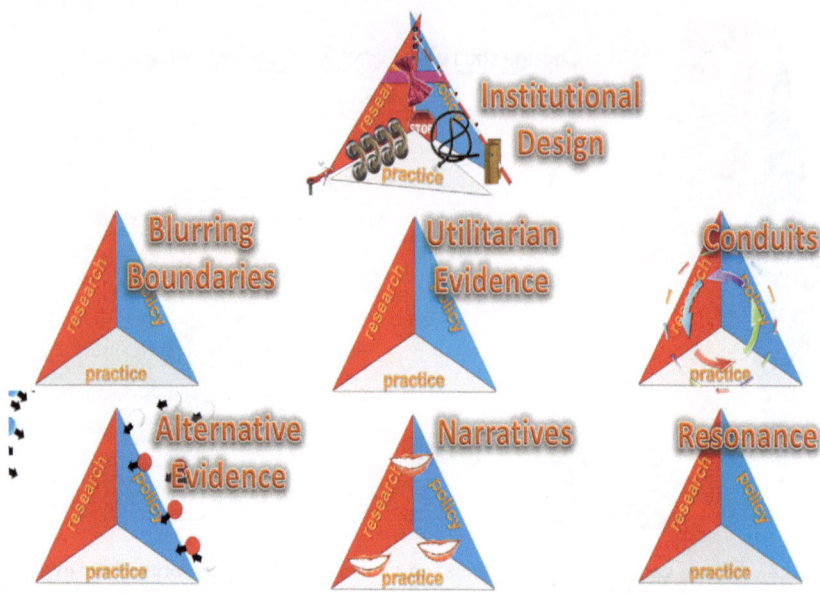

Fig. 3 Graphical representation of seven categories of acting at the nexus between research, policy and practice

immediacy and relevance. In the policy toolbox (with instruments in the areas of communicative, facilitative and regulatory intervention), we see a 'Least Coercion Rule' (Bemelmans-Videc et al., 2011)—policymakers tend to turn to rules that restrict behaviour only as a last resort. But Klijn and Koppenjan (2006), two policy network theorists, show that in particular network dynamics, the 'rules' can be changed. Actors engaged in policy networking may at times want to change the rules that formally or informally apply to the nature of, and the access to, the network, thus influencing policy outcomes. They may attempt to influence the shape of the network (by changing or consolidating actor relations, adding or changing procedures for access, or shifting external determinants of actor positions through, for instance, regulation), network outcomes (by changing performance indicators) and network interactions

given a guaranteed income which is reduced relative to the incidence of disease in their service area?

(by laying down instructions on conflict regulation or the governance of interaction). Hill and Hupe (2006) who see policy development and implementation mainly as a network governance challenge suggest that shifting rules is more easily achieved in local and other lower-level jurisdictions. This assertion resonates with the potency of street-level bureaucrats (see the updated Lipsky, 2010).

The *Blurring the Boundaries* model claims that it is possible to work towards evidence use in harmonious rather than conflictual ways, through trust, understanding and confidence between researchers, along with enhancing opportunities for research uptake. This model rejects the idea that there is a separation between scholars, practitioners and policy developers. Ideally, understanding 'the other' facilitates the development of shared understandings between these communities. By deliberately obfuscating organisational accountabilities and governance parameters this model would allow for true co-owning of research and policy processes (e.g., van Buuren & Edelenbos, 2004). Nahapiet and Ghoshal (1998) show that deliberate blurring of organisational and conceptual boundaries in the long run creates joint language and vocabulary that facilitates easier joint policy development and implementation.

The *Utilitarian Evidence* model states that only research products that are seen to be useful will be applied in policy and practice. This model describes how principles for the utility of research are different between researchers, practitioners and policymakers. It is important to recognise that utility is a dynamically perceptual quality and that its framing is as important as the 'factual' usefulness (see de Leeuw et al., 2018).

Fourth is the *Conduit* model. The 'conduit' informs different communities—policy communities, practice communities, the 'general' community—of research developments and outcomes. The conduit can be a person, agency or structure. A 'conduit' works to disseminate new knowledge in a format that is accessible and acceptable across groups (e.g., using more common, every-day terms, using graphs, avoiding jargon). The 'conduit' agent facilitates collaboration between the communities for the ongoing engagement of all partners in research (Bernier et al., 2006). The 'conduit' is an advocate and provides a platform for communities to express their concerns, in particular those who have fewer material and symbolic (e.g., skills and resilience) resources. Also, in disseminating new knowledge in an accessible manner, 'conduits' are at the ready to feed knowledge into fertile ground.

Sometimes research outcomes are not at all consistent with current political agendas or organisational practice. *Alternative Evidence* says that if research findings run counter to current political agendas/paradigms, its immediate potential impact will be muted. However, there may come a time where the volume of counter evidence can no longer be ignored— or at least not without creating organisational and political upsets or outrage (Hanney et al., 2003). In any event, researchers should also keep in mind that 'at the end of the day, policies...are constantly framed and reframed in response to changing contexts' (Choi et al., 2005). This model suggests that scholars and policy entrepreneurs should arm themselves with a repertoire/arsenal of evidence that can be inserted into the policy process when the opportunity arises.

Research Narratives aim to create a human dimension to research by including personal stories. Through personal stories, they inject 'common man' experiences into research outcomes (Sutton, 1999). The narratives humanise the research, but can also bring a sense of immediacy to the research topic that a 'dry' presentation of results might otherwise lack. Given policymakers' wish to include experience and common sense (over esoteric science) in their 'selection' of evidence (Booth, 1988), the inclusion of narratives in the overall presentation of research would be appropriate. The narratives support the research, and they highlight practitioner experiences. *Research Narratives* approaches provide an additional layer to the previous four models.

The *Resonance* model works on the idea that researchers, policy entrepreneurs or evidence conduits should have their 'finger on the pulse' of belief systems. In doing so, they can link their research outcomes with popular or emergent belief systems (e.g., 'social inclusion', a 'safe environment for all individuals'). When research resonates with what people believe, they find it easier to accept evidence.

Discourses around 'morally fraught' issues such as HIV/AIDS, birth control or euthanasia have often been framed from a religious starting point. It would not be helpful to argue that moral foundations are 'wrong' (and thereby polarise the policy discourse), as they are strongly connected to people's life worlds. However, trying to make the evidence resonate with other belief systems could advance the application of new knowledge. The Research Resonance model argues, for instance, that connecting the HIV/AIDS discourse to issues of 'safety', and the euthanasia discourse to 'dignity', rather than to 'morality', is helpful in integrating research, policy and practice. Issues of safety and dignity are issues that any individual, irrespective of their belief system, can identify with. The Research Resonance model demonstrates how the 'spin' which promotes research can influence the level of public and organisational interest in the research.

Is local better in this particular view of 'acting at the nexus' (rather than 'knowledge translation')? Our suite of studies suggests it is—even at the institutional redesign level. The other six models are exquisitely well-tuned to the particular context of street-level engagement, short lines of accountability and communication between research agents and policy actors, and practical blurred boundary spanning. But even at the institutional redesign level (which most would conceptualise as a state effort), we see that, through Hill and Hupe's (2006) gaze of multi-level governance, there is prominence and legitimacy for local types of governance (see, e.g., de Leeuw, 2015).

4   POLICY TRANSFER: SCALING UP AND SCALING WIDE

Earlier I illustrated policy agenda setting with work that applied Cobb and Elder (1971). A different perspective on how policies come about is provided by the policy transfer perspective. The suite of policy transfer theories and conceptual frameworks continues to be much debated and refined. The first comprehensive theory was proposed by Dolowitz and Marsh (1996). They argued that policy transfer occurs as 'a result of strategic decisions taken by actors inside and outside of government' (1996, p. 343). They saw that diffusion theory, policy learning and adaptation were all part of a bigger policy transfer process that describes the travel of policy ambitions through larger systems. Their most widely cited definition of policy transfer is:

> ... a process in which knowledge about policies, administrative arrangements, institutions etc. in one time and/or place is used in the development of policies, administrative arrangements and institutions in another time and/or place. (Dolowitz & Marsh, 1996, p. 344)

Such policy transfer may happen 'voluntarily' or 'coercively' (terms applied by Dolowitz and Marsh—for local policy we might think of a slightly different casting, e.g., 'internally' vs 'externally motivated'). The coercive model happens where a government or supra-local agency 'forces' another government to adopt a particular policy that is in their interests, explicitly highlighting the importance of agency (or lack thereof) in their framework.

Making the distinction between voluntary and coercive transfer the core issue, Dolowitz and Marsh (1996) argue that voluntary transfer is the policymakers' motivational result of some form of dissatisfaction or problem with the status quo. Perceived policy 'failure' creates incentives to identify new policies that can be borrowed from elsewhere—and at the local level, policy failure (a burst sewerage line; persistent health inequities among particular groups; etc.) is always more urgent and visible. Coercive transfer, while rarer, comes about through supranational mechanisms such as international treaties, trade and investment agreements, or the actions of international organisations such as the World Bank or International Monetary Fund (IMF). On occasion, the enforcement is carried by civil society through lawsuits, for instance in the Netherlands. Here, climate change advocacy group *Urgenda* successfully sued the state to act on its commitment to international agreements (Mayer, 2019). Law scholars see this case as deeply influential and suggest it will eventually impact on every level of government and force governance adherence to global standards—which then become local norms. This also works the other way around. The moment former President Trump withdrew the United States from the climate change accords, hundreds of state and local governments signed up to them—often with much more significant ambitions (e.g., Murthy, 2019).

Stone et al. (2020) suggest that policy substance can be instrumental in the transfer dynamic, and not just institutional politicking. An example of this dimension of policy learning and transfer can be identified in European Healthy Cities. The strict designation and accreditation processes are factors in 'externally motivated' policy development (de Leeuw & Skovgaard, 2005). Our analysis showed that the imposition of a designation process itself significantly strengthens adherence to local health policy objectives and processes. Interestingly, WHO maintains its position as an international collaborative member organisation and at best might facilitate coercion—except in cases where strong Treaty powers have been established (such as, for instance, the International Health Regulations, and less coercively, the Framework Convention on Tobacco Control [FCTC]). Indirect coercive transfer can be forced upon governments through other externalities, such as environmental damage, or through technological progress or economic integration, which compel governments to work together to solve supranational problems. How these commitments trickle down to local policymaking is as yet doubtful, but the increasing presence of networks of local governments in formal international forums suggests that we are on the brink of a glocal governance shift (see also Acuto & Leffel, 2020).

The literature identifies nine categories of transfer actors, some directly involved in the transfer process, and some who are external 'influencers': elected officials; political parties; bureaucrats/civil servants; pressure groups; policy entrepreneurs and experts; transnational corporations; think tanks; and supranational governmental and non-governmental institutions and consultants. This final group seems to have gained a particular power in recent years. Network governance and management concepts now show that policymaking is ever more becoming a non-state actor (including civil society and industry entities) enterprise. Provan and Kenis (2008) show the organisational and accountability mechanisms associated with this reality—and argue that lower-level government and organisational-level engagement are more elegantly suited to get this right.

Back to 'policy transfer'—what precisely is transferred: the policy; its intervention package; an idea; institutional arrangements; or ambitions? Answering this question depends on our view of the nature of policy and the policy process. Dolowitz and Marsh (1996) seek to move away from narrow conceptualisations of policy and policy transfer and seek to incorporate broader macro-objects of transfer such as ideology, ideas and negative lessons. This seems to be a pertinent point to our Healthy Cities perspectives.

'Transfer' assumes a source and a destination. Although the destination may well be clearly identified (e.g., a particular level of government with clear governance arrangements), the source may be more diffuse. It is argued that policy actors can turn to different levels of governance—the international, national and local—to draw inspiration, which provides opportunities for both horizontal transfer (between nations, geographical areas or sectors) and vertical transfer (through different levels of governance).

This more diffuse image of the policy transfer endeavour also offers a spectrum of policy transfer modalities, from 'carbon copying' at one end of the scale to 'inspiration' at the other, where policymakers do not adopt all aspects of a policy or seek to achieve identical outcomes.

Dolowitz and Marsh (1996) emphasise that policies are not imported into a vacuum, and the contextual, institutional and political arrangements of the borrowing jurisdiction and the specific motivations and objectives of decision makers influence the success or failure of introducing policy and its implementation. Closely related to this issue, three elements of the transfer process have been identified that are critical for 'successful' transfer outcomes: information deficit, 'cherry-picking' and contextual factors. If a borrowing jurisdiction does not have full information about the policy itself and the institutional arrangement within which it sits, this leads to 'uninformed' transfers. Where a policy and the institutional aspects that make it a success are not transferred in their entirety, then there is the risk of 'incomplete' transfer. Finally, the differences between the original and borrowing jurisdiction can result in 'inappropriate' transfer. From our earlier research in Healthy Cities, it appears that the mere requirement of European cities to be active members of a national and the international WHO network was influential for its success and survival (Camagni & Capello, 2004): the more they networked, the better they seemed able to deliver on Healthy City qualities.

The Dolowitz and Marsh model faced criticism of its status as a mere heuristic device rather than an explanatory theory of policy change (Evans & Davies, 1999; James & Lodge, 2003). Evans and Davies (1999) elevated these ideas and merged them into a perspective that embraced a connected and nested approach to policy movement through multi-scalar systems. They see five dimensions:

1. International structure and agency;
2. Domestic structure and agency;
3. Policy network analysis;
4. Policy transfer analysis; and
5. Epistemic community approaches.

Of these, in Healthy Cities evaluation work that I have led and carried out, we adopted (1), (3) and (5). Evans and Davies also focus on the 'spatial' dimension of policy transfer within and between different levels of governance. They identify 25 transfer pathways, working *horizontally* and *vertically* between the five different levels of governance (the transnational, regional, international, national and local levels). They argue that economic, technological, ideological and institutional structures of the 'borrowing' and 'lending' jurisdictions must be analysed in order to establish how they facilitate policy transfer and the impact on the transfer process.

They end up with a model of twelve stages. In these, the transfer process is broken up into discrete (but connected) actions:

- *Recognition*: whereby a decision-making elite, politician or bureaucrat (known as the 'client') identifies a policy problem;
- *Search*: which is undertaken if an obvious acceptable policy response is not available;
- *Contact*: whereby a policy transfer 'agent' (e.g., an epistemic community within an international organisation) is identified;
- *Emergence of an information feeder network*: whereby the 'client' is provided with an increase in volume and detail of information regarding the potential for transfer;
- *Cognition, reception and the emergence of a transfer network*: whereby the client evaluates the information provided by the information feeder network, with cognition and reception depending on a common value system existing between the client and the network;
- *Elite and cognitive mobilisation*: whereby the transfer agent's information and networks are tested, as they are expected to provide robust information on programmes or policies that address similar problems to those experienced by the client at the 'recognition' stage;
- *Interaction*: whereby the transfer agent organises forums for the exchange of ideas between the client and knowledge elites with policy-relevant knowledge;
- *Evaluation*: whereby the client evaluates the intelligence gathered by the agent relating to the object of transfer (e.g., policy goals, content, instruments, institutions, ideology), the degree of transfer (e.g., copying, hybridisation or inspiration) and the prerequisites of transfer (e.g., political feasibility and institutional conditions);
- *Decision*: whereby the chosen policy is tested against other competing ideas arising in the borrowing jurisdiction, within what Kingdon (1984) describes as the 'policy primeval soup';
- *Implementation:* whereby the policy is adopted by the client country, often by implementers who are different people to those who formulated the policy.

In the peer-reviewed and more narrative accounts of Healthy Cities success (e.g., Farrington et al., 2015; Tsouros, 1991), these action areas are clearly identifiable. Interestingly, they may not have resulted in a longer lasting or even permanent institutionalisation of local movements for health—they are morphing and shifting, as always. de Leeuw et al. (2020) in fact describe how the health generating potential of other glocal networks (notably *Citta Slow* and *Sustainable Cities*) may be more significant than *Healthy Cities a l'Europe*.

5   FRAMING AND ENTREPRENEURSHIP FOR NETWORK AND SYSTEMS CHANGE

This, then, brings us to the next political science-inspired question: how do Evans and Davies' (1999) twelve actions create enduring and meaningful policy change for local health? In a theoretical and method-ological 'proof-of-concept' paper (de Leeuw et al., 2018), we attempted to demonstrate and map some of the cognitive-informational and network dimensions of their approach. We wrote that actor networks and frame networks could (or should) be interleaved to identify opportunities for boundary spanning and policy transfer entrepreneurship.

The policy network map or configuration does not necessarily indicate which dynamics of the policy process will create new opportunities for policy development or voluntary transfer. Evidence-informed (or based) policy change does not just depend on network structure, but also on actions to shape the dimensions of the network. That is, the processes of negotiation and cooperation which result in the identification and pursuit of new ambitions to resolve social issues must also be examined (cf Left-wich, 1994). In other words: what do individuals and organisations *do* to change the network configuration to their (policy preference) advantage?

This is not the place to systematically review the body of litera-ture around policy change actions, and I will necessarily remain brief and eclectic. Laumann and Knoke (1987) mapped two policy domains in the United States (health and energy). They found that actors that deploy more personnel to scan and anticipate organisational behaviour and particular policy process interventions of the other network elements are better able to realise their ambitions—they anticipate, pre-empt and counter policy process change. John Kingdon (1984) famously identified 'policy entrepreneurs' who engage in processes of 'alternative specifica-tion' to connect actors and events in the eponymous Multiple Streams.

Those individuals, who well may be functions of social and political entrepreneurial institutions, are variously described (e.g., Skok, 1995) as 'issue initiator', 'policy broker', 'strategist' or 'caretaker' in addition to 'boundary worker' and 'issue manager'—they connect, disconnect and reconnect the players in the network around particular versions of the same reality (Knight & Lyall, 2013). The local health policy research that I cover in this chapter (e.g., also de Leeuw & Lin, 2017; Hoeijmakers et al., 2007) shows that these perspectives and roles are both more astute and tangible at the local level than they can be at the national or global level.

Common to this dimension of policy agency is the capacity to deploy relevant language. This, again, is not a new theoretical proposition in the evidence-policy-practice discourse. Stone (1997) dwells extensively on the power of the word, rhetoric and symbolism in policy processes; Khayatzadeh-Mahani et al. (2017) recently showed that words can act as 'collaboration magnets', and the novel behavioural economics units springing up around the world to nudge the citizenry to adopt preferred government action (Frain & Tame, 2017) use language—rather than monetary incentive or other 'hard' policy instruments—as their most prominent change tool. In fact, the particular framing of (perceived) reality is a key technique for individuals, groups, communities and political systems to make sense of the world (Entman, 1993). The art of mastering discourse, framing and storytelling may well be key to successfully bridging the nexus between whatever is construed as 'the evidence' and the negotiated endeavour to resolve social problems (i.e., 'policy') as Davidson (2017) astutely demonstrates. He quotes a tweet by Advocate Thuli Madonsela, former Public Protector of South Africa (4 July 2017):

"For people who want the truth adequate evidence is enough but for those who don't want the truth overwhelming evidence is inadequate" which echoes an almost proverbial insight by famed economist John Maynard Keynes: *"There is nothing a Government hates more than to be well-informed; for it makes the process of arriving at decisions much more complicated and difficult".* (Keynes & Moggridge, 1982)

To use an ancient Greek perspective on 'knowing', it may just be episteme 'the facts', but also regna 'wisdom', phronesis 'political astuteness', techne 'skill' or even parrhesia 'speaking truth to power' and combinations thereof (Sharpe, 2007) that create the urge for policy change. It appears that effective operators, notably at the local level, recognise two things:

- We are dealing with complex, dynamic, interdependent and interrelated groups of actors driving or affected by the policy process;
- Among the many tools in the process of shaping policy processes, the understanding of the discourse and the mobilisation and resonance of language and symbols are key (Pearce et al., 2014).

Drawing on a symbolic interactionist perspective, I posit that cliques or clusters identifiable through policy network analyses also share world views constructed in language, symbols and frames. For instance, in the policy network that would describe public choice around particular diagnostics in internal medicine, the clusters might comprise radiographers, gastroenterologists, hospital administrators, laboratory personnel and health economists. They each have their views of what creates 'evidence'. In the context of the discussion above of five dimensions of policy transfer, theorists like Haas (1992) would call them an epistemic community; Laumann and Knoke (1987) would simply frame them as a policy sub-domain. Each group has their particular training, disciplinary grounding, professional affiliations and accreditation mechanisms, and views of what constitutes 'truth'. The feasibility of a policy development process to yield tangible policy outcomes would be greatly enhanced if significant chunks of language/symbols/frames are shared across the structure of the network.

In our proof-of-concept work, we showed that policy network structure and agency can be separated and then interleaved, to show how diverse positions in policy network elites can connect for policy change. In the nexus categories, I described earlier that we encountered boundary spanners and policy entrepreneurs. Effective ones can see both the structure (network configuration) and engage with the discourse (the set of frames pertinent to the policy network domain) of a policy development environment: if the unique language representations of each clique would not share any commonality, there would be no reason or opportunity to meaningfully engage in any policy discourse. In short, we would be interested in both the boundaries and the spanning parameters of what only seems to be a messy enterprise (Rütten et al., 2017).

The extant literature on boundary spanning tends to focus on complex issues of public service provision, in the words of Williams (2011, p. 27) involving:

> *"people and organizations working together to manage and tackle common issues, to promote better co-ordination and integration of public services, to reduce duplication, to make the best use of scarce resources and to meet gaps in service provision and to satisfy unmet needs."* Boundary spanners – in service provision or policy engagement – occupy interconnected roles of reticulist, entrepreneur, interpreter/communicator and organizer. (Williams, 2002)

Our proof-of-concept analysis, based on a single health policy case study, demonstrated the feasibility of integrating the analysis of network structure and one form of network agency (Browne et al., 2017). An important area for future research is the role of the boundary spanners/policy entrepreneurs/policy brokers, identified using these network approaches. Based on our analysis, we hypothesised that the points at which frames overlap represent opportunities for boundary spanners to shift the policy discourse and, in turn, reconfigure the network. Now that we have demonstrated that dual analysis of the structure and agency of policy networks is feasible, the potential for boundary spanners to bridge the policy-evidence nexus needs to be tested empirically. Such research would be valuable for advancing policy network theory and may assist grassroots organisations engaging in advocacy to more effectively influence the policy agenda and to integrate evidence into policymaking.

The terrain of moving 'evidence' into 'policy' is not a one-dimensional map that cannot be navigated with traditional scientific insight alone, as the core of the Knowledge Translation perspective claims. Its landscape is multidimensional and can only be fully appreciated when its ever-changing nature is taken into account. Our efforts of overlaying the network structures and agencies of the policy narrative topography add a potentially important compass to the toolkit of the boundary spanner and policy entrepreneur.

6 How is Local Better?

Local is better. It is not just where the garbage is collected (Barber, 2013). Policy failure and success are more easily identified and communicated. The diversity of stakeholders is potentially more easily identifiable and to be engaged. The nexus between research, policy and practice becomes visible and potentially more acute. Problems need solving, and policies can be made. The organisation of network governance and management is more straightforward, and policy transfer can happen between stops on a bus route or metro line as jurisdictions are closer and tighter. Nations-states are beholden to rigid welfare state paradigms, and localities have the potential to break free (de Leeuw, 2021b).

Of course, this is a rosy casting of the issue. Many challenges remain, with local institutions failing to be transparent and/or retreating into hermetic bureaucratic walled compounds. Society itself may also fail to embrace and exploit its opportunities. With the ever-reducing degrees of social capital (Putnam, 2000), a stifling indolence has descended on communities around the world, where inward-looking egotism has replaced a sense and belief in community. Community engagement in policymaking, participation in democratic institutions and having one's voice heard for systems change seem to be more remote ideals than ever. The internet age has driven many into the arms of clicktivism and hacktivism as most individual expressions of social concern (George & Leidner, 2019). The research dimension of the nexus has come under pressure of framings on alternative facts and fake news (de Leeuw, 2018). And yet, local is better.

Local government and local institutions (like sports clubs, dog parks, cafes and restaurants, hairdressers) are still the flashpoints of political organisation and the exchange of social and political emotion. There is a role for everyone at those physical and virtual venues. They create and sustain health—very much in the spirit of the Ottawa Charter's 'settings' gaze. Good local government—and good local governance—still has an opportunity to challenge, build and exploit the potential of civil society. This even extends beyond what is regularly labelled as 'the citizenry': we tend to forget (and in fact have assumed as implicit in our preceding argument) that 'locals' are 'citizens'. But in many parts of the world the locals do not have rights and very limited visibility. They live, as slum dwellers, in hidden cities (WHO & UN Habitat, 2010). But for them, without local government support, technology comes to the rescue through IT-enhanced mobile phone applications that generate data and create voice (Corburn & Karanja, 2014).

Local is better—because of sharper policy agenda setting, opportunities of making power differentials more visible, exposure to policy learning and transfer, and the mere fact that everyone has a better opportunity to be heard. We can engage in better policies for better local health through mutual respect in open governance networks and through the systematic development and application of theoretical and empirical frameworks from political science.

REFERENCES

Acuto, M., & Leffel, B. (2020). Understanding the global ecosystem of city networks. *Urban Studies*, 0042098020929261.

Acuto, M., Kosovac, A., Pejic, D., & Jones, T. L. (2021). The city as actor in UN frameworks: Formalizing 'urban agency' in the international system? *Territory, Politics, Governance*. https://doi.org/10.1080/21622671.2020.1860810

Barber, B. R. (2013). *If mayors ruled the world: Dysfunctional nations, rising cities*. Yale University Press.

Bemelmans-Videc, M. L., Rist, R. C., & Vedung, E. O. (Eds.). (2011). *Carrots, sticks, and sermons: Policy instruments and their evaluation* (Vol. 1). Transaction Publishers.

Bernier, J., Rock, M., Roy, M., Bujold, R., & Potvin, L. (2006). Structuring an inter-sector research partnership: A negotiated zone—Reply to commentaries. *Soz Praventiv Medicine, 51*, 352–354.

Booth, T. (1988). *Developing policy research*. Gower Publishing Company Limited.

Brenner, N. (2019). *New urban spaces: Urban theory and the scale question*. Oxford University Press.

Browne, J., de Leeuw, E., Gleeson, D., Adams, K., Atkinson, P., & Hayes, R. (2017). A network approach to policy framing: A case study of the National Aboriginal and Torres Strait Islander Health Plan. *Social Science & Medicine, 172*, 10–18.

Cairney, P. (2013). Standing on the shoulders of giants: How do we combine the insights of multiple theories in public policy studies? *Policy Studies Journal, 41*(1), 1–21.

Cairney, P., & Oliver, K. (2020). How should academics engage in policymaking to achieve impact? *Political Studies Review, 18*(2), 228–244.

Camagni, R., & Capello, R. (2004). The city network paradigm: Theory and empirical evidence. *Contributions to Economic Analysis, 266*, 495–529.

Choi, C. K., Pang, T., Lin, V., Puska, P., Sherman, G., Goddard, M., Ackland, M. J., Sainbury, P., Stachenko, S., Morrison, M., & Clottey, C. (2005). Can scientists and policy-makers work together? *Journal of Epidemiology and Community Health, 59*(8), 632–637.

Cobb, R. W., & Elder, C. D. (1983). *Participation in American politics: The dynamics of agenda-building*. The Johns Hopkins University Press.

Cobb, R. W., & Elder, C. D. (1971). The politics of agenda-building: An alternative perspective for modern democratic theory. *The Journal of Politics, 33*(4), 892–915.

Corburn, J., & Karanja, I. (2014). Informal settlements and a relational view of health in Nairobi, Kenya: Sanitation, gender and dignity. *Health Promotion International, 31*(2), 258–269.

Davidson, B. (2017). Storytelling and evidence-based policy: Lessons from the grey literature. *Palgrave Communications, 3*, 17093.

Davies, W. K. D. (Ed.). (2015). *Theme cities: Solutions for urban problems.* Springer.

de Leeuw, E. (2015). Intersectoral action, policy and governance in European Healthy Cities. *Public Health Panorama, 1*(2), 175–182.

de Leeuw, E. (2017). Cities and health from the neolithic to the anthropocene. In E. De Leeuw & J. Simos (Eds.), *Healthy cities—The theory, policy, and practice of value-based urban planning* (pp. 3–30). Springer.

de Leeuw, E. (2018). The short-sighted sycophant's selfie. *Health Promotion International, 33*(1), 1–5.

de Leeuw, E. (2021a, August 25). *Intersectoral action.* Oxford Bibliographies. https://doi.org/10.1093/OBO/9780199756797-0203. https://www.oxfordbibliographies.com/view/document/obo-9780199756797/obo-9780199756797-0203.xml

de Leeuw, E. (2021b, August 27). *Inequity in health—We can't handle the truth.* Croakey (editor: J. Doggett). https://www.croakey.org/inequity-in-health-we-cant-handle-the-truth/

de Leeuw, E., & Lin, V. (2017). Local health planning and governance. In E. de Leeuw & J. Simos (Eds.), *Healthy cities—The theory, policy, and practice of value-based urban planning* (pp. 395–405). Springer.

de Leeuw, E., & Polman, L. (1995). Health policy making: The Dutch experience. *Social Science & Medicine, 40*(3), 331–338.

de Leeuw, E., & Simos, J. (Eds.). (2017). *Healthy cities—The theory, policy, and practice of value-based urban planning.* Springer.

de Leeuw, E., & Skovgaard, T. (2005). Utility-driven evidence for healthy cities: Problems with evidence generation and application. *Social Science & Medicine, 61*, 1331–1341.

de Leeuw, E., Browne, J., & Gleeson, D. (2018). Overlaying structure and frames in policy networks to enable effective boundary spanning. *Evidence & Policy: A Journal of Research, Debate and Practice, 14*(3), 537–547.

de Leeuw, E., McNess, A., Crisp, A. B., & Stagnitti, K. (2008). Theoretical reflections on the nexus between research, policy and practice. *Critical Public Health, 18*(1), 5–20.

de Leeuw, E., McNess, A., Stagnitti, K., & Crisp, B. (2007). It's research, Jim, but not as we know it. In *Acting at the nexus. Integration of research, policy and practice*. Deakin University.

de Leeuw, E., Simos, J., & Forbat, J. (2020). Urban health and healthy cities today. In D. McQueen (Ed.), *Oxford research encyclopedia of global public health*. Oxford University Press.

de Leeuw, E. J. (1989). *Health policy: An exploratory inquiry into the development of policy for the new public health in the Netherlands*. Maastricht University.

Dolowitz, D., & Marsh, D. (1996). Who learns what from whom: A review of the policy transfer literature. *Political Studies, 44*(2), 343–357.

Entman, R. M. (1993). Framing: Toward clarification of a fractured paradigm. *Communication, 43*(4), 51–58.

Evans, M., & Davies, J. (1999). Understanding policy transfer: A Multi-level, multi-disciplinary perspective. *Public Administration, 77*(2), 361–385.

Farrington, J. L., Faskunger, J., & Mackiewicz, K. (2015). Evaluation of risk factor reduction in a European City Network. *Health Promotion International, 30*(suppl_1), i86–i98.

Frain, A., & Tame., R. (2017, July 4). *Government behavioural economics 'nudge unit' needs a shove in a new direction*. The Conversation Australia. https://theconversation.Com/government-behavioural-economics-nudge-unit-needs-a-shove-in-a-newdirection-80390

Gaißert, E. (1909). Gesundheitspolizei. In *Leitfaden für Polizeibeamte in Frage- und Antwortform* (pp. 72–86). Springer.

George, J. J., & Leidner, D. E. (2019). From clicktivism to hacktivism: Understanding digital activism. *Information and Organization, 29*(3), 100249.

Glasgow, S., & Schrecker, T. (2016). The double burden of neoliberalism? Noncommunicable disease policies and the global political economy of risk. *Health & Place, 39*, 204–211.

Goumans, M., & Springett, J. (1997). From projects to policy: 'Healthy Cities' as a mechanism for policy change for health? *Health Promotion International, 12*(4), 311–322.

Greenhalgh, T., & Wieringa, S. (2011). Is it time to drop the 'knowledge translation' metaphor? A critical literature review. *Journal of the Royal Society of Medicine, 104*(12), 501–509.

Haas, P. M. (1992). Introduction: Epistemic communities and international policy coordination. *International Organization, 46*(1), 1–35.

Hancock, T., & Duhl, L. (1986). *Promoting health in the urban context* (WHO Healthy Cities Papers No. 1). FADL Publishers.

Hancock, T. (2017). Healthy cities emerge: Toronto–Ottawa–Copenhagen. In E. De Leeuw & J. Simos (Eds.), *Healthy cities—The theory, policy, and practice of value-based urban planning* (pp. 63–73). Springer.

Hanney, S.R., Gonzalez-Block, M. A., Buxton, M. J., & Kogan, M. (2003). The utilisation of health research in policy-making: Concepts, examples and methods of assessment. *Health Research Policy and Systems, 1*(2). http://www.health-policy-systems.com/content/1/1/2. Accessed 15 August 2006.

Harris, P., Baum, F., Friel, S., Mackean, T., Schram, A., & Townsend, B. (2020). A glossary of theories for understanding power and policy for health equity. *Journal of Epidemiology and Community Health, 74*(6), 548–552.

Hawkins, B., Holden, C., & Mackinder, S. (2020). Policy transfer in the context of multi-level governance. In *The Battle for standardised cigarette packaging in Europe* (pp. 17–44). Palgrave Pivot.

Hill, M., & Hupe, P. (2006). Analysing policy processes as multiple governance: Accountability in social policy. *Policy & Politics, 34*(3), 557–573.

Hoeijmakers, M., de Leeuw, E., Kenis, P., & De Vries, N. K. (2007). Local health policy development processes in the Netherlands: An expanded toolbox for health promotion. *Health Promotion International, 22*(2), 112–121.

James, O., & Lodge, M. (2003). The limitations of 'policy transfer' and 'lesson drawing' for public policy research. *Political Studies Review, 1*(2), 179–193.

Jayne, M., Hubbard, P., & Bell, D. (2011). Worlding a city: Twinning and urban theory. *City, 15*(1), 25–41.

Keynes, J. M., & Moggridge, D. (1982). *The collected writings of John Maynard Keynes. Volume 21. Activities 1931–1939; world crisis and policies in Britain and America.* Macmillan and Cambridge University Press for the Royal Economic Society.

Khayatzadeh-Mahani, A., Labonté, R., Ruckert, A., & de Leeuw, E. (2017). Using sustainability as a collaboration magnet to encourage multi-sector collaborations for health. *Global Health Promotion.* https://doi.org/10.1177/1757975916683387

Kim, J., de Leeuw, E., Harris-Roxas, B., & Sainsbury, P. (2020). The three paradigms on urban health. *European Journal of Public Health, 30*(Suppl 5). https://doi.org/10.1093/eurpub/ckaa166.155

Kingdon, J. W. (1984). *Agendas, alternatives, and public policies.* Little, Brown.

Klijn, E.-H., & Koppenjan, J. F. M. (2006). Institutional design. Changing institutional features of networks. *Public Management Review, 8*(1) 141–160

Knight, C., & Lyall, C. (2013). Knowledge brokers: The role of intermediaries in producing research impact. *Evidence & Policy, 9*, 309–316.

Laframboise, H. (1990). Non-participative policy development: The genesis of "A New Perspective on the Health of Canadians." *Journal of Public Health Policy, 11*(3), 316–322.

Laumann, E. O., & Knoke, D. (1987). *The organizational state: Social choice in national policy domains.* University of Wisconsin Press.

Leftwich, A. (1994). Governance, the state and the politics of development. *Development and Change, 25*, 363–386.

Lin, V., & Gibson, B. (2003). *Evidence-based health policy: Problems and possibilities*. Oxford University Press.

Lipsky, M. (2010). *Street-level bureaucracy: Dilemmas of the individual in public service*. Russell Sage Foundation.

Mayer, B. (2019). The state of the Netherlands v. Urgenda Foundation: Ruling of the court of appeal of The Hague (9 October 2018). *Transnational Environmental Law, 8*(1), 167–192.

McKeown, T. (1976). *The role of medicine: Dream, mirage, or nemesis?* Princeton University Press.

Milio, N. (1981a). *Promoting health through public policy Philadelphia*. FA Davis.

Milio, N. (1981b). Promoting health through structural change: Analysis of the origins and implementation of Norway's farm-food-nutrition policy. *Social Science & Medicine. Part A: Medical Psychology & Medical Sociology, 15*(5), 721–734.

Mulder, M. (1977). *The daily power game*. Martinus Nijhoff.

Murthy, S. L. (2019). States and cities as norm sustainers: A role for subnational actors in the Paris Agreement on climate change. *Virginia Environmental Law Journal, 37*, 1.

Nahapiet, J., & Ghoshal, S. (1998). Social capital, intellectual capital, and the organizational advantage. *Academy of Management Review, 23*(2), 242–266.

Nilsen, P., Ståhl, C., Roback, K., & Cairney, P. (2013). Never the twain shall meet?—A comparison of implementation science and policy implementation research. *Implementation Science, 8*(1), 63.

Nutbeam, D., & Catford, J. (1987). The Welsh Heart Programme evaluation strategy: Progress, plans and possibilities. *Health Promotion International, 2*(1), 5–18.

Pearce, W., Wesselink, A., & Colebatch, H. (2014). Evidence and meaning in policymaking. *Evidence & Policy, 10*(2), 161–165.

Pinto, M., Macedo, M., Macedo, P., Almeida, C., & Silva, M. (2015). The lifecycle of a voluntary policy innovation: The case of local Agenda 21. *Journal of Management and Sustainability, 5*, 69.

Provan, K. G., & Kenis, P. (2008). Modes of network governance: Structure, management, and effectiveness. *Journal of Public Administration Research and Theory, 18*(2), 229–252.

Puska, P. (2002). Successful prevention of non-communicable diseases: 25 year experiences with North Karelia Project in Finland. *Public Health Medicine, 4*(1), 5–7.

Putnam, R. D. (2000). *Bowling alone: The collapse and revival of American community*. Simon & Schuster.

Richter, R., Giroldi, E., Jansen, J., & van der Weijden, T. (2020). A qualitative exploration of clinicians' strategies to communicate risks to patients in the complex reality of clinical practice. *PloS One, 15*(8), e0236751.

Rodríguez, M. A., Marmot, M. G., de Snyder, V. N. S., Galvão, L. A., Avellaneda, X., del Rocio Saenz, M., Dubois, A. M., Tarzibachi, E., Ritterbusch, A. E., Castro, A., & Plough, A. (2019). The transformative potential of strategic partnerships to form a Health Equity Network of the Americas. *Ethnicity & Disease, 29*(Suppl 1), 153–158.

Rütten, A., Frahsa, A., Abel, T., Bergmann, M., de Leeuw, E., Hunter, D., Jansen, M., King, A., & Potvin, L. (2017). Co-producing active lifestyles as whole-system-approach: Theory, intervention and knowledge-to-action implications. *Health Promotion International*. https://doi.org/10.1093/heapro/dax053

Sabatier, P. A. (1999). Introduction: The need for better theories. In P. A. Sabatier (Ed.), *Theories of the policy process*.

Sharpe, M. (2007). A question of two truths? Remarks on parrhesia and the 'political-philosophical' difference. *Parrhesia, 2*, 89–108.

Skok, J. E. (1995). Policy issue networks and the public policy cycle: A structural-functional framework for public administration. *Public Administration Review, 55*, 325–332.

Snow, J. (1855). *On the mode of communication of cholera*. John Churchill.

Stone, D. A. (1997). *Policy paradox: The art of political decision making* (Vol. 13). WW Norton.

Stone, D., Porto de Oliveira, O., & Pal, L. A. (2020). Transnational policy transfer: The circulation of ideas, power and development models. *Policy and Society, 39*(1), 1–18. https://doi.org/10.1080/14494035.2019.1619325

Straus, S. E., Tetroe, J., & Graham, I. (2009). Defining knowledge translation. *Canadian Medical Association Journal, 181*(3–4), 165–168.

Studlar, D. T. (2015). Punching above their weight through policy learning Tobacco control policies in Ireland. *Irish Political Studies, 30*(1), 41–78.

Sutton, R. (1999). *The policy process: An overview*. Overseas Development Institute.

True, J. L., Jones, B. D., & Baumgartner, F. R. (2019). Punctuated-equilibrium theory: Explaining stability and change in public policymaking. In *Theories of the policy process* (pp. 155–187). Routledge.

Tsouros, A. D. (1991). *World Health Organization Healthy Cities project: A project becomes a movement, review of progress 1987 to 1990*. World Health Organization Regional Office for Europe.

Van Buuren, M. W., & Edelenbos, J. (2004). Conflicting knowledge: Why is joint knowledge such a problem? *Science and Public Policy, 31*(4), 289–299.

Villermé, L.-R. (1840). Tableau de l'état physique et moral des ouvriers employés dans les manufactures de coton, de laine et de soie (Study of the Physical Condition of Cotton, Wool and Silk workers). Forgotten Books Classic Reprint.

WHO. (1978). *Alma-Ata 1978: Primary health care.* World Health Organization.

WHO & UN Habitat. (2010). *Hidden cities: Unmasking and overcoming health inequities in urban settings.* WHO & UN Habitat.

Williams, P. (2002). The competent boundary spanner. *Public Administration, 80,* 103–124.

Williams, P. (2011). The life and times of a boundary spanner. *Integrated Care, 19*(3), 26–33.

World Health Organization, Canada, H., & Association, C. P. H. (1986). Ottawa charter for health promotion. *Bulletin of the Pan American Health Organization (PAHO), 21*(2), 200–204.

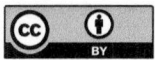

Select Committee Governance and the Production of Evidence: The Case of UK E-cigarettes Policy

Benjamin Hawkins and Kathryn Oliver

1 INTRODUCTION

The House of Commons select committees were introduced to the UK (UK) parliament in 1979 and have existed in the current form since the 'Wright reforms' of 2010 (see Russell & Grover 2017: 205–233). They exist alongside six permanent (and other ad hoc) House of Lords Committee and various bicameral joint committees in the overall parliamentary architecture. Within the Commons, select committees are thematically organised reflecting either the key competences of government and key ministerial functions (e.g. the Health and Social

B. Hawkins (✉)
MRC Epidemiology Unit, University of Cambridge, Cambridge, UK
e-mail: brh28@cam.ac.uk

K. Oliver
Faculty of Public Health and Policy, London School of Hygiene and Tropical Medicine, London, UK

© The Author(s) 2022   187
P. Fafard et al. (eds.), *Integrating Science and Politics for Public Health*,
Palgrave Studies in Public Health Policy Research,
https://doi.org/10.1007/978-3-030-98985-9_9

Care Committee), or on cross-cutting issues relating to parliamentary or governmental business (e.g. the Members' Expenses Committee). The activities of the Commons select committees are overseen by the Liaison Committee, made up of each individual committee chair.

Commons select committees exhibit a high degree of independence from the machinery of government and opposition around which the Westminster system is structured. While the membership (usually totalling 11, but on occasion more to accommodate smaller parties) reflects the number of MPs each party has, the particular MPs occupying these positions are elected by ballots within their party groups. This may lead to experienced or interested individuals on a given topic but who diverge from their party line, taking up positions. Likewise, the Chairs of each committee are elected, with the number of Chairs allocated to each party again reflecting the balance of the Commons. This invests the Chairs not only with an independent democratic mandate, but also with a platform from which ambitious politicians outside government can establish their reputation in a specific policy area and their wider credentials for high office.

The committee system of the UK parliament differs from those in many other comparable democratic systems in that the legislative and executive scrutiny functions are split between different forums. Select committees do not play a role in the legislative process, which is overseen instead by ad hoc committees established for each Bill, whose membership reflecting the government majority in the Commons. The role of select committees is instead to monitor the activities of government by scrutinising issues of importance to both government and wider society (see, e.g., Benton & Russell, 2012; Geddes et al., 2018; Russell & Benton, 2011; Russell & Gover, 2017). Committees are able to appoint specialist advisors, hear evidence and produce reports, which solicit governmental responses, usually within two months of the publication of a report. Thus, their key function is that of knowledge generators and disseminators within parliament and the wider polity. Since select committees enjoy high levels of credibility, both amongst policy actors and the wider public, their reports represent potentially important and influential interventions within policy debates.

Yet relatively little attention has been paid to the governance mechanisms which oversee their activities. The main focus of the existing literature is on the role of such committees in holding governments to account as opposed to the mechanisms through which their own activities should be scrutinised (see, e.g., Benton & Russell, 2012). More recent studies have analysed the representativeness of witnesses called to give evidence before committees (Geddes, 2017), but wider analyses of the processes and oversight of committee enquiries remain rare. Given the very high degree of autonomy given to committees in terms of the focus (i.e. what to research), the conduct of their enquiries and the drafting of their reports and recommendations, this is an important gap in the literature. This is particularly the case where these issues are viewed in light of the now extensive literature on the corporate determinants of health and, most notably, the policy influencing strategies of the transnational tobacco industry (Hurt et al., 2009). These include extensive and continually evolving efforts to influence scientific research and shape the evidentiary content of policy debates in ways designed to achieve favourable (or at least less unfavourable) regulatory environments for their products (Brandt, 2012).

Identifying, interpreting and synthesising evidence poses potentially significant the challenges for non-specialist MPs and committee staff in what are often complex and highly technical regulatory issues. The opaque governance structures and lines of accountability creates an opportunity for motivated and well-resourced policy actors, such as transnational corporations, to be able to influence the outputs from such committees in ways amendable to their interest and policy objectives.

This chapter seeks to highlight these issues through the example of UK e-cigarette policy debates and the Commons Science & Technology Committee's, 2018 enquiry into their regulation and use. We do not seek to identify the appropriate regulatory regime for e-cigarettes or to evaluate the underlying evidence in support of different policy regimes. Instead, we focus on what this contentious policy debate tells us about the politics and governance of evidence-informed policy within the Westminster system, and the potential opportunities which the select committee system affords policy actors to shape the evidential content of policy debates and potentially, therefore, regulatory outcomes. The issue of e-cigarettes was chosen since the questions raised here about select committee governance may be particularly relevant in contexts in which policy debates are framed in evidentiary terms, where evidence base is immature or contested and where key actors, like the tobacco sector, are excluded from other forms of engagement in the policy process (Hawkins & Ettelt, 2019). As such, the debate around a novel product such as e-cigarettes, and the role of the tobacco industry within this, provides an ideal context in which to explore these issues.

The chapter builds on previous studies of the 'good governance' of evidence, extending its focus to the role of select committees in the production, evaluation, synthesis and dissemination of policy-relevant evidence (Hawkins & Parkhurst, 2016; Parkhurst & Abeysinghe, 2016). It seeks also to expand the literature on the commercial determinants of health (Mialon, 2020) and to add additional insights into the evidence management component corporate political strategies (Brandt, 2012). Our analysis here has implications for our understanding of the governance of evidence within policy-making processes, and the role and oversight of parliamentary committees, in both the UK and in other contexts and will be of particular relevance for understanding the evidentiary content of e-cigarette policy debates in various policy settings.

2   Select Committees' Impact on Policy

Despite scepticism about the importance of parliament as a policy actor in the Westminster polity (King & Crewe, 2014), both parliament (Russell & Cowley, 2016) and parliamentary committees (Hindmoor et al., 2009; Russell & Benton, 2011) have been identified as important components within the policy system, and there is a limited but growing literature on their policy impact. Russell and Benton (2011) studied the work of 7 House of Commons select committees between 1997 and 2010, tracing the passage of recommendations from committee enquiry reports into policy and identifying less tangible forms of influence. Overall, they found select committee influence is significant with around 40% of recommendations taken up by government and implemented and smaller changes and requests for information disclosure even more likely to be accepted (see also Russell & Gover, 2017; Yowell, 2012). Hindmoor et al. (2009) found that 20 out of 93 proposals in government education bills demonstrated similarities with proposals emanating from the Education Select Committee. Perhaps counter-intuitively, recommendations from committees with opposition Chairs were more likely to be taken on board, reflecting the efforts made by these actors to foster cross-party consensus for their proposals. Indeed, the cross-party nature of select committees is identified as a key source of the authority and influence over policy-makers (Russell & Gover, 2017). Similarly, it is often backbench MPs, as opposed to members of the government, who take up select committee reports and act as a conduit for their impact on government (Russell & Gover, 2017). In a small number of cases—around 5% of reports—select committees are asked to undertake pre-legislative scrutiny of draft legislation. While select committees cannot amend bills formally, existing studies have found evidence of committee impact on the resulting legislation (see Mulley & Kinghorn, 2016; Smookler, 2006).

However, conceptualising influence in narrow, transactional and quantitative terms, focussing solely on traceable recommendations in formal policy documents, misses both the myriad forms which policy-making takes and the complex and nuanced ways in which influence may occur (see Benton & Russell, 2012). Committee influence extends beyond uptake of recommendations in policy, with Russel and Benton (2011: 8) identifying seven more indirect or less readily quantifiable forms of committee influence: contributing to debate, drawing together evidence, spotlighting issues, brokering between actors in government, improving the quality of government decision-making through accountability, exposing failures and, perhaps most importantly, 'generating fear' about how things might look if examined by a select committee.

The latter represents an important mechanism of 'soft power' through which select committees can shape the thinking of government in the development of policy. Select committee outputs and members (particularly committee Chairs) are also identified as sources of authority in policy debates, for example, through references to their work in parliamentary debates and policy evaluation (see Russell & Gover, 2017). Both criticism and endorsement by select committees—whether anticipated or actual—can shape policy-makers' behaviour. The latter may feel compelled to take committee Chairs seriously given their capacity to 'make life difficult' for government if they so choose (Russell & Gover, 2017: 228). Hawes (1992) identified how influence can be subtle and indirect and may take the form of simply raising the profile of a given policy issue: the 'delayed drop' effect, perhaps analogous to Carol Weiss' (1979) enlightenment model of knowledge transfer and diffusion.

In addition to their function within parliament, select committees have become a prominent component of the policy space, with committee chairs enjoying an increasing media profile (Gaines et al., 2019). The generally favourable perception of their work (Gaines et al., 2019) means the activities of committees, including their hearings and evidence sessions, can be a means of promoting public as well as a parliamentary consciousness about policy issues and particular framings and accounts of these.

3   SELECT COMMITTEES AS EVIDENCE SYNTHESISERS AND PRODUCERS

Select committees are both consumers and producers of policy-relevant information and evidence within the Westminster system. They function as evidence gathering tools for parliamentarians (Geddes, 2020), while the reports and other documents they generate exist as independent, policy-relevant artefacts within the information environment. A small but emerging literature has begun to examine the processes through which parliamentary committees gather, interpret and synthesise information (Benton & Russell, 2012; Geddes, 2016, 2017, 2020), identifying common knowledge translation barriers (Geddes et al., 2018) and examining the type and representativeness of witnesses (Geddes, 2017). The tight timetables to which UK parliamentary committees work, and their geographical location, potentially skews inputs towards those who can be physically present in London (to give personal testimony) and/or who have the resources and expertise to be able respond to evidence calls at short notice and in forms most accessible to/likely to influence parliamentarians. Pedersen et al. (2015) found similar issues in a comparative study of Denmark, the Netherlands and the UK. Perhaps counter-intuitively, they identified that closed calls led to a wider variety of actors being involved and a more even distribution of evidence being received by the committee. Geddes et al. (2018) also highlight the value which parliamentarians place on 'consensual knowledge' and 'generalised findings' with clear policy relevance versus the more 'cutting edge' or 'boundary pushing' research which academics often seek to promote. Select committees thus emphasise breadth of evidence and notions of balance in their evidence gathering and reporting. This norm of inclusivity is likely to create a significant opportunity for well-resourced industry actors to feed into these processes.

While select committees may be perceived to be led by the evidence, in reality committees and MPs on them face a competing range of priorities, including political expediency and agendas as well as the 'performative' nature of committee hearings. This means there may be a trade-off between style and substance in selecting witnesses who will be able to engage and explain evidence to committee members (and their wider audience) (Geddes, 2019). Similarly, the desire to produce impactful reports and influence policy may shape the content of committee outputs given the types of information likely to be most impactful on fellow parliamentarians and the government.

The evidence produced by select committees, in terms of reports and the recommendations, is often highly regarded by ministers in relation to other sources of policy-relevant information. Bates and colleagues (2017: 783) argue that select committees are seen by policy actors as a 'source of unbiased information, rational debate, and constructive ideas' (see also Geddes, 2019). According to Benton and Russell (2012: 789), ministers may take recommendations from a committee more seriously than proposals from civil servants or outside groups, since committees apply 'a political filter' to the evidence collected and usually present reports on a unanimous cross-party basis. More generally, scholars agree that the form in which evidence is presented influences the likelihood that findings will be taken up by policy-makers, with researchers encouraged to present findings in accessible forms. Stevens (2010) found that outputs with clear, unequivocal findings represented in certain forms (i.e. 'killer charts') from which clear policy directions could be derived were often favoured over other types of evidence. This may sway policy actors towards outputs such as select committee reports over more equivocal and less readily accessible findings in the peer reviewed academic literature. If select committees are identified as important sources of clear, reliable, policy-relevant (and politically road-tested) evidence by policy-makers—able to influence the content of policy in the ways identified above—then assessing the quality of their evidentiary output, the processes through which it is produced and the mechanisms which oversee this, is of paramount importance to a policy science committed to effective, evidence-informed decision-making.

Select committees thus offer a potentially important point of contact and opportunity for knowledge exchangebetween legislators on the one hand, and researchers, experts and policy stakeholders on the other. However, key questions arise about who has access to these committees and the relative weight afforded to their inputs by members in their role as knowledge conduits for parliament as a whole. While, as noted above, the focus to date has been largely on the social make up of committee witnesses, it is necessary to focus not just on diversity and democratic representativeness, but on power politics and vested interests. Given the asymmetric resource distribution between different policy actors, for example, between trans-national corporations and civil society organisations, they may be able to obtain disproportionate access (and thus potential to influence) to committees. This is particularly important as corporations in certain sectors are increasingly positioning themselves as legitimate producers of policy-relevant evidence and participants in evidence evaluation processes. This potential conflict between democratic norms of inclusivity and those of scientific rigour and independence reflects the wider tensions within select committees between the desire to be led by the relevant evidence and the political realities of parliament and the priorities of individual committee members. This in turn raises important questions about the governance of select committees and the mechanisms in place to protect their procedures from capture by vested interests.

4   SELECT COMMITTEE GOVERNANCE

Select committees are formally established, and their role set out, in House of Commons Standing Order 152. However, the governance mechanisms surrounding select committees depend to a large degree on convention and afford a high degree of autonomy to the membership, and particularly select committee Chairs, in deciding the focus of enquiries, the appointment of expert advisors, evidence collection and interpretation, and the drafting of reports and recommendations. Considering the salience given to select committee reports, questions arise about the basis on which these decisions are taken and the oversight mechanisms which govern them.

Parliamentarians often have long-term commitments to specific policy issues and in-depth understanding of the issues and actors involved in the areas of focus of their committees. However, given the potentially wide-ranging remit of a committee such as the Health and Social Care Select Committee, it is unrealistic that committee members will be equally conversant with every issue that may come before the committee or indeed demonstrate the same level of interest and engagement with each of these.

In addition, while select committee members may have specialist *knowledge* in a certain subject, it does not necessarily follow that they have the specialist *skills* to undertake all aspects of select committee including the collection, interpretation, synthesis and production of policy-relevant evidence involved in committee enquiries. This includes a range of relevant competence including the forensic interviewing or cross-examination skills required for the successful questioning of witnesses appearing before committees. This may be the lifeblood of the many barristers populating the House of Commons but may come less naturally to those from different professional backgrounds. Equally, most parliamentarians will have limited training in the methodological norms of conducting research in different disciplines and contexts. This includes an ability to assess the conflicts of interest which may affect some policy actors and sources of information with which the committee may be confronted. In this context, the clerks to the committee and the expert advisers will play an important role in guiding the work of the committee. However, while committee support staff may be able to advise and support MPs on these matters, the resources available to them and timescales for producing committee reports, mean they may able unable to search for and assess evidence in a way that would be considered systematic, exhaustive and robust by specialist researchers. While academic researchers do not have a monopoly on the production of legitimate, policy-relevant evidence, research outputs of different kinds and provenance nevertheless have a different epistemological status and must be handled appropriately in the context of policy deliberations.

5   Corporate Actors and Policy Influence

The inherently political nature of evidence use in (health) policy-making perhaps comes most obviously to the fore in contexts in which both the nature of the policy problem—and thus the objectives of government interventions—and the underlying evidence bases are highly contested. There is a long and well-documented history of tobacco industry attempts to shape regulation of their products and the policy-making process more generally (Apollonio & Bero, 2007; Cairney et al., 2011; Fooks et al., 2011; Hawkins et al., 2018; Hurt et al., 2009; Peeters et al., 2015; Savell et al., 2014; Smith et al., 2013). The release of internal tobacco industry documents into the public domain as a result of whistle-blower leaks and court-mandated document releases following litigation in the USA in the 1990s revealed the extent of industry attempts to shape the policy environment through political lobbying; financial donations to politicians, parties and agencies; and other influencing strategies (Hurt et al., 2009). A key component of industry strategy focussed on the development of an allegedly 'reduced risk' through innovations such as filtered cigarettes and lower tar products, which studies reveal to be no safer than conventional or preceding products (Gilmore & Peeters, 2013; Peeters & Gilmore, 2013, 2015). We refer to product development as the industry's *technological strategy*.

In addition, trans-national tobacco corporations (TTCs) invested significant resources in the production and dissemination of scientific research related to their products and associated harms with the objective of influencing both public perceptions of the harmfulness of their products and the evidentiary content of regulatory debates (Bero, 2005; Brandt, 2012; Grüning et al., 2006; Muggli et al., 2001, 2003; Oreskes & Conway, 2014). We term this component of industry activities their *epistemic strategy*. A key component of their epistemic strategy centred on the funding of apparently independent researchers and the formation of front organisations (Apollonio & Bero, 2007), which offered the veneer of independence and scientific integrity to industry funded research (Cash et al., 2002) in order to shape the evidentiary content of policy deliberations and the wider information environment informing public debate. This strategy led Brandt (2012) to conclude that the tobacco industry practically invented the concept of (conflict of interest) COI in health policy research.

These now infamous examples of the tobacco industry placing narrow corporate interests over those of public health have led to unprecedented moves by tobacco control (and wider public health) researchers and advocates to press for regulation of the sale, marketing and consumption of tobacco products, culminating in the adoption of the Framework Convention on Tobacco Control (FCTC) (World Health Organization, 2003). In particular, Article 5.3 of the FCTC requires signatories to take active measures to protect public policies 'from the commercial and vested interests of the tobacco industry', leading to the effective exclusion of the tobacco industry from decision-making in many policy contexts (World Health Organization, 2003, 2008). Notwithstanding ongoing issues of implementation (Fooks et al., 2017; Hawkins & Holden, 2018), the TI's ability to engage policy-makers or promote favourable research is limited by FCTC Article 5.3 (Malone, 2013; McKee & Allebeck, 2014).

These developments have led TTCs to evolve and seek new ways to advance their business objectives by adapting their epistemic and technological strategies, leading to an important symbiosis between these two strands of industry strategy. In terms of their technological strategy, TTCs have invested significantly in new nicotine delivery systems, particularly e-cigarettes but also heat not burn technology (Mathers et al., 2019). This has included the formation by TTCs of wholly owned subsidiary companies dedicated to their 'next generation' products. Investment in e-cigarettes has conferred significant benefits to the industry by blurring the edges of restrictions on advertising and promotion and undermining clear air legislation while maintaining nicotine dependence in users (MacKenzie & Hawkins, 2016). The emergence of e-cigarettes has fostered division within the tobacco control research and advocacy communities whose unity was a key factor in delivering previous policy successes (Gneiting, 2015). This has been particularly marked in the UK, which is a strategically important context for tobacco control debates (Gornall, 2015; Hawkins & Ettelt, 2019). In addition, attempts by TTCs to rebrand themselves as nicotine technology companies offer a pretext for engagement with policy-makers, circumnavigating FCTC restrictions on meetings with the tobacco industry TI and giving them a seat at the table for the development of regulatory responses to these novel products under the auspices of being technical experts. As will be discussed below, this includes using deliberation of e-cigarette policy as a means of engaging with parliamentarians in ways which would be deemed highly problematic in other areas of tobacco control.

Closely related to this, TTCs have sought to promote their technological strategy through funding and promoting research sympathetic to their new nicotine delivery devices and their favoured policy agenda. The most obvious manifestation of this strategy is the creation of the Philip Morris Foundation for a Smoke-Free World (FSFW), with an endowment of $1 billion. The conflict of interest associated with this is reflected in the decision by researchers and institutions, including the authors' own employer, not to accept funding from the FSFW and to enact policies of non-engagement with a tobacco industry body (Piot, 2018), as well as the decision by leading scientific journals to refuse to publish tobacco industry funded research (Cohen et al., 2017). However, strategies to promote e-cigarettes have not been limited to this global initiative. A number of industry friendly e-cigarette conferences and events have been established and have succeeded in developing networks amongst prominent and highly regarded scholars in the field of public health (Hawkins & Gornall, 2015; Lee, 2013).

6   UK E-cigarette Policy and the Science and Technology Committee Enquiry

Previous studies of UK e-cigarettes policy have identified a strong rhetorical commitment to evidence based (or evidence informed) policy-making within a policy context characterised by an absence of robust, policy-relevant evidence (Ettelt & Hawkins, 2018; Hawkins & Ettelt, 2019). The still limited, but rapidly expanding, evidence-base on the health effects of e-cigarettes, and thus the appropriate policy regime which should apply to them, remains highly contested (Newman, 2019). In keeping with this, governments countries across the globe have taken greatly differing regulatory approaches to e-cigarettes (Campus et al., 2021).

In the UK, significant divisions emerged within the tobacco control and public health communities between e-cigarette proponents and sceptics (Hawkins & Ettelt, 2019). Although recent studies identify the existence of a sizeable 'middle ground' of policy actors with still evolving or undecided positions of different aspects of e-cigarette regulation, these sit between the more sedimented and ardent bodies of opinion at either end of the spectrum (Smith et al., 2021). These cleavages have been exacerbated by the increasing presence of the global tobacco industry within the e-cigarette sector (Mathers et al., 2019), and the controversy arising from their potential engagement in policy-making and implementation in this context despite the limitations placed on this by Article 5.3 of the FCTC. No significant divergences in approach were identified between the main political parties on this topic and much of the debate centred instead of the research and public health communities.

Debates between the 'pro' and 'anti' e-cigarette camps are often articulated in terms of a failure of the other side to recognise 'the evidence' and the policy regimes that follow from this (Hawkins & Ettelt, 2019). However, this misrecognises the fundamentally political nature of the policy process and the function of evidence within it. Arguments which purport to be about facts are often actually arguments about competing values, ideologies and political priorities (Stone, 1997). Consequently, the ability to shape the information environment in which policy debates are conducted becomes a powerful means for policy advocates to achieve their desired outcomes. This includes the public health actors identified above, but also other vested interests such as the tobacco industry which has a well-documented history of attempting to influence scientific research and evidence related to the regulation of its products industry actors in a variety of ways.

As noted above, UK e-cigarette policy has been framed principally in terms of evidence and competing claims about what constitutes an evidence-based approach. Consequently, debates have evolved principally through the production, identification and promotion of new evidence supportive of policy advocates' favoured position. Most notably, Public Health England (PHE) commissioned an evidence review, the findings of which are often reduced to the claim that e-cigarettes are '95% safer' than conventional tobacco products (McNeill et al., 2015). However, this widely repeated figure has been consistently challenged in other quarters (Fairchild et al., 2019; McKee, 2019).

Subsequently, the UK Parliament's Science and Technology Committee (STC) opened an enquiry into e-cigarettes with a call for written evidence published in October 2017 setting the deadline for submissions as the 8 December that year. This was followed by 5 oral evidence sessions between January and May 2018. The resulting report was published in August 2018. The UK Government published its response to the report in December 2018, which accepted the main recommendations of the report (Science & Technology Committee, 2018). In keeping with PHE's report, the STC adopted a largely positive framing of the health impact of e-cigarettes, arguing in favour of a less restrictive regulatory model and appeared to prioritise the potential of e-cigarettes as smoking cessations aids over concerns about their wider effects on population health, including their gateway effect on non-smokers and the possibility that dual use may actually undermine quit attempts. In addition, the report called into question the rationale for bans on their use in various public spaces in order to facilitate e-cigarette uptake amongst a greater number of smokers and lead to reduction in smoking rates. The report does not advocate a reversal of bans on vaping in all public spaces, calling instead for a debate on this subject as a prelude to possible policy change. However, it implies that current exclusions are unjustifiable on the basis of evidence about the relative harms if vapour and cigarette smoke (Paragraph 60). The report does, however, call more clearly for a repeal of such bans in mental health facilitates—arguing the default should be for vaping to be permitted (Paragraph 57)—and raises the potential of their use being facilitated in the prison estate (Paragraphs 53, 54). While the report acknowledges the 'uncertainty about long-term effects' of e-cigarettes—and in a specific section of the report under that heading—this was presented in equivocal terms in which it was explicitly and repeatedly argued that any potential risks to users must be offset again the risks of harms associated with not promoting e-cigarettes as quit aids (Paragraph 29).

The approach to e-cigarettes exemplified by this report has been criticised by some public health actors for failing to sufficiently reflect the equivocal nature of the research evidence on both the effectiveness of e-cigarettes in smoking cassations and on their potentially adverse health effects (Lancet, 2018; cf. Lamb, 2019). Others, meanwhile, have highlighted that this approach to e-cigarettes, and the framing of the policy debate more generally, is seemingly at odds with the consensus towards a more precautionary approach adopted by regulators beyond the UK (Campus et al., 2021; McKee, 2019). Thus, while e-cigarettes may be useful quit aids for some smokers, offering an additional option in the smoking cessation toolkit, it is at least open to doubt, on the basis of current evidence, that they are the 'disruptive technology' or game changer for smoking cessation which industry actors and other advocates claim they are. Moreover, we are simply unable on the basis of current evidence to accurately assess the long-term health effects of such a novel product, only recently entering into use.

The tone of the STC report, while in keeping with the tenor of much of the UK debate, raises a number of questions about the provenance and conduct of the enquiry. Firstly, how and why was it decided to hold the enquiry when it was? How were the terms of reference for the enquiry and the parameters for the call for evidence set? Were independent expert advisors appointed to oversee the enquiry and, if so, through what process? How was it decided who should be called to give oral evidence? How were evidence submissions and testimony analysed and the expertise and credibility of the respondents evaluated? How was the report drafted and reviewed? How were any disagreements about the content of the report (if any) managed and the final text agreed? All of these issues are central to understanding the governance of the enquiry and thus the way in which the report should be interpreted and used.

Perhaps the questions of greatest concern arise about the way in which the STC sought to comply with Article 5.3 of the FCTC and how decisions were taken to take evidence, in both written and oral forms, from TTCs. Of a total of 25 witnesses who gave evidence to the STC e-cigarette enquiry four were from TTCs and/or their e-cigarette subsidiaries and two more were from the e-cigarette trade associations, including one with TTC members meaning almost 25% of oral testimony came from industry actors and 20% from the tobacco industry or TTC-associated bodies. There is an obvious tension between the desire of select committees' desire to gain a comprehensive range of perspectives, on the one hand, and their obligation to adhere to the UK's international commitments, on the other. Moreover, there is some debate about whether engagement with tobacco companies in the capacity as e-cigarette producers or with e-cigarette companies largely or wholly owned by TTCs falls within the remit of Article 5.3. Yet the degree of access gained by the tobacco sector is noteworthy in any instance. How did the committee decide to afford such a large percentage of the time for oral evidence to these actors? How did they interpret their responses and what emphasis did they place on these? Did the committee differentiate between TTCs, their e-cigarette subsidiaries and associations, and independent e-cigarette companies? Given the ongoing commitment of TTCs to their core combustible nicotine products, and their robust defence their right to sell and market these across the globe, this type of engagement with tobacco industry actors represents a potential conflict of interest.

The case of the e-cigarettes enquiry thus raises important questions about the interpretation and implementation of the FCTC and how to define and engage with the modern, evolving tobacco industry which is now heavily invested not only in the nicotine technology' sector but is now moving into the pharmaceutical sector with the purchase by Philip Morris International (PMI) of the UK based company Vectura, which specialises in inhaled medications. The potential synergies for PMI, but also the conflicts of interests to which this move gives rise, warrant scrutiny and may be indicative of wider strategic objectives of the sector.

7 Conclusion

The political standing of select committees and their opaque accountability mechanisms create a significant opportunity for advocates seeking to influence the content of regulation to influence policy debates. Given select committees' wish to solicit evidence from a wide range of stakeholders, corporate actors may be able to gain access in the policy process and to shape the evidence and information environment within which policy is scrutinised. The kudos enjoyed by select committees and their effectiveness in influencing policy makes them potentially important targets for the epistemic strategies of corporate political actors. This may be particularly the case in policy-making contexts with long-standing, established commitments to 'evidence-based policy' such as the UK, and on policy issues about which the relevant body of research remains limited and/ or contested, as is the case with e-cigarette regulation.

The role of health-harming industries such as the tobacco industry in shaping policy has been well documented in health policy (Hurt et al., 2009) and in other sectors (see Kenworthy et al., 2016). A key component of corporate political strategy is to shape the information environment in which policies are made via the funding, conduct and promotion of research (Brandt, 2012; McCambridge et al., 2018). Given the resources available to such corporations they are able to engage in all aspects and stages of the policy process. Studies of the tobacco (Apollonio & Bero, 2007) and other industries (Hawkins & McCambridge, 2014; McCambridge & Mialon, 2018; McCambridge et al., 2013) identify a long-standing strategy of seeking to 'capture' (Katz, 2015) apparently independent bodies to produce research amenable to their underlying policy objectives. Such outputs enjoy the added benefit of both disassociation with the industry and the credibility associated with established bodies at the heart of the body politic. TTCs, excluded from many aspects of the policy process as a result of the FCTC, have consistently sought to identify new ways to influence policy and new forums in which to engage government. Most recently their investment in e-cigarettes has offered them a novel pretext for meeting with policy-makers in their guise as the nicotine technology industry in ways previously precluded by the FCTC.

While there is no suggestion that any of the actors involved in the conduct of the STC enquiry were compromised in any way, they received submissions and took evidence from a number of tobacco industry actors. This demonstrates the way in which select enquiries offer controversial industries a forum for engagement with decision-makers, which is a potentially powerful component of corporate political strategy (Baron, 1995) and raises important questions about the oversight of evidence production by government bodies. It is vital to understand how evidence is produced, managed and evaluated within these bodies. Who is able to submit written evidence? Who gets called to testify in person? How is the expertise of different respondents evaluated and their inputs emphasised or ignored? What is the relative weight given to written versus oral evidence?

This chapter argues that there is currently a lack of clearly defined governance mechanisms and lines of accountability surrounding the work of UK parliamentary select committees. There is a tacit understanding amongst policy scholars that the function and character of select committees are to think independently and to hold government to account. Yet we have little understanding of the mechanisms which are in place, or should be established, to oversee the conduct of the committees' own work. This creates a 'regulatory vacuum' in which the best resourced policy advocates are potentially able to shape the framing development of key policy debates and processes by influencing the work of select committees. The current gap in the research literature is a particularly pressing concern given the highly sophisticated and rapidly evolving strategies of corporate political actors in health-harming industries such as tobacco to maintain their influence in increasingly hostile regulatory environments.

REFERENCES

Apollonio, D. E., & Bero, L. A. (2007). The creation of industry front groups: The tobacco industry and "get government off our back." *American Journal of Public Health, 97*, 419.

Baron, D. P. (1995). Integrated strategy: Market and nonmarket components. *California Management Review, 37*, 47–65.

Bates, S., Goodwin, M., & Mckay, S. (2017). Do UK MPS engage more with select committees since the wright reforms? An interrupted time series analysis, 1979–2016. *Parliamentary Affairs, 70*, 780–800.

Benton, M., & Russell, M. (2012). Assessing the impact of parliamentary oversight committees: The select committees in the British House of Commons. *Parliamentary Affairs, 66*, 772–797.

Bero, L. A. (2005). Tobacco industry manipulation of research. *Public Health Reports, 120*, 200.

Brandt, A. M. (2012). Inventing conflicts of interest: A history of tobacco industry tactics. *American Journal of Public Health, 102*, 63–71.

Cairney, P., Studlar, D., & Mamudu, H. M. (2011). *Global tobacco control: Power, policy, governance, and transfer*. Palgrave Macmillan.

Campus, B., Fafard, P., St Pierre, J., & Hoffman, S. J. (2021). Comparing the regulation and incentivization of e-cigarettes across 97 countries. *Social Science & Medicine, 291*, 114187.

Cash, D., Clark, W. C., Alcock, F., Dickson, N. M., Eckley, N., & Jäger, J. (2002). *Salience, credibility, legitimacy and boundaries: Linking research, assessment and decision making*.

Cohen, C. G., Henriksen, L., Hill, S., Malone, R. E. & O'Connor, R. (2017). *Why tobacco control still won't publish tobacco industry funded work, even if the funding is laundered through PMI's new 'independent' foundation.*

Ettelt, S., & Hawkins, B. (2018). Scientific controversy, issue salience, and e-cigarette regulation: A comparative study of policy debates in Germany and England. *European Policy Analysis, 4*, 255–274.

Fairchild, A. L., Bayer, R., & Lee, J. S. (2019). The e-cigarette debate: What counts as evidence? *American Journal of Public Health, 109*, 1000–1006.

Fooks, G., Smith, J., Lee, K., & Holden, C. (2017). Controlling corporate influence in health policy making? An assessment of the implementation of article 5.3 of the world health organization framework convention on tobacco control. *Globalization and Health, 13*, 1–20.

Fooks, G. J., Gilmore, A. B., Smith, K. E., Collin, J., Holden, C., & Lee, K. (2011). Corporate social responsibility and access to policy élites: An analysis of tobacco industry documents. *PLoS Medicine, 8*, E1001076.

Gaines, B., Goodwin, M., Bates, S., & Sin, G. (2019). A bouncy house? UK select committee newsworthiness, 2015–18. *Journal of Legislative Studies, 25*(3), 409–433.

Geddes, M. (2016). *Interpreting parliamentary scrutiny: An enquiry concerning everyday practices of parliamentary actors in select committees of the house of commons.* University of Sheffield.

Geddes, M. (2017). Committee hearings of the UK Parliament: Who gives evidence and does this matter? *Parliamentary Affairs, 71*, 283–304.

Geddes, M. (2019, October). Performing scrutiny along the committee corridor of the UK house of commons. *Parliamentary Affairs, 72*(4), 821–840. https://doi.org.ezp.lib.cam.ac.uk/10.1093/pa/gsz037

Geddes, M. (2020). The webs of belief around 'evidence' in legislatures: The case of select committees in the UK house of commons. *Public Administration.*

Geddes, M., Dommett, K., & Prosser, B. (2018). A recipe for impact? Exploring knowledge requirements in the UK Parliament and beyond. *Evidence & Policy: A Journal of Research, Debate and Practice, 14*, 259–276.

Gilmore, A. B., & Peeters, S. (2013). Understanding corporations to inform public health policy: The example of tobacco industry interests in harm reduction and reduced risk products. *The Lancet, 382*, S14.

Gneiting, U. (2015). From global agenda-setting to domestic implementation: successes and challenges of the global health network on tobacco control. *Health Policy and Planning, 31*, Czv001.

Gornall, J. (2015). Why e-cigarettes are dividing the public health community. *BMJ, 350*, h3317.

Grüning, T., Gilmore, A. B., & Mckee, M. (2006). Tobacco industry influence on science and scientists in Germany. *American Journal of Public Health, 96*, 20–32.

Hawes, D. (1992). Parliamentary select committees: Some case studies in contingent influence. *Policy & Politics, 20*, 227–236.

Hawkins, B., & Ettelt, S. (2019). The strategic uses of evidence in UK e-cigarettes policy debates. *Evidence & Policy: A Journal of Research, Debate and Practice, 5*, 579–596.

Hawkins, B., & Holden, C. (2018). European Union implementation of article 5.3 of the framework convention on tobacco control. *Globalization and Health, 14*, 79.

Hawkins, B., Holden, C., & Mackinder, S. (2018). A multi-level, multi-jurisdictional strategy: transnational tobacco companies' attempts to obstruct tobacco packaging restrictions. *Global Public Health, 13*, 1–14.

Hawkins, B., & Lee, K. (2013). Tobacco industry & e-cigarettes: new issue, familiar tactics. *Tobacco Control, 22*(6), 365

Hawkins, B., & Mccambridge, J. (2014). Industry actors, think tanks, and alcohol policy in the United Kingdom. *American Journal of Public Health, 104*, 1363–1369.

Hawkins, B., & Parkhurst, J. (2016). The 'good governance' of evidence in health policy. *Evidence & Policy: A Journal of Research, Debate and Practice, 12*(4), 575–592.

Helboe Pedersen, H., Halpin, D., & Rasmussen, A. (2015). Who gives evidence to parliamentary committees? A comparative investigation of parliamentary committees and their constituencies. *The Journal of Legislative Studies, 21*, 408–427.

Hindmoor, A., Larkin, P., & Kennon, A. (2009). Assessing the influence of select committees in the UK: The education and skills committee, 1997–2005. *The Journal of Legislative Studies, 15*, 71–89.

Hurt, R. D., Ebbert, J. O., Muggli, M. E., Lockhart, N. J., & Robertson, C. R. (2009). Open doorway to truth: Legacy of the Minnesota tobacco trial. *Mayo Clinic Proceedings. Mayo Clinic, 84*, 446–456.

Katz, A. (2015). *The influence machine: The US chamber of commerce and the corporate capture of American life*. Spiegel and Grau.

Kenworthy, N., Mackenzie, R., & Lee, K. (2016). *Case Studies on corporations and global health governance: impacts, influence and accountability*. Pickering & Chatto Publishers.

King, A., & Crewe, I. (2014). *The blunders of our governments*. Simon And Schuster.

Lamb, N. (2019). E-cigarettes. *The Lancet, 393*, 876.

Lancet. (2018). E-cigarettes-is the UK throwing caution to the wind? *Lancet (London, England), 392*, 614.

Mackenzie, R., & Hawkins, B. (2016). How e-cigarettes could 'health wash' the tobacco industry [Online]. *The Conversation*. https://theconversation.com/how-e-cigarettes-could-health-wash-the-tobacco-industry-68428. Accessed 22 May 2017.

Malone, R. E. (2013). Changing tobacco control's policy on tobacco industry-funded research. *Tobacco Control, 22*, 1–2.

Mathers, A., Hawkins, B., & Lee, K. (2019). Transnational tobacco companies and new nicotine delivery systems. *American Journal of Public Health, 109*, 227–235.

Mccambridge, J., Kypri, K., Miller, P., Hawkins, B., & Hastings, G. (2013). Be aware of drinkaware. *Addiction* [Online]. https://onlinelibrary.wiley.com/doi/full/10.1111/Add.12356

Mccambridge, J., & Mialon, M. (2018). Alcohol industry involvement in science: A systematic review of the perspectives of the alcohol research community. *Drug and Alcohol Review, 37*, 565–579.

Mccambridge, J., Mialon, M., & Hawkins, B. (2018). Alcohol industry involvement in policymaking: A systematic review. *Addiction, 113*, 1571–1584.

Mckee, M. (2019). Evidence and e-cigarettes: Explaining Exceptionalism exceptionalism. *American Journal of Public Health, 109*, 965–966.

Mckee, M., & Allebeck, P. (2014). Why the European Journal of Public Health will no longer publish tobacco industry-supported research. *The European Journal of Public Health, 24*, 182–182.

Mcneill, A., Brose, L., Calder, R., Hitchman, S., Hajek, P., & Mcrobbie, H. (2015). E-cigarettes: An evidence update. *Public Health England, 3*.

Mialon, M. (2020). An overview of the commercial determinants of health. *Globalization and Health, 16*, 1–7.

Muggli, M., Hurt, R. & Blanke J. D., D. D. (2003). Science for hire: A tobacco industry strategy to influence public opinion on secondhand smoke. *Nicotine & Tobacco Research, 5*, 303–314.

Muggli, M. E., Forster, J. L., Hurt, R. D., & Repace, J. L. (2001). The smoke you don't see: Uncovering tobacco industry scientific strategies aimed against environmental tobacco smoke policies. *American Journal of Public Health, 91*, 1419–1423.

Mulley, J., & Kinghorn, H. (2016). Pre-legislative scrutiny in parliament. In A. Horne & A. Le Sueur (Eds.), *Parliament: Legislation and accountability*. Bloomsbury Publishing.

Newman, J. (2019). The role of uncertainty in regulating e-cigarettes: The emergence of a regulatory regime, 2005–15. *Politics & Policy, 47*, 407–429.

Oreskes, N., & Conway, E. M. (2014). *Merchants of doubt*. Bloomsbury Publishing.

Parkhurst, J. O., & Abeysinghe, S. (2016). What constitutes "good" evidence for public health and social policy-making? From hierarchies to appropriateness. *Social Epistemology, 30*, 1–15.

Peeters, S., Costa, H., Stuckler, D., Mckee, M., & Gilmore, A. B. (2015). The revision of the 2014 European tobacco products directive: an analysis of the tobacco industry's attempts to 'break the health silo'. *Tobacco Control.* https://doi.org/10.1136/tobaccocontrol-2014-051919

Peeters, S., & Gilmore, A. B. (2013). Transnational tobacco company interests in smokeless tobacco in Europe: Analysis of internal industry documents and contemporary industry materials. *PLoS Medicine, 10*, E1001506.

Peeters, S., & Gilmore, A. B. (2015). Understanding the emergence of the tobacco industry's use of the term tobacco harm reduction in order to inform public health policy. *Tobacco Control, 24*, 182–189.

Piot, P. (2018). *LSHTM policy on contact with the tobacco industry* [Online]. https://www.lshtm.ac.uk/sites/default/files/statement_on_working_with_the_tobacco_industry.pdf. Accessed 19 June 2019.

Russell, M., & Benton, M. (2011). *Selective influence: The policy impact of house of commons select committees.* Constitution Unit London.

Russell, M., & Cowley, P. (2016). The policy power of the Westminster parliament: The "parliamentary state" and the empirical evidence. *Governance, 29*, 121–137.

Russell, M., & Gover, D. (2017). *Legislation at Westminster: Parliamentary actors and influence in the making of British Law.* Oxford University Press.

Savell, E., Gilmore, A. B., & Fooks, G. (2014). How does the tobacco industry attempt to influence marketing regulations? A Systematic Review. *PLoS ONE, 9*, E87389.

Science and Technology Committee. (2018). *E-cigarettes: 7th Report of the session 2017–2019* [Online]. House of Commons. https://publications.parliament.uk/Pa/Cm201719/Cmselect/Cmsctech/505/505.Pdf. Accessed 20 June 2019.

Smith, K. E., Ikegwuonu, T., Weishaar, H., & Hilton, S. (2021). Evidence use in e-cigarettes debates: Scientific showdowns in a 'wild west' of research. *BMC Public Health, 21*, 1–16.

Smith, K. E., Savell, E., & Gilmore, A. B. (2013). What is known about tobacco industry efforts to influence tobacco tax? A systematic review of empirical studies. *Tobacco Control, 22*, E1–E1.

Smookler, J. (2006). Making a difference? The effectiveness of pre-legislative scrutiny. *Parliamentary Affairs, 59*, 522–535.

Stevens, A. (2010). Telling policy stories: An ethnographic study of the use of evidence in policy-making in the UK. *Journal of Social Policy, 40*, 237–255.

Stone, D. A. (1997). *Policy paradox: The art of political decision making.* W. W. Norton.

Weiss, C. H. (1979). The many meanings of research utilization. *Public Administration Review, 39*, 426–431.

World Health Organization. (2003). *Who framework convention on tobacco control* [Online]. http://whqlibdoc.who.int/publications/2003/9241591013.pdf?ua=1. Accessed 4 June 2018.

World Health Organization. (2008). *Guidelines for implementation of article 5.3 of the who framework convention on tobacco control* [Online]. https://www.who.int/fctc/guidelines/article_5_3.pdf. Accessed 4 June 2018.

Yowell, P. (2012). The impact of the joint committee on human rights on legislative deliberation. In M. Hunt, H. Hooper, & P. Yowell (Eds.), *Parliaments and human rights: Redressing the democratic deficit.* Bloomsbury.

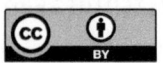

PART III

Making Public Health Policy: Insights from Political Science

The Policy and Politics of Public Health in Pandemics

Katherine Fierlbeck, Kevin McNamara,
and Maureen MacDonald

1   INTRODUCTION

The utility of political science insight and methodology for public health has become increasingly apparent in discussions over policy implementation. In areas such as tobacco regulation (Jarmon, 2018), sugary beverage taxation (Nestle, 2015), and healthy urban design (Corburn, 2009), the

Kevin McNamara: Former Deputy Minister of Health for the Province of Nova Scotia and Chair of the Council of Canadian Provincial and Territorial Deputy Ministers of Health, Canada; **Maureen MacDonald**: Former Minister of Health for the Province of Nova Scotia, Canada.

K. Fierlbeck (✉)
McCulloch Chair of Political Science, Dalhousie University, Halifax, NS, Canada
e-mail: K.Fierlbeck@dal.ca

K. McNamara · M. MacDonald
Halifax, NS, Canada

© The Author(s) 2022   211
P. Fafard et al. (eds.), *Integrating Science and Politics for Public Health*,
Palgrave Studies in Public Health Policy Research,
https://doi.org/10.1007/978-3-030-98985-9_10

issue is how to mobilize decision-makers in order to bring about particular kinds of legislation or policy initiatives. Analytical frameworks such
as Kingdon's multiple-stream approach (1984) or Sabatier and Jenkins-
Smith's Advocacy Coalition Framework (1993) have been particularly
useful in helping public health advocates understand how best to navigate the policy-making realm and to push public health initiatives on to
the agenda.

These discussions of policy implementation are quite interesting for
political scientists because they utilize accounts of agency and advocacy
that sit firmly within the discipline. Public health responses to pandemics
are qualitatively different, as they are essentially reactive. Pandemic planning requires getting the right goods and services to the right places at
the right time. It necessitates clear lines of accurate communication. But it
also means decision-making in a context of limited information, a rapidly-
changing base of evidence, thoroughgoing uncertainty, and heightened
public anxiety.

This chapter was originally presented in June 2019. Its focal point
was the claim that the political analysis of public health was too focused
on the implementation of health promotion policies, and that it could
be useful to think more carefully about another public health context—
pandemics—to prepare us better in the off-chance that another pandemic
manifested itself. As such, the paper showed remarkable foresight. In the
subsequent two years between presentation and publication, however, the
focus of this chapter has shifted to an analysis of the ways in which understanding the political response to previous pandemics could have prepared
us much better for COVID-19, had there been more interest in this topic.
For example, previous pandemics showed us that the crucial aspects of
pandemic governance included the coordination of roles and responsibilities within and between jurisdictions; the importance of coordinating
messaging across jurisdictions; the need to provide clear information in
a context of rapidly-changing scientific understanding; the prioritization
of which groups would be vaccinated first; the determination of relative
effectiveness and safety of vaccines; and the issue of how to deal with the
vaccine-hesitant. But, given the context of limited access to primary and
acute care across provinces, an analysis of how to deal with what *might*
happen was given low priority compared to those areas generating immediate political dissatisfaction. Neither policy-makers nor policy analysts
invested the time to consider events that might or might not occur.

The overarching claim in this chapter is that the evidence-policy-politics nexus in public health differs substantially between the fields of "health promotion" and "disease surveillance and mitigation". In the former, there is often much solid evidence supporting a public health intervention; the difficulty is in getting it on the political agenda. In the latter, the issue is squarely on the political agenda, but the evidentiary base is limited, in flux, and often contradictory. While we discuss the larger decision-making context that characterized the influenza A (H1N1) pandemic (itself a product of the brief Severe Acute Respiratory Syndrome [SARS] pandemic), we will focus more sharply on the decision-making surrounding vaccines and antivirals developed for H1N1. We note that, while pandemic preparedness has increasingly addressed the conditions of hyper-bounded rationality that decision-makers face by establishing clear practices in many areas, the protocols that arose in response to the H1N1 pandemic had many limitations.

2   THE H1N1 PANDEMIC IN NOVA SCOTIA

The 2009 global pandemic was caused by the influenza A (H1N1) strain. It was formally identified on 18 March 2009 as originating in central Mexico. A student on a school trip to the Yucatan Peninsula during the first week of April infected three other students at a residential boarding school in Nova Scotia. These were Canada's first confirmed cases of H1N1. On 25 April, the World Health Organization (WHO) declared a Public Health Emergency of International Concern. Two days later, it raised the pandemic alert level to phase four (sustained human-to-human transmission); after two further days, this was raised again to phase five (widespread human infection and imminent pandemic). By this point, there were 13 confirmed cases of H1N1 across Canada. On 9 June 2009, Nova Scotia elected its first NDP government which, in addition to the logistics of governance transition, now had a virulent pathogen to manage. Two days later, on 11 June, the WHO raised its pandemic alert to level six, the highest level, indicating a global outbreak.

The 2009 influenza pandemic manifested itself in two waves: the peak period for the first was between 31 May and 20 June; the second was between 25 October and 14 November. The second wave was much larger than the first, resulting in almost five times more hospitalizations and deaths (Public Health Agency of Canada, 2010). Altogether, 40,185 cases of H1N1 influenza in Canada would be formally confirmed by laboratory testing: of these, 16.9% would be admitted to an intensive care unit, and 428 people would die (Standing Senate Committee on Social Affairs, Science, and Technology, 2010). In terms of straightforward mortality, the H1N1 pandemic was considered much less severe than the previous 1918 ("Spanish flu"), 1957 ("Asian flu"), and 1968 ("Hong Kong flu") pandemics. However, because many older individuals had been exposed to similar strains in the past, those more likely to be severely infected by H1N1 were younger individuals. Over three-quarters of cases of H1N1 occurred in those under 30, and those between 10 and 19 seemed especially vulnerable (Fineberg, 2014, 1336; Low & McGeer, 2010, 1874). This meant that, calculated in terms of estimated years of life lost, the severity of the H1N1 became more considerable. Worldwide, more than 214 jurisdictions reported over 18,000 lab-confirmed cases of H1N1 resulting in death (Public Health Agency of Canada [PHAC], 2010); estimates for H1N1 deaths not confirmed by lab results have been placed at 201,200 respiratory disease deaths and 83,000 cardiovascular deaths globally (Dawood et al., 2012).

In Nova Scotia, there were 1,334 lab-confirmed cases of H1N1 between April 2009 and January 2010. As only the most serious cases were being lab-tested, it is likely that the number of actual cases was much higher. During the same period, there were 291 hospitalizations resulting from H1N1; of these, 50 were in intensive care units. Seven deaths in the province over this period were directly due to H1N1 (Government of Nova Scotia, 2010, p. 3).

From a public health perspective, the 2009 pandemic was a significant test of the protocol put into place after the 2003 Severe Acute Respiratory Syndrome (SARS) outbreak. Internationally, the 2005 International Health Regulations (which came into effect in 2007) tested the leadership role of the WHO in managing and coordinating an international pandemic. The H1N1 outbreak was also notable insofar as it was the first pandemic where antivirals were widely used, and it was the first time that adjuvanted influenza vaccines were employed in North America. Both of these points will be discussed in more detail below. 50 million doses of the H1N1 vaccine were purchased by PHAC on behalf of the provincial, territorial, and federal governments. Canada's overall vaccination rate was 40%, which was, next to Sweden, the highest vaccination rate for H1N1 in the world. Nonetheless, there were considerable disparities between regions, with Québec, the Atlantic provinces, and the territories achieving vaccination rates of over 50%, and rates in Alberta, Manitoba, and Ontario hovering around 30% (Low & McGeer, 2010).

3   HOW WAS THE H1N1 PANDEMIC *Political*?

After 10 August 2010, when the WHO declared that the H1N1 pandemic was officially over, agencies and academics alike evaluated the official response to the pandemic (Fineberg, 2014; Low & McGeer, 2010; Moghadas et al., 2010; Public Health Agency of Canada, 2010; Standing Senate Committee on Social Affairs, Science and Technology, 2010). The assessments generally fell into three categories: decision-making processes, communication, and institutional readiness.

The assessment of decision-making processes focused both on effective vertical command-and-control planning and on horizontal collaboration between units. The overarching strategic plan for the H1N1 pandemic was based on the Canadian Pandemic Influenza Plan, initially developed in 2006 (with the active participation of provinces and territories) in the wake of the SARS epidemic. This document focused on the roles and responsibilities of key players. The overall evaluation was that Canada had acquitted itself during the H1N1 pandemic much better than it had throughout the 2003 SARS epidemic. Nonetheless, given the inherent uncertainty of pandemics, several epidemiological post-mortems agreed on the need for adaptability and scalability in response plans. There was also some recognition in these reports that more stakeholders (such as physicians) would have to be involved more directly in the planning process, and that all jurisdictions would have to endeavour to maintain vigilance and readiness (e.g. through monitoring readiness plans and by committing public health funding for pandemic preparedness) when immediate threats had disappeared.

The analysis of how effective the communication had been was more critical. A major theme in the formal review documents was consistency in information over time, between jurisdictions, and across all units involved in pandemic management both provincially and federally (e.g. in offering a consistent definition of "severity"). In retrospect, many decisions that were made for sound reasons seemed arbitrary and unfair when proclaimed without clear explanations. Several decisions by provincial or federal authorities seemed peremptory and unreasonable when they were announced but, as the review documents noted, when the full reasoning for these decisions was given, there was a clear (although contestable) logic for these choices. There were also examples of mixed messages that seemed to work at counter-purposes. This was, for example, because long-term and short-term objectives were not clearly specified.

Why, for example, was a prioritization schema for vaccinations imposed when PHAC was stating that vaccines would be available for *all* Canadians who wanted them? The answer was that vaccines would eventually be available, but that in the *immediate* term the most vulnerable groups should be prioritized. If adjuvanted vaccines were safe, why were they not being given to pregnant women? The answer to this was that adjuvanted vaccines were not clearly *unsafe* for pregnant women; merely that the safety studies had not involved pregnant women, and so this group was excluded on precautionary grounds until the safety information was better established (see WHO, 2014). Why were first responders not given immediate priority for vaccination? The position here was that vulnerable groups with a high risk of mortality took precedence over first responders; this point had been clearly developed by PHAC in accordance with WHO guidelines. However, critics noted that these stipulations were merely guidelines, and that jurisdictions did have the authority to deviate from them. They also argued that this prioritization, while justifiable in terms of being "evidence-based", was quite "difficult to implement on the ground" (Standing Senate Committee on Social Affairs, Science, and Technology, 2010, p. 34). This illustrates the ambiguous use of "evidence" as the pandemic evolved: given the disparate contexts within which the pandemic was played out, evidence of "good practice" could be (and was) quite variable across locations.

In non-crisis times, the evidence base for best practices can be established gradually and iteratively. The demand for collegial input in the establishment of these practices means that they generally require time for discussion and for widespread input. Crisis management is largely based on the principle of command-and-control, which is effectively top-down decision-making. Yet, to instil confidence in front-line workers, there must be an opportunity for them to advise on whether the accepted evidence-based practices work for *them*. With H1N1, not only was this grassroots input missing, but even the top-down flow of communication was patchy. In some northern and remote areas, for example, providers reported receiving important information via their car radio during their drive in to work (Hodge, 2014).

Because so much attention had been placed on vaccines and antivirals, most evaluations of institutional readiness focused on access to these drugs. In fact, Canada's performance was, in comparative perspective, relatively impressive. As the vaccine used in Canada—Arepanrix—was manufactured in Québec, both the provincial and federal leads were in constant contact with the company. Thus, Canada was able to negotiate contracts with pharmaceutical manufacturers that ensured that, notwithstanding a few wrinkles (such as packaging), the country had reasonably direct access to these drugs, at lower cost than many other jurisdictions were paying. Yet the provision of vaccines was not straightforward: GlaxoSmithKline (GSK), which produced the vaccine, was also selling to larger markets, and Canada was not always the preferred customer.

Other aspects of institutional readiness included epidemiological planning capacity, the logistics of implementing mass vaccination clinics, health human resources planning (including the way in which the scope of practice for professions such as pharmacists and paramedics could be utilized more effectively during pandemics), the establishment of electronic health IT (such as vaccination records), and the monitoring of pandemic surge capacity.

Nonetheless, none of the pandemic post-mortems squarely addressed the *political* dynamics that made the attempt to negotiate pandemic planning so difficult notwithstanding the existence of the thorough and detailed pandemic planning protocol that had been established post-SARS. Planning protocols are usually based on very quantitative information: how many vaccine doses, syringes, and respirators will be needed? Are there sufficient health care providers with the required skills at the right place at the right time? Are the roles and responsibilities for all responders and decision-makers set out clearly enough? There is in pandemic planning an implicit assumption that the context within which these features are measured and evaluated is operationally neutral; there is little sense of the underlying political dynamics upon which these planning specifications are imposed. Yet establishing emergency measures on a system with underlying tensions can limit the effectiveness of even the best-considered strategies. It is, in fact, when crises descend that the fault lines for such political stressors truly become visible. By understanding where these tensions exist, and how these dynamics manifest themselves, pandemic planning processes can better anticipate where and why established protocol may not be effectively implemented. Even where some of these political dynamics are chronic and intractable, advance recognition of these circumstances can permit greater attention and monitoring in real time.

3.1   Structures and Institutions

The most apparent manifestation of political conflict is influenced by (and reflected in) formal institutional structures. These can include national, provincial, or organizational structural frameworks. At the national level, one obvious tension is related to the distribution of the vaccine and antivirals. Because of the time required to manufacture the products, distribution had to be prioritized. The negotiation for the procurement of vaccines was a federal responsibility, but it was the provinces which were to allocate the vaccines to individuals. But on what basis? Manitoba, for example, was quickly overwhelmed by the H1N1 virus, and the Winnipeg Regional Health Authority declared a state of emergency on 7 June 2009. The province was hit particularly hard because of the high numbers of First Nations residents, who were disproportionately vulnerable to the virus, with a rate of infection 2.8 times higher than non-indigenous populations (Charania & Tsuji, 2010; Hodge, 2014; Kumar et al., 2009; Zarychanski et al., 2010). British Columbia, where the second wave of H1N1 influenza manifested itself more quickly as well, asked to (but did not) receive vaccinations before less-affected provinces (Moghadas et al., 2010). The H1N1 vaccination was, at this point, the largest single vaccination programme in the country's history. Ottawa did provide distribution projections for all provinces, but production challenges meant that the number of doses each province received was subject to change at short notice, with little communication providing forewarning of shortages (Standing Senate Committee on Social Affairs, Science, and Technology, 2010). However, formal distributional protocol was also buttressed by informal collaboration between provinces. After the initial interprovincial allotment of vaccines was determined, for example, extensive discussion amongst the provinces led to a willingness on the part of many provinces to give up part of their allotments to provinces (especially Saskatchewan and Manitoba) with higher Indigenous populations (who were more vulnerable to H1N1).

The federal structure led to tensions in unanticipated ways as well. An attempt was made by the federal government to establish a pan-provincial electronic health registry for vaccinations, as provinces were recording vaccination records on hard copy only. British Columbia was designated as the lead on this initiative, and each province was asked to contribute. Nova Scotia's Department of Health Promotion gave $1 million, but not all provinces would contribute. Québec, as with other ventures (such as Canadian Blood Services), preferred to develop their own system parallel to, but distinct from, pan-Canadian ventures. And, as other larger provinces contributed a greater proportion of the funding (while enjoying limited control), they calculated that they could develop their own systems with the money that it could cost them (and even do so more cheaply). In the end, the funds collected were retained by British Columbia and eventually used towards the development of that province's own IT systems.

The tracking of adverse events in pharmaceuticals is a complicated and highly political issue in its own right. As Lexchin (2006) notes, the problems with reporting adverse events are well known: "poor quality of submitted reports; significant underreporting of adverse reactions; difficulty in calculating rates because of incomplete numerator data along with unreliable denominators; and limited ability to establish cause and effect". And, as explained below, influenza vaccines—because of the particular way in which they are designed—cannot be tested as rigorously as non-biologic drugs. While the provisional "base" for the vaccines is standard, the "added on" component for each specific variant of influenza is novel. Strain-specific vaccines cannot be produced without the existence of the strain; yet once the strain is identified, there is a serious time-pressure to produce and distribute the vaccine to curb its prevalence. But adverse event reporting with vaccines in general, and during pandemics in particular, is even more fraught with political difficulties. Generally, with adverse events, the precautionary principle—assume a potential problem identified is serious, until proven otherwise—is applied. With vaccines, however, the precautionary principle can heighten public anxiety, undermine public trust, and lead to greater vaccine hesitation. At the same time, epidemiologists have expressed concern that "the five current methods of vaccine vigilance (case reports, case–control studies, active and passive surveillance and randomized controlled trials) are insufficient and further developmental work should be undertaken" (Jefferson, 2000, 402). Thus, good science would, in normal times, dictate an abundance of caution, but in a pandemic such a strategy can inflame public anxiety, leading to depressed uptake of vaccines and the concomitant rise of virus spread. Fragmentation also existed horizontally between federal agencies: for example, during the provision of H1N1 vaccines, Health Canada was responsible for approving the vaccine in an expedited manner. Thus, the H1N1 vaccine was approved on a "rolling" basis, where data was examined as it became available, with "a greater emphasis on post-marketing commitments" (PHAC, 2010, 67). But, as noted above, post-market collection of possible adverse events is quite poor at the best of times, and in Canada, it was not Health Canada but rather the Public Health Agency of Canada (PHAC) which was responsible for tracking the adverse effects of the vaccine (Standing Senate Committee on Social Affairs, Science, and Technology, 2010, 36). Yet most adverse events tracked were those that appeared within hours or days of vaccination; the problem, as Jefferson (2021) argues, is that there was little careful scrutiny of possible longer-term adverse events, such as neurological damage.

Within Nova Scotia, institutional fragmentation, both vertical and horizontal, tested the capacity of the province to deal effectively with the H1N1 outbreak. When Nova Scotia established nine district health authorities (DHAs) in 2001, these regional units were given the responsibility of managing responses to potential pandemics, with the province becoming involved only when a DHA "could no longer adequately respond to the situation" (Nova Scotia Auditor General, 2009, p. 12). Yet, as there was no central review of district health authority plans, nor a clear sense of whether these plans existed at all, a situation existed which could permit DHAs and provincial departments to attempt to offload responsibility to each other. Because there were regular communication sessions between the Deputy Ministers for the Departments of Health and Health Promotion and the CEOs of the DHAs, there was generally effective cooperation between units on implementation strategy in the province. While some issues of coordination did surface, as this chapter describes, the province was able to contain and minimize the fallout. A somewhat more concerning issue was that information on the available stockpiles of supplies held by DHAs was not readily available, and the province was uncertain whether they could "legally require the DHAs to provide details of their supplies on hand and costs for those supplies" (ibid., 20).

A separate issue was the unclear division of authority between the province's Department of Health and the Department of Health Promotion and Protection. The nature of acute health care demands on the health care system makes it difficult to protect stable, long-term funding for public health and, in a novel administrative move, the Progressive Conservative administration developed a cabinet portfolio for health promotion in 2002. This guaranteed a discrete budget as well as a separate voice for public health in cabinet discussions. The aim of this restructuring was to give public health an opportunity to develop and flourish without competing with acute health services for direct funding. Ironically, it was precisely a public health crisis which led to the dissolution of the Department and Health Promotion and Protection, and its ultimate reabsorption in a consolidated Department of Health and Wellness in 2012.

The problem, as outlined by the Nova Scotia Auditor General, was that there was no clear command-and-control structure of authority between the Department of Health, the Department of Health Promotion and Protection, and the Emergency Management Office, such that it was "not clear who will be involved in decisions once the response is being managed by multiple entities" (Nova Scotia Auditor General, 2009, p. 10). Communication and planning between the two units were indeed lacking on important matters. On one occasion, for example, the Department of Health Promotion and Protection neither consulted with the Department of Health, nor even gave them advance warning, when they announced a policy of offering free (regular season) flu shots. This had budget implications for the Department of Health, as well as some staffing implications, due to this unknown announcement that had not been anticipated by the Department of Health. However, both departments reported to the Minister of Finance, who was, after this, able to maintain a degree of oversight over the coordination between departments. This underscores the fundamental tension involved in promoting public health objectives: a policy that clearly ring-fences resources for public health and provides a conduit for public health policy champions to achieve long-term goals can, if not carefully monitored, also interfere with immediate public health planning objectives in emergency situations.

Another example of horizontal tensions between institutions was in the competition for scarce resources. Formally, H1N1 vaccines and antivirals were purchased by PHAC on behalf of the Government of Canada and distributed to the provinces and territories, which would then allocate these drugs to their respective populations on their own authority, taking into account guidelines on prioritization that had been developed in consultation between federal, provincial, and territorial representatives. In practice, however, the provinces (as in the case of Nova Scotia) could be circumvented by the DHAs, which were able directly to access the drugs. The IWK Health Centre in Halifax, for example, was able to purchase the antiviral Tamiflu directly, without consultation with the province, leading to considerable tension between agencies.

3.2   Interests

The political tensions between stakeholder interests are less obvious than those at an institutional level, yet arguably led to more acrimony and tension. The most evident tension during the H1N1 pandemic again focused on drugs and addressed the prioritization of recipients for vaccination. The production of the H1N1 vaccine, once it was developed, was first delayed because (following WHO guidelines) companies were asked to complete their production of the seasonal influenza vaccine (which could likely be circulating simultaneously with the H1N1 variant). Thus, while the H1N1 virus was first identified in April 2009, production of the vaccine began in September 2009. The H1N1 vaccine being produced contained an adjuvant, or booster, which was designed to increase the effectiveness of each dose. However, the WHO had advised that pregnant women, a designated highly-vulnerable group, should receive a unadjuvanted vaccine, and so production of the adjuvanted vaccine was halted again to allow for production of the unadjuvanted variant.

The doses that were released thus had to be distributed to designated priority groups first. Priority for vaccination was initially given to children 6 months to five years of age, pregnant women, individuals with certain underlying or chronic medical conditions, and individuals living in rural and remote settings. PHAC's Pandemic Vaccine Task Group collaborated with the provinces and territories to develop these prioritization guidelines, but the provinces and territories were not strictly obliged to follow these guidelines, and so the implementation of the sequencing guidelines varied across regions. This led to public confusion regarding who had first call on the limited number of vaccines. Public health nurses reported that the criteria for priority groups shifted quickly "sometimes changing by the hour during immunization clinics" (Hodge, 2014; Long, 2013, cited in Hodge, 2014).

Across Canada, the media exacerbated the tension, reporting that inmates in penitentiaries and professional sports teams were being allowed to gain preferential access. Another source of controversy was the choice not to include first responders in the initial priority groups. This upset many health care providers, who worried that they were at high risk to contract the virus given that they were in contact with many infected patients, and could not only be infected themselves, but also risked passing the influenza virus on to their families (Hodge, 2014). The decision was a deliberate and arguably defensible one, and it focused on minimizing illness and death of those most vulnerable in the first instance (Standing Senate Committee on Social Affairs, Science, and Technology, 2010, 34). The prioritization schema, based on WHO protocol, was established fairly quickly at the federal level, but they were simply guidelines, and provinces had full authority to make their own prioritization decisions. Because the vaccines came onstream just before the second peak in October 2009, it was important to vaccinate as many individuals as possible as quickly as possible as "very rapid delivery of vaccination was the only means of optimizing program impact" and, for this reason, some provinces at the outset simply "attempted to get the vaccine out to as many people and as soon as possible, and did not enforce the priorities of the Public Health Agency of Canada" (Low & McGeer, 2010, p. 1876). Nonetheless, the explanation for why certain groups were or were not given precedence was not clearly communicated, leading to considerable resentment and criticism.

The acrimony over prioritization underscored another source of conflict, again focused on vaccines. Physicians in Canada are accorded a relatively high level of autonomy in medical decision-making. The command-and-control protocol of pandemic governance, however, strongly constrained the ability of doctors to make decisions in areas they had historically considered to be within their purview (Nhan et al., 2012). They particularly wanted to determine for themselves who amongst their patients could receive a vaccination, claiming that they were the best judge of who was most vulnerable to the virus. Public health nurses in more remote areas also expressed a level of frustration, based on the observation that they knew more about their geographic areas of practice and the inhabitants within them (Hodge, 2014). Health care providers, in turn, often had to address the antagonism of individuals who were refused vaccinations based on protocol with which the providers themselves did not support.

In Nova Scotia, the discord between physicians and the province was especially fraught, as the province made the decision to direct allotted vaccine supplies to large-scale immunization clinics, run by public health nurses, rather than to GPs' offices, which was standard protocol for seasonal influenza vaccines (Standing Senate Committee on Social Affairs, Science, and Technology, 2010, 34). The doctors took issue with this measure and openly criticized the provincial government's strategy to maximize vaccination rates. In response to this criticism, the Minister of Health responded that:

Some people have criticized us for not just doing a doctor-based program; I want to explain why that is, why we didn't do a doctor-based program. First of all, it's not what we do traditionally in terms of influenza. Secondly, we want our doctors doing what we need them to do most - treat sick people, number one. Number two, for example if we just took the Capital District Health Authority, 270 doctors times, let's say they can do 50 vaccines a day - at the end of the week, we would have vaccinated 13,500-some-odd people. With the mass community-based clinics, staffed by nurses and docs - we have docs in some of those clinics - we can do 1,000 people per clinic in a day. We have roughly maybe six clinics - 6,000 people a day versus 1,350 people in a week. (Hansard Nova Scotia, 2009)

At the same time, the front-line workers—mainly public health nurses in the immunization clinics—were employed by the District Health Authorities, yet accountable to the Department of Health Promotion (and had no relationship whatsoever with the Department of Health). This leads to a disconnect where Public Health staff were seen as a priority during the pandemic, which resulted in the manifestation of resentment on the part of other health care providers. When the immunization clinic project was completed, for example, the Department of Health Promotion sent each public health office a sum of money to be used on a "thank you" event for staff. This was, however, not well received by those in either the Department of Health or the DHAs. Such tensions contributed to the eventual reintegration of the Departments of Health and Promotion into the new Department of Health and Wellness. The province was engaged in a separate but equally charged political tussle with the health unions. Certain provisions of the unions' collective bargaining provisions were subject to suspension in the event of a pandemic. To address the concerns of the unions, the province negotiated a "Good Neighbour Protocol" to deal with human resource issues during the pandemic period. This protocol addressed issues such as where health workers could be sent, quarantine, liability, temporary licensing, and compensation (Nova Scotia Auditor General, 2009). The protocol, which involved seven unions representing close to 50,000 workers, was expected to be signed in May 2009 (ibid.). However, while the unions accepted in principle the need to facilitate flexibility in the labour supply and to suspend collective bargaining, they were nonetheless concerned about provisions that might require them to drive long distances across the province to report to work. In the end, the parties finally came to an historic agreement—the first of its kind in

Canada—but not until 27 October 2009 (Government of Nova Scotia, 2010).

On another front, the province also had to deal with the Auditor General's Office (AGO). The AGO had begun its audits of the province's pandemic preparedness plans early in the spring, under the Conservative government. The intention of the AGO had been to submit its evaluation in its regular fall report, but subsequent to the April 2009 outbreak, and the declaration of a pandemic in June, the AGO decided to issue a Special Report in July 2009 in order to assist the province to take measures to ensure adequate preparedness (Nova Scotia Auditor General, 2009). Yet the report was a public document, and it was quite critical of some aspects of the province's readiness to deal with the pandemic. Key points included the absence of a central provincial agency responsible for central planning and the lack of an adequate stockpile of supplies needed to address the pandemic. The new NDP government, which was presented with a draft of the AGO's report weeks after assuming office, was concerned that the report would have an incendiary effect on a population that was already alarmed by the growing tide of H1N1, including the first death in the province attributed to H1N1 on 24 July. How much information was it responsible to release in the middle of a pandemic? The original point of the AGO's report was to determine how well placed the province was to deal with another SARS-like epidemic. But health care workers had died in the SARS outbreak in Ontario, and the province was concerned that if the public conflated SARS with the H1N1 pandemic, it would create widespread panic. The province requested that the AGO tone down the report and remove references to SARS and, four days after the province's first H1N1 fatality, the AGO's report was published. While a fairly rare occurrence, the AGO agreed, given the quite exceptional circumstances, to comply with this request.

3.3   Discourses and Narratives

Another level at which political dynamics are played out is in the construction of narratives of reality, which can influence public sentiment to serve the ends of specific stakeholders. The context of a pandemic is particularly precarious, as the volatility of the public mood combined with scientific uncertainty about the nature and extent of the virus (as well as the disruption occasioned by the demands of coordinating a major response) permits interests subtly to frame narratives to their advantage.

One underlying problem with H1N1 was the nature of the new influenza virus. While the scientific community had been preparing for an influenza pandemic for some time, the expected threat was from avian H5N1 influenza, which can lead to a mortality rate of 50% in humans (Fineberg, 2014). A major influenza pandemic was thus anticipated to be one of considerable severity. As the first six months of the H1N1 outbreak began to show far fewer major effects than expected, many Canadians began to exhibit a pronounced indifference to vaccination once the vaccine became available. Then, the same week that the vaccines began to arrive on stream, a healthy, hockey-playing 13-year-old died suddenly. The death was clearly attributable to H1N1, and the public mood suddenly shifted from nonchalance back to panic.

The darker possibility of a *deliberately*-constructed narrative—a narrative of fear—has been suggested by researchers tracking the development of the vaccines and antivirals used in the H1N1 pandemic (Doshi, 2011). In this account, the demand for speed of production and distribution of a pandemic vaccine introduces a higher level of uncertainty regarding safety and effectiveness. But, because of relative risk calculations (the severity of a pandemic outweighing the limited testing of the vaccine) as well as public pressure for governments to take action, most states were willing to enter into confidential advance purchase agreements (APAs) that locked purchasers in, yet exonerated pharmaceutical companies from liability should problems be identified with the vaccines after the fact.

4   How Were Vaccines and Antivirals Addressed by Policy-Makers During H1N1 pandemic, and What Lessons are Relevant for the COVID-19 Pandemic?

The H1N1 influenza was formally identified in Mexico in March 2009. By July 2009, it was clear that the threat level of the virus had been overestimated. H1N1 had nowhere near the mortality rates that had been projected for a H5N1 pandemic. Nonetheless, governments who had entered into APAs with pharmaceutical companies were locked into payment for production, and the vaccines came onstream in October 2009, in time for the "second wave" of the pandemic. Ironically, those countries which—like Canada—were amongst the best-prepared for a pandemic (by virtue of having a purchasing agreement negotiated well in advance) were also those countries least able to make adjustments as the nature of the H1N1 virus became more apparent.

A major problem with the H1N1 vaccine was that initial risk assessments by Health Canada and other regulators determined that the limited clinical evidence for the safety and effectiveness was outweighed by the potential severity of a novel influenza strain (based on assumptions derived from the H5N1 influenza). Yet, once the mildness of H1N1 had been noted, the regulatory "short cuts" taken to bring the new vaccine into production should have been recalibrated against the reduced mortality threat of the new influenza strain. They were not. It is important to stress that the H1N1 vaccine was largely untested: all H1N1 studies began in September 2009, so that at registration no direct evidence of the effects of the vaccine was available (Jefferson, 2021). Rather, *indirect* markers which inferred effectiveness were used, as was common for the evaluation of regular seasonal influenza vaccines:

> By the definition of the time, the pandemic virus would be a novel virus, against which there was little or no immunity in the population. With no knowledge of what was coming and with the urgency impelled by the doomsday scenario, regulators used serological surrogates (antibodies) as correlates of field protection against influenza, i.e. markers of effectiveness, to kick start production of the vaccines. This was a standard procedure at the time for seasonal influenza vaccines. However, regulators themselves were unsure of the significance of the antibody response surrogate used as a proxy for field effectiveness estimation. These doubts are supported by the observed modest field performance of seasonal vaccines, registered yearly using the same surrogates of effectiveness ... None of these doubts were allowed to interfere with the juggernaut unleashed by the pandemic declaration. (ibid.)

Complicating the matter was the use of an adjuvant for most of the vaccines (with a unadjuvanted version produced for specific subgroups, such as pregnant women). Adjuvants, or compounds added to normal vaccines to enhance their effectiveness, "had never been tested in trials against an inert substance in humans", so their relative toxicity was unknown (ibid.). The specific adjuvant used in the H1N1 vaccine had never been used in any licensed vaccines (Low & McGeer, 2010, p. 1877).

How important were these effectiveness and safety concerns? It is instructive to note that levels of vaccination did not correlate with levels of mortality from H1N1. In Canada, where vaccination rates were high in comparison with other countries (40% overall), the mortality rate was 1.3 per 100,000 population (IPAC, 2014). In France, where vaccine scepticism is quite high, the overall vaccination rate was only 7.1% amongst those 18–60 (Schwarzinger et al., 2010). Nonetheless, the overall mortality rate for H1N1 in France (0.98 per 100,00) was *lower* than that in Canada (Lemaitre et al., 2012). In addition to vaccines, there is considerable evidence to show that the effectiveness of the oseltamivir antiviral stockpiled for use during the H1N1 pandemic ("Tamiflu") was quite minimal (e.g. Kmietowicz, 2017; Jefferson et al., 2014). A Cochrane review of oseltamivir in 2009 determined that the drug reduced complications of illness, but researchers subsequently discovered that this evaluation was based on a small, selective set of the available evidence. A protracted freedom of information request eventually provided 20,000 pages of data on the drug and, when this data was analysed, a 2014 Cochrane review found that there was "insufficient evidence to support claims that oseltamivir reduced lower respiratory tract complications or impeded viral transmission" (Dyer, 2020).

Even more concerning was evidence of toxicity of the Pandemrix H1N1 vaccine. The initial registration trials used to license the H1N1 vaccine employed only a few hundred people. By 2012, when millions of individuals had been vaccinated, a sensitivity analysis found a link between the Pandemrix vaccine (produced in Dresden) and narcolepsy in adults (Schnirring, 2012; Song et al., 2016). Overall, more than 1300 individuals in Europe developed narcolepsy after receiving the Glaxo-SmithKline's Pandemrix vaccine (Vogel, 2015). But narcolepsy was not the only adverse event identified:

> Pandemrix manufactured in Dresden was associated with a higher cumulative rate of harms, serious adverse events, deaths, anaphylaxis, facial palsy, convulsions and miscarriages … Data for these indicators of rare but serious toxicity were available since the end of October 2009, and should have led to immediate action by the competent authorities, either switching to a less toxic pandemic or seasonal influenza vaccine or halting the programme. (Jefferson, 2021)

In the end, there was little investigation of the relative risks posed by the H1N1 vaccine (or the antivirals) in Canada. During the pandemic, the only discussion of medical risk centred on pregnancy. After the pandemic, Canada's federal structure meant that the agencies responsible for distributing and administering the vaccines—the provinces—had no interest and little authority in the area of drug safety, which comes under the purview of the federal government. But because the federal government was not largely responsible for administering the drug, its main concern was (and remains) adequate supply, not long-term health effects. The federal body responsible for monitoring adverse events related to pandemic drugs, the Public Health Agency of Canada is, formally, charged with the collection of health data related to pandemic vaccines. However, in the case of H1N1, the system was merely a passive one "which only collects adverse event reports that have been submitted by health care professionals, the manufacturer, and in some cases the public" (Standing Senate Committee on Social Affairs, Science, and Technology, 2010, p. 36).

A key lesson of H1N1 is thus that caution should be exercised when developing and approving treatment interventions for COVID-19. There is little likelihood that this lesson will be heeded. The pressing political imperative to develop treatments has led to a greater willingness to sanction shortcuts in data gathering, as well as approval based on limited data. Pfizer's study protocol permitted an interim analysis after 32 cases of COVID-19 occurred in the study population. This meant that it could potentially determine the vaccine to be effective if only six individuals testing positive for the virus were given the vaccine (along with 26 cases in the placebo group): thus, expedited approval could conceivably have occurred if only six people responded favourably to the vaccine (Herper, 2020). Moreover, the definition of "effectiveness" outlined in these protocols had set the bar quite low: for both the Pfizer and Moderna trials, for example, very mild cases of COVID-19 were included. This meant that these vaccines would be considered "successful" even if they only worked on mild cases, and had no effect at all on preventing moderate or serious cases. Any vaccine approved on these terms would give individuals a sense of immunity while providing no protection against severe cases of COVID-19. Beyond the *definition* of effectiveness, the *level* of effectiveness of a vaccine is generally considered, and in the case of potential COVID-19 vaccines, regulators in the United States and Canada have stated publicly that a vaccine showing just 30% effectiveness in reducing symptomatic cases of COVID-19 would be considered to be "beneficial" (Herder & Graham, 2020). Thus, the initial authorization for the vaccines was made, as these authors have noted, on very limited grounds. As uptake of the vaccines allowed greater corroboration of initial positive statistics, the evidence base provided increasing confidence in the relative safety and effectiveness of the vaccine. But pandemic conditions do underscore the need to provide vaccines (arguably as much for political reasons as medical ones), and the imperative to vaccinate populations as quickly as possible increases the willingness to risk authorization with a much smaller evidence base. Governments have the unenviable task of securing vaccines as quickly as possible while convincing the public (and the larger scientific community) of the safety of these products. Complicating the situation, public trust (especially on the part of the scientific establishment) might have been won had all test data been released to the public. But many pharmaceutical firms (such as Pfizer) rejected this, arguing that it would destroy confidential commercial information. Governments, in no position to negotiate, gave in to the demand for data protection, thereby losing the opportunity to secure wider public trust in the process.

Another concern is that expedited approval for vaccines does not provide sufficient time to establish adverse events that may arise: in the case of Pandemrix, for example, there was a long lag between wide-scale vaccination and the onset of symptoms of narcolepsy. There is also a further issue that pandemic interventions are not tested on the very groups who are the most vulnerable to the disease. Is a vaccine just as effective on the elderly cohort as it is on the young? Are risks to pregnant women greater from the disease or from the vaccine? Again, the assumption that efficacy calculations from full trial populations can be extrapolated to a frailer cohort could lead to serious health outcomes. It is here, too, that a clinical trial protocol, even when made public in its entirely, does not provide sufficient information on the potential effectiveness of a drug, as the trial may have difficulty enrolling participants from these cohorts in practice, notwithstanding an articulation in the protocol that these cohorts should be represented. In such cases, decision-makers are forced to make judgements with limited information. And, while decisions can be made with greater certainty as more data is processed, the about-turns in official public health positions can itself undermine the public trust.

Wider political contexts are also important to consider. Early in the pandemic, most of the focus on expedited approval focused on the United States because of the imperative faced by the executive branch to show immediate progress on COVID-19 interventions. Moreover, regulatory decisions made in some jurisdictions will have an impact on others: as data is so limited, regulators will keep an eye on progress in other jurisdictions (but some regulators will privilege some information, and other regulators will ignore it, leading to differences in regulatory decisions across jurisdictions). In Canada, the antiviral remdesivir was given expedited approval through the Special Access Program, even though Health Canada did not have access to the manufacturer's clinical study reports that are normally used as the evidentiary basis for drug approval (Edmonds et al., 2021). Another pathway for rapid approval in Canada, the Interim Order, allows the Minister of Health to provide expedited authorization if the treatment has received an authorization for sale in a foreign jurisdiction.

Not only does Canada in this way authorize COVID-19 treatments with a much less robust evidence base than normally expected for drug approval in non-crisis contexts, but it tolerates conflicts of interest in the use of experts used to provide guidance on COVID-19 interventions. This, again, is an echo of the H1N1 experience. Critics point out that the WHO's policy position on the use of antivirals for H1N1 was authored by an influenza expert who was receiving payments from the drug's manufacturer (Godlee, 2010). Similarly, Canada's COVID-19 vaccine task force is co-chaired by one individual who has received funding from three of the major vaccine developers (Novavax, Pfizer, and Johnson & Johnson) and another individual who was CEO of another company competing to develop a vaccine (Sanofi). These commercial relationships were not disclosed until a member of the federal task force resigned due to the lack of transparency governing the task force (Dougherty, 2020).

Thus, the issues underlying the development and regulation of vaccines and antivirals in a pandemic situation are fundamentally political issues which require a sophisticated form of political analysis to comprehend. What is the structural and institutional context through which these interventions are developed, approved, and distributed? How does this institutional framework affect the safety and effectiveness of such treatments in an atmosphere of desperate public demand and (sometimes opportunistic) political response? Who are the agents playing key roles in the roll-out of these interventions, and what interests do they have in pushing one agenda rather than another? How can these interests use context-framing and selective narratives in order effectively to achieve their respective objectives? While the immediate response to pandemics seems to be the development and crystallization of scientific principles, the wider political context within which this scientific discussion emerges will subtly but substantially shape this discussion.

5   CONCLUSION

Pandemics pose particular problems for public health. The dynamics of public health politics under pandemic conditions are quite different from the kinds of political dynamics that inform policies geared to health promotion activities. On the one hand, public health actors in pandemic conditions enjoy an obvious advantage, as crises involving virulent pathogens have an immediacy that places them directly on the political agenda, often with the promise of generous funding to match policy initiatives. On the other hand, public health decision-making in pandemic conditions must be formulated in an atmosphere of heightened intensity, with limited or contradictory evidence; and the consequences of these decisions will be serious and immediate. Canada has had the opportunity to think about modern pandemic policy-making in slightly more depth than many other jurisdictions because of two pandemic events that occurred prior to COVID-19. These two events—SARS and H1N1—did establish a useful blueprint for dealing with pandemics. Key points that emerged were the need to develop structures and processes that addressed Canada's decentralized federal model and ensured the clear assignment of roles and responsibilities as well as consistent messaging within and between jurisdictions (Fierlbeck & Hardcastle, 2020).

But a key area of complexity for pandemic management that has *not* been effectively addressed is the development and utilization of pharmaceutical interventions for pandemic diseases. The emergence of SARS in 2003 was quite limited in scope, and the dominant strategy was containment. H1N1 was novel insofar as it was the first time pandemic management included both antivirals and vaccines. The development and utilization of these drugs, as noted above, were problematic for various reasons, but the virulence of H1N1 was relatively limited. With COVID-19, the stakes were much higher. There was a much greater political imperative for governments to be seen to be providing solutions to the crises, and this urgency established a tension with the need to ensure a solid and expansive evidence base for the safety and effectiveness of any intervention.

Political tensions underlie many aspects of the formal response to COVID-19 (Flood et al., 2020), but the pharmaceutical interventions that many feel hold the key to controlling the disease involve a complex assortment of political relationships that must be scrutinized carefully. The experience of H1N1 gave us a good sense of the kinds of political problems that arise in the development of a pharmaceutical response to pandemics. These include the procurement and distribution of vaccines at the federal level; establishing the precedence for vaccination across groups; setting out the most effective means to administer vaccinations; and monitoring vaccination rates across regions (which, interestingly, were consistent from H1N1 to COVID-19, with the Atlantic provinces and Québec with the highest uptake rates, and the prairie provinces and Ontario having amongst the lowest). To address these issues, one must have a clear sense of the kinds of tensions and obstacles that arise due to the particular institutional structure of the country (e.g. the constraints posed by Canada's federal system of health care governance, or the degree of decentralization in provincial health care institutions). One must also understand the competing interests involved in pandemic management, including competition for vaccines, disagreement over who is best placed to determine prioritization or administration of vaccines, and differences over the relative safety or efficiency of vaccines and antivirals. And one should anticipate the various kinds of narratives, built both on power relationships and more ineffable cultural dynamics, that can influence public behaviour during pandemic situations. The tools of political science, from the analysis of institutional relationships to the illumination of latent power dynamics, can be very useful in navigating these tumultuous waters.

REFERENCES

Charania, N. A., & Tsuji, L. J. S. (2010). The 2009 H1N1 pandemic response in remote First Nations communities or Subarctic Ontario: Barriers and improvements from a health care services perspective. *International Journal of Circumpolar Health, 70*(5), 564–575.

Corburn, J. (2009). *Toward the healthy city: People, places, and the politics of urban planning.* MIT Press.

Dawood, F., Iuliano, A. D., Reed, C., Meltzer, M. I., Shay, D. K., Cheng, P.-Y., Bandaranayake, D., Breiman, R. F., Brooks, W. A., Buchy, P., Feikin, D. R., Fowler, K. B., Gordon, A., Hien, N. T., Horby, P., Huang, Q. S., Katz, M. A., Krishnan, A., Lal, R., ... Widdowson, M.-A. (2012). Estimated global mortality associated with the first 12 months of 2009 pandemic influenza A

H1N1 virus circulation: A modelling study. *Lancet Infectious Diseases, 12*(9), 687–695.

Doshi, P. (2011). *Influenza: A study of contemporary medical politics.* 2011 PhD thesis. http://hdl.handle.net/1721.1/69811

Dougherty, K. (2020, September 21). Leading vaccine developer walks out on federal vaccine task force. *iPolitics.* https://ipolitics.ca/2020/09/21/lea ding-vaccine-developer-walks-out-on-federal-vaccine-task-force/

Dyer, O. (2020). What did we learn from Tamiflu? *British Medical Journal, 368*, m626. https://doi.org/10.1136/bmj.m626

Edmonds, S., MacGregor, A., Doll, A., Lexchin, J., Eren Vural, I., Graham, J., Fierlbeck, K., Fierlbeck, K., Lexchin, J., Doshi, P., & Herder, M. (2021). Transparency too late? Why and how Health Canada should make clinical data and regulatory decision-making open to scrutiny in the face of COVID-19. *Journal of Law and the Biosciences, 7*, lsaa083.

Fierlbeck, K., & Hardcastle, L. (2020). Have the post-SARS reforms prepared us for COVID-19? Mapping the institutional landscape. In C. Flood, V. MacDonnell, J. Philpott, S. Theriault, & S. Venkatapuram (Eds.), *Vulnerable: The law, policy, and ethics of COVID-19* (pp. 31–48). University of Ottawa Press.

Fineberg, H. (2014, April 3). Pandemic preparedness and response—Lessons from the H1N1 influenza of 2009. *The New England Journal of Medicine, 370*(14), 1335–1342

Flood, C., MacDonnell V., Philpott J., Theriault S., & Venkatapuram S. (Eds.). (2020). *Vulnerable: The law, policy, and ethics of COVID-19* (pp. 31–48). University of Ottawa Press.

Godlee, F. (2010). Conflicts of interest and pandemic flu. *British Medical Journal, 340*(7759), 1256–1257.

Government of Nova Scotia. (2010). *Nova Scotia's response to H1N1: Summary report.* https://novascotia.ca/dhw/publications/H1N1-Summary-Report.pdf

Hansard Nova Scotia. (2009). https://nslegislature.ca/legislative-business/han sard-debates/assembly-61-session-1/61_1_house_09nov03.htm

Herder, M., & Graham, J. (2020, September 15). Canadians need and deserve transparency on COVID-19 vaccines. *Ottawa Citizen.* https://ottawacitizen. com/opinion/herder-and-graham-canadians-need-and-deserve-transparency-on-covid-19-vaccines

Herper, M. (2020, September 28). A layperson's guide to how—And when—A Covid-19 vaccine could be authorized. *STATnews.* https://www.statnews. com/2020/09/28/a-laypersons-guide-to-how-and-when-a-covid-19-vac cine-could-be-authorized/

Hodge, J. (2014). *Canadian healthcare workers' experiences during pandemic H1N1 influenza: Lessons from Canada's response.* National Collaborating

Centre for Infectious Diseases. https://nccid.ca/publications/canadian-hea lthcare-workers-experiences-during-pandemic-h1n1-influenza/

IPAC. (2014). *2009 H1N1 pandemic.* https://ipac-canada.org/pandemic-h1n1-resources.php

Jarmon, H. (2018). Legalism and tobacco control in the EU. *European Journal of Public Health, 28*(S1), 26–29. https://doi.org/10.1093/eurpub/cky154

Jefferson, T. (2000). Real or perceive adverse effects of vaccines and the media—A tale for our times. *Journal of Epidemiology & Community Health, 54*(6), 402–403.

Jefferson, T. (2021).The European registration of the pandemic influenza vaccine Pandemrix: rushing an untested vaccine to market. In K. Fierlbeck, M. Herder, & J. Graham (Eds.), *Policy gain or confidence game? Transparency, power, and influence in the pharmaceutical industry: Policy gain or confidence game?* University of Toronto Press.

Jefferson, T., Jones M., Doshi P., & Spencer, E. (2014). Oseltamivir for influenza in adults and children: Systematic review of clinical study reports and summary of regulatory comments. *British Medical Journal, 348,* g2545. https://doi.org/10.1136/bmj.g2545

Lexchin, J. (2006, January 17). Is there still a role for spontaneous reporting of adverse drug reactions? *The Canadian Medical Association Journal, 174*(2), 191–192. https://doi.org/10.1503/cmaj.050971

Kingdon, J. (1984). *Agendas, alternatives, and public policy.* Little, Brown.

Kmietowicz, Z. (2017, June 12). WHO downgrades oseltamivir on drugs list after reviewing evidence. *British Medical Journal, 357.* https://doi.org/10.1136/bmj.j2841

Kumar, A., Zarychanski, R., Pinto,R., Cook, D. J., Marshall, J., Lacroix, J., Stelfox, T., Bagshaw, S., Choong, K., Lamontagne, F., Turgeon, A. F., Lapinsky, S., Ahern, S. P., Smith, O., Siddiqui, F., Jouvet, P., Khwaja, K., McIntyre, L., Menon, K., ... Canadian Critical Care Trials Group H1N1 Collaborative. (2009). Critically ill patients with 2009 influenza A (H1N1) infection in Canada. *The Journal of the American Medical Association, 302*(17), 1872–1879.

Lemaitre, M., Carrat F., Rey G., Miller M., Simonsen, L., & Viboud, C. (2012). Mortality burden on the 2009 A/H1N1 influenza pandemic in France: comparison to seasonal influenza and the A/H3N2 pandemic. *PLoS One.* https://journals.plos.org/plosone/article?id=10.1371/journal.pone.0045051

Low, D., & McGeer, A. (2010). Pandemic (H1N1) 2009: Assessing the response. *The Canadian Medical Association Journal, 182*(17), 1874–1878.

Moghadas, S., Pizzi, N., Wu, J., Tamblyn, S., & Fisman, D. (2010). Canada in the face of the 2009 H1N1 pandemic. *Influenza and Other Respiratory Viruses, 5,* 83–88.

Nestle, M. (2015). *Soda politics: Taking on big soda (and winning)*. Oxford University Press.

Nhan, C., Laprise, R., Douville-Frader, M., Macdonald, M. E., & Quach, C. (2012). Coordination and resource-related difficulties encountered by Québec's public health specialists and infectious diseases/medical microbiologists in the management of A (H1N1). *BMC Public Health, 12*, 115.

Nova Scotia, Auditor General. (2009). *Pandemic preparedness*. https://oag-ns.ca/sites/default/files/publications/2009%20-%20Special%20Report%20-%20Pandemic%20Preparedness.pdf

Public Health Agency of Canada. (2010). *Lessons learned review: Public Health Agency of Canada and Health Canada Response to the 2009 H1N1 pandemic*. https://www.canada.ca/en/public-health/corporate/mandate/about-agency/office-evaluation/evaluation-reports/lessons-learned-review-public-health-agency-canada-health-canada-response-2009-h1n1-pandemic.html

Sabatier, P., & Jenkins-Smith, H. (1993). *Policy change and learning: An advocacy coalition approach*. Routledge.

Schnirring, L. (2012). *French study finds narcolepsy link to H1N1 vaccine in adults*. Center for Infectious Disease Research and Policy, University of Minnesota http://www.cidrap.umn.edu/news-perspective/2012/09/french-study-finds-narcolepsy-link-h1n1-vaccine-adults

Schwarzinger, M., Flicoteaux, R., Cortarenoda, S., Obadia, Y., & Maotti, H.-P. (2010). Low acceptability of A/H1N1 pandemic vaccination in French adult population: Did public health policy fuel public dissonance? *PLOS One*. https://journals.plos.org/plosone/article?id=10.1371/journal.pone.0010199

Standing Senate Committee on Social Affairs, Science, and Technology. (2010). *Canada's response to the 2009 H1N1 influenza pandemic*. https://sencanada.ca/content/sen/committee/403/soci/rep/rep15dec10-e.pdf

Song, J. H., Kim, T. W., Um, Y. H., & Hong, S. C. (2016). Narcolepsy: Association with H1N1 infection and vaccination. *Sleep Medicine Research, 7*(2), 43–47.

Vogel, G. (2015). Why a pandemic flu shot caused narcolepsy. *Science*. https://www.sciencemag.org/news/2015/07/why-pandemic-flu-shot-caused-narcolepsy. https://doi.org/10.1126/science.aac8792

WHO. (2014). *Safety of immunization during pregnancy: A review of the evidence*. https://www.who.int/vaccine_safety/publications/safety_pregnancy_nov2014.pdf

Zarychanski, R., Stuart, T. L., Kumar, A., Doucette, S., Elliott, L., Kettner, J., & Plummer, F. (2010). Correlates of severe disease in patients with 2009 pandemic influenza (H1N1) virus infection. *The Canadian Medical Association Journal, 182*(3), 257–264.

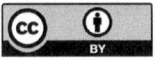

CHAPTER 11

How Can Policy Theory Help to Address the Expectations Gap in Preventive Public Health and 'Health in All Policies'?

Paul Cairney, Emily St. Denny, and Heather Mitchell

1 Introduction: The Search for Political Science Within Public Health

This book explores how to combine insights from public health and political science. In Chapter 2, Fafard et al. (2022) present the crucial distinction between different roles for political science in this collaboration, used: *instrumentally* to help public health advocates improve their political strategies (research *for* public health) or *empirically* to explain the lack of public health policy progress (research *of* public health). Our collective ambition may be to encourage a third, more collaborative and integrated role (political science *with* public health) while accepting that few studies of public health policymaking achieve this aim (yet).

P. Cairney (✉)
Division of History, Heritage, and Politics,
University of Stirling, Stirling, Scotland, UK
e-mail: p.a.cairney@stir.ac.uk

© The Author(s) 2022   239
P. Fafard et al. (eds.), *Integrating Science and Politics for Public Health*,
Palgrave Studies in Public Health Policy Research,
https://doi.org/10.1007/978-3-030-98985-9_11

In that context, this chapter explores not only the consequences of the lack of public health and political science integration but also the possibilities for collaboration. To do so, it focuses on preventive public health policy in general and the global public health strategy 'Health in All Policies' (HiAP) in particular. First, we describe exemplars of public health approaches to policy change which are not informed heavily by political science. Such studies identify the large amount of scientific evidence on the social determinants of health and seek an amount of public policy change that is consistent with the size of the policy problem. One key theme is the need to pursue some variant of 'evidence-based policymaking' (EBPM) in which public health advocates identify and seek to close an evidence-policy gap (Cairney, 2016). Another is the need for high strategic commitment and 'political will' behind health equity policies.

Second, we describe and explain the gap between public health expectations and public policy. Governments often use the right language to signal their sincere commitment to preventive approaches and public health policy, but there remains a major gap between policy and outcomes. Public policy theories help to explain this gap, with reference to the ambiguity of preventive policy initiatives exacerbated by policymaking complexity in which no actor or organisation has strong coordinative capacity. Political science accounts connect major or minor policy change to two key limits to individuals and governments: the role of *bounded rationality* in limiting attention to, and understanding of, policy problems; and *complex policymaking environments* over which policymakers have low knowledge and even less control (Cairney, 2020; Cairney et al., 2019). Both factors explain ever-present limits to policy change. They apply to policymakers regardless of their sincerity or commitment. A vague focus on the 'political will' of policymakers distracts us from a focus on the limits to their resources in relation to their policymaking environments.

E. St. Denny
Department of Political Science, University of Copenhagen, Copenhagen, Denmark

H. Mitchell
Institute for Social Marketing, University of Stirling, Stirling, Scotland, UK

Third, it relates these discussions to key themes to emerge from our qualitative systematic review of HiAP research (Cairney et al., 2021). We focus on the small proportion of HiAP articles that use policy theories to explain policymaking. This 'best case' analysis highlights an enduring obstacle to political science *with* public health: the tendency to use theories instrumentally to improve (a) practical advice to advocates as part of a HiAP playbook, or (b) a HiAP programme logic in the service of better policymaking. Most policy theories were not designed for this specific purpose. Their practical lessons come from critical reflection on the limits to political actor agency in various policymaking contexts (Weible & Cairney, 2021). As such, an integrated public health/political science would foster deliberation on policymaking dilemmas rather than simply identifying political obstacles to overcome.

2   Public Health Provides a Coherent Narrative on Policy Change

'Public health' is an umbrella term covering different approaches, professional backgrounds, and practices. Still, it is possible to highlight a small number of elements to emerge from published public health research, such as a common focus on health equity and addressing the 'social determinants of health', coupled with common references to the same texts, including:

- The working definition of social determinants promoted by the World Health Organization (WHO) (2019), describing 'the unfair and avoidable differences in health status' that are 'shaped by the distribution of money, power and resources' and 'the conditions in which people are born, grow, live, work and age'.
- Whitehead and Dahlgren's (2006, p. 4) argument that 'all systematic differences in health between different socioeconomic groups within a country' are unfair and avoidable, since 'there is no biological reason for their existence' and 'systematic differences in lifestyles between socioeconomic groups are to a large extent shaped by structural factors'.
- Solar and Urwin's (2010, p. 6) argument that a country's socioeconomic and political context underpins variations in education, occupation, and income in relation to class, gender, and ethnicity,

which influence people's 'living and working conditions', mental health, and behaviour, which contribute to their health.

We can then show how such elements combine to produce common public health narratives regarding the policy problem, how to understand it, and the processes necessary to address it. To that end, we drew on earlier published and in-progress work—literature reviews and documentary analysis underpinning our studies of tobacco policy (Cairney et al., 2012), prevention policy (Cairney & St. Denny, 2020), and HiAP (Cairney et al., 2021)—to identify a list of assumptions and expectations among public health research. We then sought to sense-check this list in conversations with public health practitioners and academics in two workshops (at Public Health England, June 2019 ($n = 10$); at Integrating Science and Politics for Public Health workshop, June 2019 ($n = 12$)).

2.1   Public Health Provides a General Narrative of Policy and Policymaking

We were able to discern a common public health narrative on prevention policy that has the following recurring elements (Cairney & St. Denny, 2020). Most important is a focus on preventing ill health rather than treating it when it becomes too severe. For example, there is an emphasis on using health improvement (or health promotion) strategies to prevent an epidemic of non-communicable diseases (NCDs, such as heart disease, strokes, cancers, and diabetes) as well as health protection measures to prevent infectious disease pandemics. There is also a tendency to distinguish between types of prevention:

- *Primary.* Focus on the whole population to stop a problem occurring by investing early and/or modifying the social or physical environment (generally the preferred form of prevention).
- *Secondary.* Focus on at-risk groups to identify a problem at a very early stage to minimise harm (often the pragmatic approach to policy).
- *Tertiary.* Focus on affected groups to stop a problem getting worse (last resort prevention, which can be difficult to distinguish from reactive health services).

Public health accounts of prevention policy also seek to promote health equity by focusing on the social determinants of health and health inequalities. There is an ongoing effort to promote 'upstream' measures designed to improve health equity or the health of the whole population rather than 'downstream' measures targeting individuals. Similarly, there is much use of scientific evidence to identify the nature of problems and most effective solutions. There is also a resolute focus on the role of industry causing public health problems (the 'commercial determinants of health') or undermining the political will to regulate commercial activity. Thus, there is an interest in conceiving of public health and prevention as a form of social protection in which there is a moral imperative to intervene (in sharp contrast to arguments that emphasise individual responsibility for 'lifestyles', and opposition to the 'nanny state'). In that context, 'prevention' sums up an overall policy goal and 'preventive policymaking' is an approach to that end, including a focus on joined-up government, since the responsibility for health improvement goes well beyond health departments.

Our workshops explored some variations in this narrative. First, there are many approaches within this umbrella, drawing more or less on biomedical versus social perspectives on the causes of ill health, and tying arguments more or less to economic conceptions of efficient ways to foster health equity (such as via WHO 'best buys'). Second, although there is a common focus on evidence, there is not always a common definition of what counts. Some describe evidence quality in relation to methods, as part of a 'hierarchy' in which the systematic review of randomised control trials often represents the gold standard and 'systems modelling' often plays a key role (although see Cairney, 2021 on the many types of 'systems thinking'). However, others challenge that hierarchy energetically, particularly when prevention policy goes beyond health (Cairney, 2019a). Third, there remains some ambiguity about the meaning of 'upstream' in relation to the ultimate causes of health inequity (see McMahon, 2021a, 2021b, and compare Shankardass et al., 2011, p. 29; Brownson et al., 2010, p. 6). Fourth, there is more or less support for using tobacco control as a model for other specific issues (e.g. alcohol use, obesity, salt) and the prevention agenda more generally (Studlar & Cairney, 2019). Finally, some key terms remain ill-defined. Most importantly, the phrase 'political will' is central to public health accounts but remains 'hollow political rhetoric' unless operationalised (Post et al., 2010, p. 654). It appears to describe two different factors:

1. *Agency.* A sufficient number of powerful policymakers, with the same understanding of a policy problem, committed to supporting the same policy solution (2010, p. 671).

2. *Context.* Policymaking contexts influence their motivation and ability to act, with key factors including: the 'path dependency' of existing policy and policymaking, the importance of the issue to a party's election chances (and scope for cross-party action), its individualist v collectivist philosophy, and the dominant framing of policy problems (Baum et al., 2020, p. 2).

As such, in Chapter 3, Greer (2022) highlights the *potential* for 'political will' to be operationalised usefully, such as to identify 'whose political will matters and why', and the context in which political agency and leadership are used. However, Cairney et al. (2021) show that almost all accounts use the phrase 'political will' loosely, to describe the low motivation or determination of key policymakers to do the right thing, without relating willpower to context in the way recommended by Baum et al. (2020) or Greer (2022).

2.2   Health in All Policies (HiAP) Takes It One Step Further

Our review of HiAP policymaking studies (Cairney et al., 2021) finds a tighter and more coherent presentation of a similar narrative:

1. Policymakers need to focus on the social determinants of health to promote health equity (by reducing unfair health inequalities).
2. Major policy measures—to redistribute income, improve public services, reduce discrimination, and improve social, economic, and physical environments—are not in the gift of health departments.
3. An effective policymaking response requires collaboration across all sectors of government, and with key stakeholders and citizens outside of government.
4. Long-term success requires high and enduring levels of political will.

This literature also contains (what we describe as) a playbook for HiAP, in which the same advice appears frequently, including: focus on win–win solutions to foster trust-based intersectoral action; avoid projecting

a sense of 'health imperialism' in the pursuit of health equity; and identify policy champions and entrepreneurs (Baum et al., 2014). Relatively,
few articles engage critically with this HiAP story (at least in the way
pursued by De Leeuw and Clavier [2011] and De Leeuw and Peters
[2014]), and few engage with studies of politics and policy to make it
(at the level of Carey & Friel, 2015; Carey et al., 2014; Greer & Lillvis,
2014). Rather, such assumptions tend to underpin high expectations for
the role of government and provide a stylised frame of reference to assess
the overall substance and direction of policy.

3   Governments Adopt Similar Arguments, but There Is Always a Gap Between Commitments and Outcomes

Many governments adopt similar ways to discuss policy and policymaking.
For example, there is a widespread international commitment to the adoption of a specific project such as HiAP (as tracked by the WHO, 2014),
while many countries also use the broader language of prevention to
signal the use of public health ideas across government.

To demonstrate the general focus on prevention, here we draw on
Cairney and St Denny (2020) to track the extent to which the UK and
devolved governments appear to have embraced this way of thinking.
Many successive UK governments have used the general language of
prevention to describe policy agendas in health and fields such as 'families
policy' and justice. The UK Labour government (from 1997 to 2010)
used this language more seriously, included reference to the social determinants of health, and encouraged early years policies such as Sure Start.
From 2011, the Scottish Government declared a 'decisive shift to prevention' across government (2020, pp. 116–118). NHS England's (2014,
p. 3) *Forward View* argued that, 'the future health of millions of children, the sustainability of the NHS, and the economic prosperity of
Britain all now depend on a radical upgrade in prevention and public
health'. 'Prevention is better than cure' was the title of the most recent
(relevant) policy paper by the Department of Health and Social Care
(2018). The UK and Scottish governments also tied prevention policy to
policymaking, emphasising: joined-up and evidence-based policymaking,
localism, service-user-driven policymaking ('we need to make policy *with*
you, not do it to you'), partnerships between government departments

and the public sector, and support for long-term measures of quality of life (Cairney & St. Denny, 2020, pp. 10–12).

However, in each case, there is an unusually large gap between this description and outcomes. It is beyond the usual 'implementation gap' that we would expect in any policy: 'there is great potential for governments to pursue *contradictory* policies at the *complete* expense of their prevention agendas', such as when they pay lip service to prevention but devote most resources to reactive or acute services (2020, p. 2). Cairney and St Denny (2020) describe the three main steps from vague commitment to limited progress:

1. Policymakers show support for prevention policy before they attach meaning to it, beyond the vague idiom that 'prevention is better than cure'. By choosing a vague solution to an unclear problem, they 'do not appreciate the scale of their task until they define prevention while producing strategies and detailed objectives'. Then, they 'find the evidence base to be limited and no substitute for political choice' and realise that these political choices (such as on the role of the state in personal and family life) are divisive (2020, p. 221).
2. When they begin to make enough sense of prevention policy to produce specific aims and objectives, their high-level attention is fleeting. When they relate prevention to their wider agenda, it becomes a relatively low priority, often secondary to—or undermined directly by—other policy aims. When they 'encounter major trade-offs between long-term preventive aims and short-term objectives', they favour the latter and 'devote most resources to reactive services' (2020, p. 221).
3. Policymakers try to deliver governance reforms within a complex policymaking environment over which they have limited understanding and even less control. In many cases, they settle for the *appearance* of success, based on the popularity of their response or narrow indicators of outcomes, without addressing the 'root cause' of the problem they profess to be solving: 'Policymakers begin to think of problems as too 'wicked' to solve. They use prevention as a quick fix, passing on responsibility *and* less funding to delivery bodies … they focus on telling a story of their success rather than achieving it' (2020, p. 221).

In some cases, governments persevere with specific policy agendas (such as the UK government's 'Troubled Families' programme) or approaches to evidence and governance (such as the Scottish Government's support for improvement methods) (2020, p. 227; Cairney, 2017b, 2019c). Or, they set up dedicated agencies to foster preventive health (Boswell et al., 2019). In other cases, they maintain a vague commitment without going any further. As such, even a high profile and sincere commitment to prevention-style policies and policymaking can have *no effect*. Or, the projection of political will behind a new approach can act as a *substitute* for more substantive action.

4   Policy Theory Relates This Gap to Bounded Rationality and Complexity

The simplest explanation for this outcome requires minimal political science or policy theory input: policymakers act in bad faith. They *deliberately* choose a vague policy solution. They engage in strategic ambiguity. The language of prevention and EBPM helps them to depoliticise issues and generate superficial cross-party or public support. They do not intend to deliver or have no belief that they will follow through. They measure their success (in McConnell's, 2010 terms) according to how popular the policy makes them, or how easy it is to process, rather than the long-term health outcomes.

We push back against this argument largely because the assumption of bad faith can exacerbate the policy problem by drawing attention from more important explanations (Cairney & St. Denny, 2020). We argue that the problem of policy ambiguity, and a policy process over which policymakers have limited knowledge and even less control, would exist even if policymakers exhibited high sincerity, competence, commitment, energy, and will.

4.1   Bounded Rationality Causes Uncertainty and Ambiguity

Policymakers do not possess the cognitive and organisational capacity to gather and process all information relevant to their decisions and then make clear, consistent, and well-ranked choices. Rather, they face 'bounded rationality' (Simon, 1976), in which their possession and grasp of evidence, and their ability to make and implement consistent policy choices, are limited. Individuals can only pay attention to—and understand—a small number of issues. Organisations have more capacity but rely on standard operating procedures to help them ignore most information (Baumgartner et al., 2018; Cairney, 2020; Koski & Workman, 2018). Policymakers prioritise some issues, some ways to define them as problems, and some information about them, and ignore the rest. These problems do not decrease when our ability to produce more information increases (Botterill & Hindmoor, 2012, p. 367; Cairney & Kwiatkowski, 2017).

This focus on bounded rationality helps identify the important distinction between policy *uncertainty* (a lack of information on a policy problem) and *ambiguity* (a lack of agreement on how to define the problem) (Zahariadis, 2007; compare with Tuckett and Nicolic, 2017). Actors produce more information to reduce uncertainty, but exercise power to frame problems to reduce ambiguity (Cairney, 2019b). They (a) cooperate with some actors, and compete with others, to (b) limit attention to their preferred way to understand public health policy problems and possible solutions, to (c) inform policy priorities and the selection of policy instruments.

Ambiguity is crucial because, although there may be a clear consensus on how to define policy agendas such as prevention *in the abstract*, it becomes illusory in practice. At the same time, we find a tendency among a small number of people in public health to believe that *they* know the precise meaning of terms like prevention, social determinants, and HiAP. Then, when things are not going well, they reinvent phrases to sum up the same policy intent in new ways. This response becomes counterproductive if the political aim is to generate much wider understanding and agreement. Resolving ambiguity is a contested process to address *policy choice* (e.g. on what problems do we focus?) and *policymaking trade-offs* (e.g. what should be the balance of funding between preventive/reactive services?). The process is political rather than technical, and generating vague agreement is like kicking the can down the road.

4.2   Complex Policymaking Environments Constrain and Facilitate Action

Policy theories identify five conceptual elements—Fig. 1—to describe the 'environment' in which this competition takes place (Heikkila & Cairney,

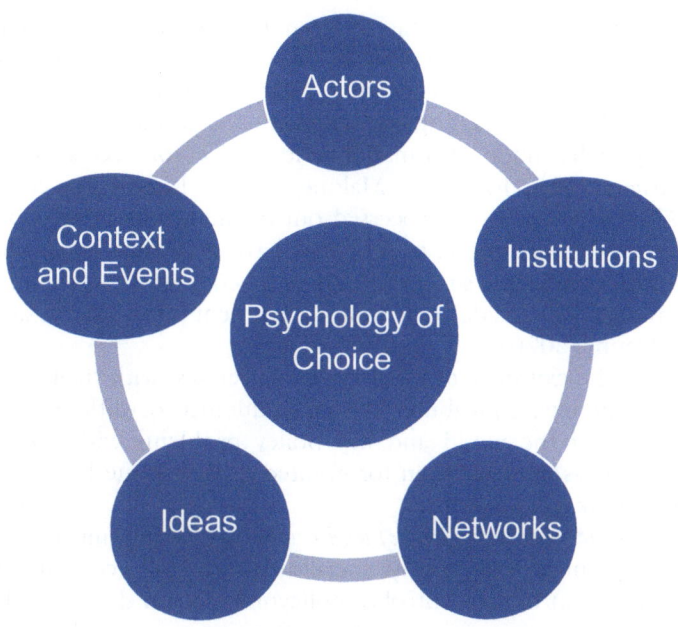

Fig. 1 Key elements of the policy process (Cairney, 2017a)

2018; John, 2003; compare with elements of complex policymaking 'systems'—Cairney, 2012):

1. *Actors*. A huge number of people and organisations make and influence policy across many levels and types of government. There are many 'centres' or policymaking 'venues' (defined as arenas for authoritative choice) (Cairney et al., 2019).

2. *Institutions*. This proliferation of actors contributes to a myriad of formal and informal rules (institutions) across many venues. Some rules are written and understood widely. Others are implicit and may not even be communicated verbally (Ostrom, 2007). In studies of EBPM, this insight is key to actors seeking to promote the same evidence in different venues with different rules (Cairney, 2016). In studies of joined-up government, it presents a challenge to the idea that different actors will use the same idea—such as prevention—in similar ways across government.

3. *Networks*. Each venue has its own relationships between policy-makers and influencers. Classic studies of 'policy communities' highlight a logic of delegating policy responsibility to relatively junior civil servants, engaged in routine consultation with interest groups who trade information and advice for access (Jordan & Cairney, 2013; Jordan & Maloney, 1997; Richardson & Jordan, 1979). Most policy is processed out of the spotlight, at a low level of central government, in silos that have their own logic. Or, policymaking reforms, such as localism, encourage the shift of policy communities outside of central government altogether (Cairney & St. Denny, 2020).

4. *Ideas*. The existence of many different venues, with their own rules and networks, contributes to the endurance of different ways to understand the world and key policy problems within it. Public health ideas may be taken for granted in one venue but seem alien or unthinkable in another.

5. *Policy context (or conditions) and events*. Socioeconomic factors such as geography, demography, social attitudes, and economic activity are often out of the control of policymakers, and they contribute to non-routine events such as 'crises'. Routine events such as elections can also produce major shifts in policy agendas or outcomes.

These factors contribute to the sense that elected policymakers or central governments are not in full control of policymaking. They set high-level aims but rely on many other actors to make sense of and deliver them. There is debate within policy studies about the extent to which central governments can control the governance of policy (compare Bevir, 2013 with Sørensen & Torfing, 2009). For example, one reading of the literatures on 'multi-level', 'polycentric', or 'complex governance' is that elected policymakers should not even try to seek control (Cairney et al., 2019). They should be pragmatic enough to diffuse policymaking responsibility across political systems to give local actors the flexibility to respond to an ever-changing context or *accept that this power diffusion will happen anyway*. Elected governments may still try to project an image of central control, but to address their need to demonstrate governing competence when held to account (particularly in Westminster systems).

Even in accounts more sympathetic to the idea of central control, we find a story that policymakers have to prioritise a small number of issues, while the delivery of their aims depends on the behaviour of a large number of actors. They can set the policy agenda, by identifying the target populations most worthy of support and directing resources towards some problems at the expense of others. However, a sole focus on these choices ignores the wider policymaking context over which they have far less control. A government's energetic focus on the implementation of specific policies helps, but at the expense of attention to other policies.

Identifying this context is crucial to any long-term consideration of prevention policies or initiatives such as HiAP. Although it is tempting to conclude that policies fail because politicians engage in bad faith, even the most sincere and committed policymakers would face major obstacles that they may never overcome. Political enthusiasm is not a good predictor of policy outcomes. Indeed, policymaker *stoicism* may reflect a more practical realisation that they can only enjoy limited success (Boswell & Corbett, 2015).

5   These Factors Help Explain: But not Close—The HiAP Implementation Gap

These discussions provide a lens through which to view the key findings and themes of our qualitative systematic review of HiAP (Cairney et al., 2021). The review includes 113 journal articles (2001–2020, research and commentary) that provide a non-trivial reference to policymaking processes. Initially, we set a low bar to allow comprehensive coverage: the HiAP article provides at least one reference to a policy theory or concept and a corresponding entry in its bibliography (compare with the higher bar set by Embrett and Randall [2014]). In this chapter, we focus on the much smaller subset of articles that use policy theories in a meaningful way. Although to policy scholars this initial bar would seem too low, and distinction too vague, it has proven useful in interdisciplinary academic fields where policy theory is used rarely and meaningful engagement jumps out (Munro & Cairney, 2020). The bigger problem is the skewing of our review towards South Australia, which accounts for over one-quarter of policy theory-informed HiAP studies and most of the examples in themes 2 and 3.

5.1   Theme 1: HiAP as a Symbol for High but Unfulfilled Expectations

The largest set of articles tells a story of *unfulfilled expectations*. Put simply, the less they draw on policy theories, the higher expectations they have for substantive policy change. Since most HiAP articles draw superficially on policy theories, they focus more on the potential than evidence for implementation success. There is a common narrative with the following elements:

1. *Problem.* A discussion of the evidence for the social determinants of health and health inequalities, often accompanied by an estimated economic cost.
2. *Solution.* A description of HiAP as a model, to represent a *solution* (a combination of policy instruments to reduce health inequalities) and *style* (joined-up and collaborative governance), bolstered by high political commitment. HiAP is an ambitious, coherent, and feasible approach. A government's HiAP strategy represents the beginning of major policy change.
3. *Implementation gap.* A report of a large gap between expectations and outcomes, even when there is initially high political will. HiAP becomes a symbol of unfulfilled expectations.

When combined with our more general discussion of preventive policy-making, this work provides a useful cautionary tale in which a government's commitment to a HiAP strategy does not tell us if it will come to fruition. HiAP proves to be an ambiguous approach, exacerbated by policymaking complexity in which no actor or organisation has strong coordinative capacity or the ability to define HiAP consistently. A consensus within one group of specialists—on the nature of policy problems, and HiAP as the solution—is not the same as wider understanding and ownership. Rather, these studies find a heterogeneous mix of experiences when many different policy actors try to make sense of HiAP in different contexts.

However, the conclusions to these articles often undermine the moral to the tale: it would be a mistake to treat HiAP as a uniform model to be implemented in full rather than to be discussed, clarified, and amended by the actors—outside of health departments—deemed crucial to its success. We argue that the 'politics' of HiAP should describe democratic processes to make sense of HiAP in the real world. Yet, too many studies either ignore the positive role of politics or imply that politicians *get in the way* of the aims of HiAP advocates.

5.2 Theme 2: Use Policy Theory Insights to Inform Programme Theory and Reframe the Evaluation of HiAP

Some studies use policy theories to inform the programme theories that underpin the design, delivery, and/or evaluation of HiAP strategies. Programme theory is akin to a theory of change to guide action (Baum et al., 2014: i135), rather than a policy theory used to explain general policy processes:

> Theory-based evaluation makes the causal assumptions behind policy inter-ventions explicit, ie, it explains how and why a program or policy is thought to work, which forms the logic that underpins an initiative. As Leeuw and others note, program theory is often drawn from stakeholder knowledge and is considered distinct from substantive social science theory, which may nevertheless inform and enrich program theory. A distinction can also be drawn between program theory and implementation theory. *Program theory is concerned with mechanisms leading to the desired changes rather than the activities per se.* Implementation theory sheds light on how a particular initiative is operating, and program theory seeks to understand how program effects are realized. (Lawless et al., 2018, p. 512)

In other words, researchers identify HiAP aims and combine their own experience with interviews or focus groups with stakeholders to identify the practices that they expect to work, including 'developing relational systems', 'joint problem identification and problem-solving', and 'gov-ernance systems that connect HiAP work with senior decision-makers' (2018, pp. 513–514). In that context, policy concepts help HiAP advo-cates recognise that the success or failure of a programme relates to factors other than the programme itself (2018, p. 511).

Six commentary articles engage with Lawless et al.'s (2018) study, and their conclusions reflect an enduring confusion about how policy theories contribute to HiAP programme theories. *To some extent*, this confusion relates to general uncertainty about how to interpret a complex world with simple-enough models and concepts, since there are so many from which to learn and it is not clear how they fit together. If so, the use of multiple policy theories can provide more obfuscation than clarity. If so, Lawless et al. (2018) help *visualise* complexity but not *navigate* complexity well enough to support and evaluate interventions (De Leeuw, 2018, pp. 763–764; Harris, 2018; Holt & Ahlmark, 2018, p. 758; Shankardass et al., 2018).

However, it also relates to two profound limitations to HiAP as a policy agenda *and* focus of study. First, there is a gulf between the *assumptions underpinning HiAP theories of change* and *actual politics and policymaking*. The former suggests that the pursuit of intersectoral action, built on win–win strategies and avoiding health imperialism, will foster more collaborative policymaking, better policy, and health equity. Yet, the current evidence does not back up these assumptions, to the extent that it is time to rethink them by drawing more on studies of political economy and power (De Leeuw, 2018, p. 765; Harris, 2018, p. 875). A focus on programme logics, structures, and systems presents HiAP as a technical project, which distracts from the power imbalances and dominant ideologies that undermine HiAP as a global political project (Holt & Ahlmark, 2018, p. 758; Labonté, 2018, p. 656; Peña, 2018, p. 761; Shankardass et al., 2018, p. 757).

5.3   Theme 3: Political Science as a Source of Practical Lessons for Public Health

Second, there is a gulf in intentions between the use of policy theories to (1) *explain policymaking and outcomes* versus (2) *facilitate new forms of policymaking and outcomes*. Many studies use political science to serve the latter: translate the insights of policy theories into practical lessons for HiAP advocates (in other words, political science *for* public health— see Chapter 2, Fafard et al., 2022). For example, some use Kingdon (1984) to present a case study of the *agency of policy entrepreneurs*, describing their role in the famous 'window of opportunity' for major policy change when problem, policy, and politics streams come together. In doing so, they omit references to modern developments in 'multiple streams' analysis, recognising that most entrepreneurs fail, or noting that an entrepreneur's success may relate primarily to their *policymaking environment* (Cairney & Jones, 2016; Cairney, 2018, 2021; Herweg et al., 2018; see also Chapter 3, Greer, 2022).

In comparison, Kickbusch et al. (2014, pp. 187–192) describe (well) Kickbusch's impact as a policy entrepreneur in South Australia. Kickbusch and others were able to convince policymakers that a strategic focus on the social determinants of health across government could help reduce the unsustainable burden on health services. This account also situates entrepreneurial action in context. Rather than simply describing the successful exploitation of a 'window of opportunity' for HiAP, they describe its establishment as an initial condition to help develop the policymaking environment conducive to specific solutions. In other words, try to establish HiAP as an approach to government and *then* work together on initiatives, rather than (as often experienced with Health Impact Assessments) being brought in after an initial decision is made (Lawless et al., 2018, p. 513). As Cairney and St Denny (2020) describe, there is a big difference between a 'window' to adopt specific policy instruments (as in experiences of tobacco policy change) and a vague solution to an unclear problem (as in prevention), but few explore the difference.

Further, some studies draw skilfully on policy theories to explore the implications for HiAP advocacy and strategy. Very few show this level of engagement with policy theories, so key articles are worth exploring as best case examples in this category. For example, Harris et al. (2018, p. 1090) seek to explain why health promotion gained a foothold in land-use policy in New South Wales, Australia. They compare explanations associated with policy theories to identify a window of opportunity, the role of advocacy coalition action, and venue shopping to challenge a monopoly of agenda setting power in one venue. In short, policy entrepreneurs exploited an opportunity caused by sudden perception in government that (a) the economic framing of the reform had fewer supporters and more opponents than expected, and (b) a focus on health benefits boosted support for policy change—the 'public mood' was against traffic jams and pollution and pro exercise amenities—while being unthreatening to most actors. Their Table 3 translates this experience into advice on advocacy:

- 'Be ready to recognize and exploit windows of opportunity',
- 'Build a broad coalition of interested actors',
- 'Know the main entrepreneurs and coalitions',
- 'Where possible, be non-threatening and co-opt their support',
- 'Ensure your issue and goal are prominent in the policy process' (or 'If it is not prominent, try to slip it in under the radar'), and
- 'If necessary, challenge the policy monopoly' (2018, p. 1098).

Similarly, Townsend et al. (2020, p. 981) reflect on the advice for HiAP advocates that they can glean from their explanation for parental leave policy change in Australia:

> Our analysis highlights the benefit of deploying multiple synergistic framings, building coalitions with non-traditional policy allies and using multiple policy venues. This is likely especially important when the dominant policy concern is economic and when public health actions directly confront private sector interest groups.

To some extent, they are reinforcing common HiAP messages on respectful collaboration, suggesting that HiAP advocates give up on health imperialism in favour of aligning their aims and frames with those of many potential allies (2019, pp. 9–10). However, the conclusions also suggest that there is a causal link between their 'game changing' strategies and policy change. As such, these articles reinforce the idea that we can use specific insights from policy theories and empirical case studies to design HiAP advocacy.

Yet, policy theories are primarily empirical tools to produce broad scientific conclusions. It is not obvious how they would translate into normative guidance or practical advice:

> relatively abstract policy theories will rarely provide concrete advice of how to act and what to do in all given contexts. There are too many variables in play to make this happen. The complexity of policy processes, its continuously changing nature, and its diversity across contexts, prevent precise prediction for policy actors seeking influence or policy change. (Weible & Cairney, 2018, p. 186)

> If we simply connect lessons from theories to 'what to do' or how to influence a policy decision or outcomes, it disposes us to overextend our conclusions to contexts where they might not apply. (Weible & Cairney, 2021, p. 202)

Theory-to-practice advice puts the agency of policy actors at centre stage. A small group of people draw lessons about policymaking systems to influence policy in them: define the HiAP policy problem, learn the 'rules of the game', show how contextual factors inform your predictions of your strategy's impact, and make informed action on that basis. In contrast, policy process research situates agency in a highly crowded and competitive political system: analysts face high uncertainty and ambiguity, there is contestation by many actors to define the policy problem, the rules of the game are unwritten and ill-understood, the audience is more important than the analyst, the same strategy can succeed with one audience and fail with another, and windows of opportunity to secure policy change can be decades apart (Cairney et al., 2022).

In that context, van Eyk et al. (2019, p. 1169) exemplify a useful way to qualify the HiAP focus on agency-based strategy, by comparing 'facilitators' to 'barriers':

1. *Recommendation.* Exploit a window of opportunity to 'create acceptance' for a HiAP approach to policy (preferably backed by legislation and a 'central mandate').

   - *Qualification.* Anticipate a 'lack of sustained commitment' particularly during changes to staffing and departments and budget cuts that shift priorities.

2. *Recommendation.* Align the HiAP response to 'existing mandates' to try to create a 'supportive authorising environment and central mandate for action'. For example, use research to show how a HiAP initiative aligns with the 'core business' of government departments, collaborate to produce joint ownership of policy aims, and make sure to avoid the 'perception that this is a top-down imposition by Health (health imperialism)'.

   - *Qualification.* Expect existing mandates to prioritise economy over health frames, with a tendency to reduce public health budgets during state retrenchment.

3. *Recommendation.* Encourage key actors to show leadership and become HiAP champions.

   - *Qualification.* Anticipate resistance to their message if it suggests 'organisational culture change and changing established ways of operating'.

Such accounts are rare in HiAP studies, but they show the potential to move away from a relative focus on the agency of key actors (such as policy champions and entrepreneurs) towards a recognition of the policymaking environments that constrain or facilitate (a) their actions and (b) policy change. Analytically, this approach would help to distinguish between the *obstacles* to policy change that can be addressed and the more enduring *dilemmas* of policymaking that we discuss in the conclusion.

6   Conclusion: What Are Policy Theories For?

Initially, policy theories provide a useful lens through which to observe public health policy implementation. Most public health studies of policymaking still emphasise the important role of models such as HiAP and identify the desire to see them implemented in practice. In that context, the policy process often represents a temporary and inconvenient barrier between expectations and outcomes, and politics is a pathological process to be overcome (French, 2012, connects the latter to a more general misunderstanding of politics among academics).

In contrast, policy theories help identify the evergreen reasons for an implementation gap, focusing on the difficulty of turning a general commitment to a vague policy agenda into actual outputs and positive outcomes in a complex policymaking environment out of the control of policymakers. As such, policy theories help close the expectations gap by reducing unrealistic expectations. Some studies of politics and public administration also draw crucial lessons on specific aspects of policymaking, such as leadership or joining-up government (Carey & Friel, 2015; Carey et al., 2014; Greer & Lillvis, 2014). However, the general role of policy theories is to explain rather than help change policy processes:

> The policy process is inherently messy and marked by a sticky resistance to change. It is also diverse across contexts and constantly changing over time. Given this complexity, there are no easy solutions. Students and policy actors looking for that simple solution to influence or improve policy processes will be disappointed. Instead, policy process theories offer a way of thinking about policymaking-related phenomena. (Weible & Cairney, 2021, p. 207)

In that context, it may be understandable that public health scholars seek to use policy theories instrumentally, to improve programme theories, or to provide practical advice to HiAP advocates. However, if theories were not designed for this purpose, we can only expect so much from this attempt to retrofit policymaking prescription from the study of policy processes.

If so, what value do policy theories offer to public health actors, and what would 'political science *with* public health' look like in the context we describe? First, like studies of public administration, policy theories help manage expectations and warn against unnecessary or counterproductive action. The ability to help policy actors avoid disheartening reform programmes should not be underestimated. Second, they help shift attention from seeing HiAP and EBPM as technical exercises, towards the inevitable role of power and (often positive) role of politics. A theory-informed public health approach can be as simple as the adoption of a research question more suited to the policymaking context, such as: *what is the policy process and how does evidence or HiAP fit in*, rather than *how can we close the evidence-policy gap or the implementation gap*? Indeed, this approach is more consistent with those of experienced policy actors who do not have the time or inclination to redesign policy processes when something goes wrong, and seek lessons more in keeping with their stoicism on the limits to their powers (Boswell & Corbett, 2015).

Finally, and perhaps most importantly, theory-informed public health studies would focus on the trade-offs that arise when public health policy actors must navigate multiple (and often contradictory) objectives. Two key examples demonstrate the tensions in public health agendas that cannot be resolved with more evidence or political will. The first is a combined commitment to EBPM *and* collaborative forms of governance. Studies should prompt difficult questions about who should participate and whose knowledge matters, and a movement away from simply declaring that obstacles to HiAP relate to 'policy-based evidence making' (see Cairney, 2017b, 2022; Cairney & Oliver, 2017). The second is a HiAP commitment to centralisation, to foster high political will and strategic commitment, *and* decentralisation, and to foster local autonomy, collaboration, and sense making. Studies should prompt difficult questions on the potential for centralisation and decentralisation to undermine each other, and away from simply declaring that any obstacle is an 'implementation gap' (see Cairney et al., 2021, pp. 25–26). Political science *with* public health would encourage critical reflection on policymaking dilemmas. Researchers and advocates would recognise, adapt to, and engage with policy processes that exist, not fantasise about how they would like politics and policymaking to be.

REFERENCES

Baum, F., Lawless, A., Delany, T., Macdougall, C., Williams, C., Broderick, D., Wildgoose, D., Harris, E., Mcdermott, D., Kickbusch, I., & Popay, J. (2014). Evaluation of health in all policies: Concept, theory and application. *Health Promotion International, 29*(Suppl_1), i130–i142.

Baum, F., Townsend, B., Fisher, M., Browne-Yung, K., Freeman, T., Ziersch, A., Harris, P., & Friel, S. (2020). Creating political will for action on health equity: Practical lessons for public health policy actors. *International Journal of Health Policy Management,* 1–14. https://doi.org/10.34172/ijhpm.202 0.233

Baumgartner, F., Jones, B., & Mortensen, P. (2018). Punctuated equilibrium theory. In C. Weible & P. Sabatier (Eds.), *Theories of the policy process* (4th ed.). Westview.

Bevir, M. (2013). *A theory of governance.* Gaia Books.

Boswell, J., & Corbett, J. (2015). Stoic democrats? Anti-politics, élite cynicism and the policy process. *Journal of European Public Policy, 22*(10), 1388–1405.

Boswell, J., Cairney, P., & St. Denny, E. (2019). The politics of institutionalizing preventative health. *Social Science and Medicine.* https://doi.org/10.1016/j. socscimed.2019.02.051

Botterill, L., & Hindmoor, A. (2012). Turtles all the way down: Bounded rationality in an evidence-based age. *Policy Studies, 33*(5), 367–379.

Brownson, R. C., Seiler, R., & Eyler, A. A. (2010). Measuring the impact of public health policy. *Preventing Chronic Disease, 7,* 4, A77, 1–7. http://www. cdc.gov/pcd/issues/2010/jul/09_0249.htm

Cairney, P. (2012). Complexity theory in political science and public policy. *Political Studies Review, 10*(3), 346–358.

Cairney, P. (2016). *The politics of evidence based policy making.* Palgrave Springer.

Cairney, P. (2017a). 5 images of the policy process. *Paul Cairney: Politics & Public Policy.* https://paulcairney.wordpress.com/2017a/07/10/5-images-of-the-policy-process/

Cairney, P. (2017b). Evidence-based best practice is more political than it looks: A case study of the "Scottish Approach." *Evidence and Policy, 13*(3), 499–515. https://doi.org/10.1332/174426416X14609261565901

Cairney, P. (2018). Three habits of successful policy entrepreneurs. *Policy and Politics, 46*(2), 199–217.

Cairney, P. (2019a). Evidence and policy making. In A. Boaz, H. Davies, A. Fraser, & S. Nutley (Eds.), *What works now?* Policy Press.

Cairney, P. (2019b). Fostering evidence-informed policy making: Uncertainty versus ambiguity. *National Collaborating Centre for Healthy Public Policy* (NCCHPP). http://www.ncchpp.ca/41/What_s_New_.ccnpps?id_art icle=1930

Cairney, P. (2019c). The UK government's imaginative use of evidence to make policy. *British Politics, 14*(1), 1–22.

Cairney, P. (2020). *Understanding public policy* (2nd ed.). Palgrave.

Cairney, P. (2021). *The politics of policy analysis*. Palgrave.

Cairney, P. (2022). The contested relationship between governance and evidence. In C. Ansell & J. Torfing (Eds.), *Handbook on theories of governance*. Edward Elgar.

Cairney, P., & Jones, M. (2016). Kingdon's multiple streams approach: What is the empirical impact of this universal theory? *Policy Studies Journal, 44*(1), 37–58.

Cairney, P., Keating, M., St. Denny, E., & Kippin, S. (2022). *Public policy to reduce inequalities across Europe: Hope versus reality*. Oxford University Press.

Cairney, P., & Kwiatkowski, R. (2017). How to communicate effectively with policymakers: Combine insights from psychology and policy studies. *Palgrave Communications, 3*, 37. https://www.nature.com/articles/s41599-017-0046-8

Cairney, P., & Oliver, K. (2017). Evidence-based policymaking is not like evidence-based medicine, so how far should you go to bridge the divide between evidence and policy? *Health Research Policy and Systems, 15*, 35. https://doi.org/10.1186/s12961-017-0192-x

Cairney, P., & St. Denny, E. (2020). *Why isn't government policy more preventive?* Oxford University Press.

Cairney, P., Heikkila, T., & Wood, M. (2019). *Making policy in a complex world*. Cambridge University Press.

Cairney, P., St. Denny, E., & Mitchell, H. (2021). The future of public health policymaking after COVID-19: A qualitative systematic review of lessons from Health in All Policies. *Open Research Europe* [version 2; peer review: Approved] *1*(23). https://doi.org/10.12688/openreseurope.13178.2

Cairney, P., Studlar, D., & Mamudu, H. (2012). *Global tobacco control: Power, policy, governance and transfer*. Palgrave Macmillan.

Carey, G., & Friel, S. (2015). Understanding the role of public administration in implementing action on the social determinants of health and health inequities. *International Journal of Health Policy and Management, 4*(12), 795–798. https://doi.org/10.15171/ijhpm.2015.185

Carey, G., Crammond, B., & Keast, R. (2014). Creating change in government to address the social determinants of health: How can efforts be improved? *BMC Public Health, 14*, 1087. https://doi.org/10.1186/1471-2458-14-1087

De Leeuw, E., & Clavier, C. (2011). Healthy public in all policies. *Health Promotion International, 26*(2), ii237, ii244. https://doi.org/10.1093/heapro/dar071

De Leeuw, E., & Peters, D. (2014). Nine questions to guide development and implementation of health in all policies. *Health Promotion International, 30*(4), 987–997. https://doi.org/10.1093/heapro/dau034

De Leeuw, E. (2018). Policy, theory, and evaluation: Stop mixing the fruit salad: Comment on "Developing a framework for a program theory-based approach to evaluating policy processes and outcomes: Health in all policies in South Australia." *International Journal of Health Policy and Management, 7*(8), 763.

Department of Health and Social Care. (2018). *Prevention is better than cure: Our vision to help you live well for longer.* Department of Health. https://ass ets.publishing.service.gov.uk/government/uploads/system/uploads/attach ment_data/file/753688/Prevention_is_better_than_cure_5-11.pdf

Embrett, M., & Randall, G. (2014). Social determinants of health and health equity policy research: Exploring the use, misuse, and nonuse of policy analysis theory. *Social Science and Medicine, 108*, 147–155.

Fafard, P., Cassola, A., & Weldon, I. (2022). Political science In, of, and with public health: Implications for the role of evidence. In P. Fafard, A. Cassola, & E. De Leeuw (Eds.), *Integrating science and politics for public health.* Palgrave Springer.

French, R. (2012). The professors on public life. *The Political Quarterly, 83*(3), 532–540. https://doi.org/10.1111/j.1467-923X.2012.02320.x

Greer, S. L., & Lillvis, D. F. (2014). Beyond leadership: Political strategies for coordination in health policies. *Health Policy, 116*, 12–17. https://doi.org/10.1016/j.healthpol.2014.01.019

Greer, S. L. (2022). Professions, data, and political will. In P. Fafard, E. De Leeuw, & A. Cassola (Eds.), *Public health political science: Integrating science and politics for public health.* Palgrave.

Harris, P. (2018). Researching healthy public policy: Navigating the 'Black Box' means thinking more about power: Comment on "Developing a framework for a program theory-based approach to evaluating policy processes and outcomes: Health in all policies in South Australia." *International Journal of Health Policy and Management, 7*(9), 874.

Harris, P., Kent, J., Sainsbury, P., Marie-Thow, A., Baum, F., Friel, S., & McCue, P. (2018). Creating 'healthy built environment' legislation in Australia; a policy analysis. *Health Promotion International, 33*(6), 1090–1100.

Heikkila, T., & Cairney, P. (2018). Comparison of theories of the policy process. In C. Weible & P. Sabatier (Eds.), *Theories of the policy process* (4th ed.). Westview.

Herweg, N., Zahariadis, N., & Zohlnhöfer, R. (2018). The multiple streams framework: Foundations, refinements, and empirical applications. In C Weible, & P. Sabatier (Eds.), *Theories of the policy process* (4th ed.). Westview Press.

Holt, D. H., & Ahlmark, N. (2018). How do we evaluate health in all policies?: Comment on "Developing a framework for a program theory-based approach to evaluating policy processes and outcomes: Health in all policies in South Australia." *International Journal of Health Policy and Management, 7*(8), 758.

John, P. (2003). Is there life after policy streams, advocacy coalitions, and punctuations: Using evolutionary theory to explain policy change? *Policy Studies Journal, 31*(4), 481–498.

Jordan, G., & Cairney, P. (2013). 'What is the 'Dominant Model' of British policy making? Comparing Majoritarian and Policy Community Ideas. *British Politics, 8*(3), 233–259.

Jordan, G., & Maloney, W. (1997). Accounting for subgovernments: Explaining the persistence of policy communities. *Administration and Society, 29*(5), 557–583.

Kickbusch, I., Williams, C., & Lawless, A. (2014). Making the most of open windows: Establishing health in all policies in South Australia. *International Journal of Health Services, 44*(1), 185–194. https://doi.org/10.2190/HS.44.1.k

Kingdon, J. (1984). *Agendas, alternatives and public policies.* HarperCollins.

Koski, C., & Workman, S. (2018). Drawing practical lessons from punctuated equilibrium theory. *Policy and Politics, 46*(2), 293–308.

Labonté, R. (2018). From mid-level policy analysis to macro-level political economy: Comment on "Developing a framework for a program theory-based approach to evaluating policy processes and outcomes: Health in all policies in South Australia." *International Journal of Health Policy and Management, 7*(7), 656.

Lawless, A., Baum, F., Delany-Crowe, T., MacDougall, C., Williams, C., McDermott, D., & van Eyk, H. (2018). Developing a framework for a program theory-based approach to evaluating policy processes and outcomes: Health in all policies in South Australia. *International Journal of Health Policy and Management, 7*(6), 510–521. https://doi.org/10.15171/ijhpm.2017.121

McMahon, N. (2021a). Framing action to reduce health inequalities: What is argued for through use of the 'upstream–downstream' metaphor? *Journal of Public Health,* 1–8. https://doi.org/10.1093/pubmed/fdab157

McMahon, N. (2021b). Working 'upstream' to reduce social inequalities in health: A qualitative study of how partners in an applied health research collaboration interpret the metaphor. *Critical Public Health.* https://doi.org/10.1080/09581596.2021.1931663

McConnell, A. (2010). *Understanding policy success: Rethinking public policy.* Palgrave Macmillan.

Munro, F., & Cairney, P. (2020, March). A systematic review of energy systems: The role of policymaking in sustainable transitions. *Renewable & Sustainable*

Energy Reviews, 119, 109598, 1–14 https://doi.org/10.1016/j.rser.2019. 109598

NHS England. (2014). *Five year forward view.* NHS England. http://www.eng land.nhs.uk/wp-content/uploads/2014/10/5yfv-web.pdf

Ostrom, E. (2007). Institutional rational choice. In P. Sabatier (Ed.), *Theories of the policy process* (Vol. 2). Westview Press.

Peña, S. (2018). Evaluating health in all policies: Comment on "Developing a framework for a program theory-based approach to evaluating policy processes and outcomes: Health in all policies in South Australia." *International Journal of Health Policy and Management, 7*(8), 761.

Post, L. A., Raile, A. N., & Raile, E. D. (2010). Defining political will. *Politics & Policy, 38*(4), 653–676.

Richardson, J. J., & Jordan, G. (1979). *Governing under pressure: The policy process in a post-parliamentary democracy.* Robertson.

Shankardass, K., O'Campo, P., Muntaner, C., Bayoumi, A. M., & Kokkinen, L. (2018). Ideas for extending the approach to evaluating health in all policies in South Australia: Comment on "Developing a framework for a program theory-based approach to evaluating policy processes and outcomes: Health in all policies in South Australia." *International Journal of Health Policy and Management, 7*(8), 755.

Shankardass, K., Solar, O., Murphy, K., Freiler, A., Bobbili, S., Bayoumi, A., & O'Campo, P. (2011). *Health in all policies: A snapshot for Ontario.* Centre for Research on Inner City Health.

Solar, O., & Urwin, A. (2010). *A conceptual framework for action on the social determinants of health.* WHO.

Simon, H. (1976). *Administrative behavior* (3rd ed.). Macmillan.

Sørensen, E., & Torfing, J. (2009). Making governance networks effective and democratic through metagovernance. *Public Administration, 87*(2), 234–258.

Studlar, D., & Cairney, P. (2019). Multilevel governance, public health and the regulation of food: Is tobacco control policy a model? *Journal of Public Health Policy, 40*(2), 147–165. https://doi.org/10.1057/s41271-019-00165-6

Townsend, B., Friel, S., Baker, P., Baum, F., & Strazdins, L. (2020). How can multiple frames enable action on social determinants? Lessons from Australia's paid parental leave. *Health Promotion International, 35*(5), 973–983. https://doi.org/10.1093/heapro/daz086

Tuckett, D., & Nicolic, M. (2017). The role of conviction and narrative in decision-making under radical uncertainty. *Theory and Psychology, 27*(4), 501–523.

van Eyk, H., Baum, F., & Delany-Crowe, T. (2019). Creating a whole-of-government approach to promoting healthy weight: What can health in all policies contribute? *International Journal of Public Health,*

64(8), 1159–1172. https://doi.org/10.1007/s00038-019-01302-4(012345
6789(),-volV)(0123456789,-().volV)
Weible, C., & Cairney, P. (2018). Practical lessons from policy theories. *Policy and Politics, 46*(2), 183–197.
Weible, C., & Cairney, P. (2021). Reflections and resolutions in drawing practical lessons from policy theories. In C. Weible, & P. Cairney (Eds.), *Practical lessons from policy theories*. Bristol University Press.
Whitehead, M., & Dahlgren, G. (2006). Concepts and principles for tackling social inequities in health: Levelling up Part 1. *World Health Organization: Studies on social and economic determinants of population health.* http://www.euro.who.int/__data/assets/pdf_file/0010/74737/E89383.pdf
WHO. (2014). *Health in all policies: Helsinki statement. Framework for country action.* World Health Organization. https://www.who.int/publications-detail/health-in-all-policies-helsinki-statement
WHO (World Health Organisation). (2019). *Social determinants of health.* https://www.who.int/gender-equity-rights/understanding/sdh-definition/en/#:~:text=Social%20determinants%20of%20health%E2%80%93The,global%2C%20national%20and%20local%20levels
Zahariadis, N. (2007). The multiple streams framework. In P. Sabatier (Ed.), *Theories of the policy process*. Westview.

CHAPTER 12

Moving Beyond Health in All Policies: Exploring How Policy Could Front and Centre the Reduction of Social Inequities in Health

Ditte Heering Holt and Katherine L. Frohlich

1 INTRODUCTION

In recent years, there has been a proliferation of concepts to understand how best to enact intersectoral health policies. Much of this work is specifically focused on the promise of Health in All Policies (HiAP), an intersectoral approach to public policy that seeks to promote action on

D. H. Holt (✉)
National Institute of Public Health, University of Southern Denmark, Copenhagen, Denmark
e-mail: dihh@sdu.dk

K. L. Frohlich
Département de médecine sociale et préventive, École de Santé Publique, Université de Montréal, Montreal, QC, Canada

© The Author(s) 2022   267
P. Fafard et al. (eds.), *Integrating Science and Politics for Public Health*,
Palgrave Studies in Public Health Policy Research,
https://doi.org/10.1007/978-3-030-98985-9_12

the Social Determinants of Health (SDH).[1] Indeed, the rapprochement of HiAP and the SDH has been viewed to be an intervention solution to reducing social inequities in health (Baum, Lawless, et al., 2013; Marmot, 2010). In practice, however, questions of health equity are often marginal in these discussions and not apparent when evaluating outcomes (Baum et al., 2017; Hall & Jacobson, 2018; Khayatzadeh-Mahani et al., 2019; van Eyk et al., 2017). Additionally, several scholars have demonstrated how governments, though paying lip service to the social determinants of health to reduce social inequities in health, often enact policies that are best described as a lifestyle drift (Fisher et al., 2017; Lynch, 2017; Smith, 2013). In this paper we develop the argument that as a policy framework, the ways in which HiAP is undertaken are insufficient to achieve reductions in social inequities in health and may even worsen them. In doing so, we believe we are demonstrating what, in practice, a political science *with* public health might look like. As discussed in Chapter 2 (Fafard et al., 2022), this involves a critical and conceptually sophisticated perspective that interrogates the inherent assumptions of public health practice while remaining sympathetic to the broader public health project.

This paper begins by discussing the distinctions between the concepts of public health policy (PHP), healthy public policy (HPP) and HiAP. We demonstrate, firstly, that the substantive concerns of these approaches differ greatly and that the blurring between these concepts may lead to inefficient public health advocacy and policy efforts. Building on this discussion, we develop a conceptual critique of HiAP that distinguishes problems of intentionality and directionality. We argue that for public policy to effectively reduce social inequities in health, it should focus desired change away from any one health issue in isolation, towards the drivers of the inequities. In order to effectively do so, new policy approaches would have to emphasize the sectoral contribution of non-health sectors. These arguments serve to clarify the disparate approaches included in the "umbrella" concept of HiAP.

As an empirical example throughout this paper, we use the last 30 years of tobacco control (as well as HiAP policy more broadly) to assist in making our point. Many would claim that tobacco control policy has been one of, if not the single-most effective public health policy in the history of modern public health. It is also highlighted as a prime example

---

[1] See Chapter 11 by Cairney et al. (2022) in this volume for a complimentary critique of HiAP.

of the need for, and potential success of, a HiAP approach. As Bettcher and Silva phrase it: "Tobacco control programmes are an example of the application of the HiAP concept as they already permeate the agendas of different sectors in different governments, resulting in a concentrated effort to improve population health" (2013, p. 203). We discuss the ways in which tobacco control policy to date does or does not fulfil the objectives of HiAP.

To conclude the paper, we draw on Amartya Sen's capability theory (1992) to develop the argument that public policy concerned with inequity in health must focus on the inequity in lack of opportunity that some may have to achieve good health due to inadequate social arrangements. We believe the use of Sen's theory may go some way to ensure that overcoming social inequities remains the focus of intersectoral policy interventions.

2   PUBLIC HEALTH POLICY, HEALTHY PUBLIC POLICY, AND HiAP

To begin to understand HiAP's shortcomings with reference to health inequity reduction, a brief historical and definitional foray into the differences between public health concepts regarding intersectoral policy approaches is necessary. We start by defining how we use the concepts of *public health policy (PHP)*, *healthy public policy (HPP)* and *HiAP* in order to clearly distinguish the implications of these different policy frameworks on equity outcomes.

Public health policy (PHP) is often used as a broad concept encompassing the total sum of policies and programmes put in place to advance public health goals. However, for the purpose of conceptual clarity, we use public health policy (PHP) more specifically to circumscribe the good number of policies concerned with "health problems" based primarily on a biomedical model (de Leeuw et al., 2013). This type of PHP is often designed to change health behaviour, either directly or indirectly, by making "unhealthy choices" less attractive. They may be directed at a structural level by changing the environment or at an individual level, but their emphasis is to reduce risk and prevent disease (Chaufan et al., 2014; Lorenc et al., 2013). Often these public health policies (PHPs) include intersectoral action. For example, in the case of tobacco control policy, justice departments have become involved to develop and enforce bans on certain kinds of tobacco products, and departments of finance have been asked to develop and implement fiscal policies that raise the price of tobacco products and thereby reduce demand. The end goal and focus of the policy, however, is to reduce the prevalence of risk factors in a population by acting on the risk factor or health behaviour itself (i.e., the reduction of cigarette smoking). There is, therefore, no intersectoral goal beyond the reduction in the prevalence of the health problem alone (tobacco smoking). As such, this kind of public health policy is characterized by a sectoral aim of better health and involves intersectoral action only to achieve this relatively narrow goal, with little or no attention to broader questions of health equity.

By contrast, we understand *healthy public policy* (HPP) to encompass policies concerned with the conditions that create a healthy society (Hancock, 1985). HPPs are based on a social model which views health to be influenced by a multitude of social, environmental, political and economic factors, often referred to as the *social* determinants of health (SDH) (Commission on Social Determinants of Health [CSDH], 2008). The concept of healthy public policy was first promoted by Nancy Milio (Milio, 1981). The Ottawa Charter for health promotion embraced the concept and argued that HPPs combine "diverse but complementary approaches including legislation, fiscal measures, taxation and organizational change. It is coordinated action that leads to health, income and social policies that foster greater equity" (World Health Organization [WHO], 1986). In other words, HPPs are public policies that involve upstream interventions with social equity as one of their goals (Oneka et al., 2017).

In contrast to public health policies, HPPs have an intersectoral aim (i.e., creating a healthy and equal society) which requires coordinated sectoral action. Examples of HPPs include, among others: giving every child the best start in life; improving education and lifelong learning; ensuring employment and good working conditions, providing a minimum income for healthy living, and healthy and sustainable communities (Marmot & Allen, 2013, p. 75). While the concept of HPP underscores the importance of coordinated policy action across sectors to achieve health equity, it has provided little guidance on how to achieve policy change in practice (de Leeuw & Clavier, 2011), and there is still little evidence on the success or failure of HPP in reducing social inequities in health through intersectoral policymaking (de Leeuw, 2017).

Since the mid-2000s, the notion of *Health in All Policies* (HiAP) has gained strong support in the public health community as a further innovation of HPP, and largely to overcome the lack of policy change provided by HPP (Baum, Lawless, et al., 2013; de Leeuw, 2015; de Leeuw et al., 2014; Kickbusch & Buckett, 2010; McQueen et al., 2012; Ollila, 2011). HiAP is often defined as: "an approach to public policies across sectors that systematically takes into account the health implications of decisions, seeks synergies, and avoids harmful health impacts in order to improve population health and health equity" (WHO, 2013). While some use HiAP interchangeably with HPP, HiAP is more often referred to as an approach (WHO, 2013, among many others), a strategy (Freiler et al., 2013; Rudolph et al., 2013), a mechanism (Baum, Ollila, et al., 2013), or a policy practice (McQueen et al., 2012), for achieving the goal of HPP (Baum, Ollila, et al., 2013). HiAP is usually understood to place a stronger emphasis on health governance than HPP does to ensure intersectoral engagement and collaboration. It also generally involves a centralized and systematic approach to considering the health effects of (all government) policies using health impact assessments or similar arrangements (Baum et al., 2014; Freiler et al., 2013; Ollila et al., 2013). While specific HiAP examples differ in terms of both governance and priorities, reflecting their local contexts, HiAP may be considered an approach that involves introducing a set of institutional arrangements to break down institutional barriers to collaboration and ensure intersectoral policymaking for better health. Carey et al. (2014) conceptualize HiAP as an instrumental process-based intervention. This means that HiAP is not understood to be inherently able to improve health as such. Instead HiAP introduces new governance structures and decision-making processes which should be instrumental in creating healthier policies (Baum et al., 2014; Carey et al., 2014; Freiler et al., 2013). Other researchers have emphasized the importance of the broader policy process to affect the uptake of HiAP and promote the use of political theory to qualify intersectoral policymaking for health (Clavier & de Leeuw, 2013; de Leeuw & Peters, 2015; Rashad & Khadr, 2014; WHO, 2015, see Chapter 11, by Cairney et al., 2022 as well). A well-recognized example of HiAP is found in South Australia (Baum, Ollila, et al., 2013) where a health lens analysis was introduced together with a dedicated HiAP unit. HiAP was supported by a mandate linked to the State Strategic Plan which was formally endorsed by Cabinet (Baum et al., 2017).

For the purpose of conceptual clarity, we thus understand HiAP to involve a change in focus from the two previous concepts. As outlined in Table 1, we use PHP and HPP as analytical concepts that circumscribe

Table 1 Definitions

Concept	Focus	Definition
Public Health Policy (PHP)	Analytical concept Circumscribing the content of policy	PHPs are concerned with health problems based primarily on biomedical determinants of health model PHPs focus on changing behaviours, reducing risk factors and preventing disease PHPs utilize individual and/or structural interventions PHPs are characterized by a sectoral health aim and intersectoral action
Healthy Public Policy (HPP)	Analytical concept Circumscribing the content of policy	HPPs are concerned with the conditions that create a healthy and equal society HPPs are based on a model of the social determinants of health HPPs entail upstream policies that support health, well-being and equity HPPs are characterized by an intersectoral aim and coordinated sectoral action
Health in All Policies (HiAP)	Approach to policymaking	HiAP is an approach to policymaking across sectors that takes into account the health implications of decisions, seeks synergies, and avoids harmful health impacts HiAP involves introducing institutional arrangements to facilitate intersectoral policymaking HiAP seeks to improve population health and health equity

end goals regarding the content of public policies. The question of their implementation is a question directed at the content of specific public policies. The question of HiAP implementation, on the other hand, refers to the introduction of health governance and decision-processes to create intersectoral policymaking for health (equity).

These definitions highlight how the substantive concerns of these three health policy concepts differ in important ways. The first two differ in terms of the content of their policy focus, and consequently their intersectoral aspirations as well as their ability to tackle inequities. HiAP differs from both of the others by focusing on the mechanisms to bring about policy change (rather than the policy content alone). However, HiAP is also routinely used synonymously with the other two, particularly HPP, which blurs the distinction between policy content and approach (Kickbusch, 2013; Ståhl, 2018).

There have been previous attempts to clarify the distinction between PHP, HPP and HiAP (Storm et al., 2007 referenced in den Broeder et al., 2015; de Leeuw et al., 2013, 2014), as well as attempts to outline the different conceptualizations of HiAP, as synonymous with HPP or as an approach involving a set of institutional arrangements (Carey et al., 2014). However, as we argue here, HiAP has at least two further shortcomings with regard to its ability to be a motor for change when concerned specifically with social inequities in health. First, the discourse on HiAP equates policies for improving population health with those concerning health equity (what we will call intentionality). Second, the discourse on HiAP lacks clarity regarding whether health is its main objective or whether health is simply part of a broader societal goal. Accordingly, this leads to confusion about the expected contribution of non-health sectors to HiAP (what we will call directionality) which, in turn, risks making public health advocacy misguided and, subsequently, the intersectoral engagement ineffective.

3   HiAP's Confused Intentionality and Ambiguous Directionality

As outlined above, a significant part of the HiAP literature argues for changes in the ways in which governments engage in intersectoral collaboration as much as it argues for changes to policy content. To ensure conceptual clarity, we use the terminology of PHP and HPP below when we refer to specific variations in HiAP policy content.

We use intentionality to refer to the (implicit or explicit) policy intention to address social inequity in health when discussing the content of HiAP policies. Taking inspiration from Bacchi's (2009) "What's the problem represented to be", intentionality involves the policy analytical question of how HiAP policies explicate how they will address social inequity in health.

By directionality we refer to the aim and scope of HiAP engagement. Directionality involves the analytical question of how HiAP constructs the role and contribution of health and non-health sectors in achieving the goal of reducing social inequities in health.

3.1   Confused Intentionality: The Shortcomings of HiAP to Address Social Inequity in Health

The first criticism of HiAP with regard to its ability to tackle social inequity in health relates to its approach to policy content, or more specifically, the ambiguity that ensues from its dual aim of both promoting population health and reducing social inequity in health (WHO, 2013). This reflects the dual meaning of the social determinants of health (SDH) as identified by Hilary Graham (2004, 2009): targeting both the social causes of health and the social factors determining the distribution of these causes. The former encompasses health promoting or impairing resources found in the social and material environments for example, the home, neighbourhood and workplace. The latter refers to the distribution of societal-level resources like income and wealth, education, employment opportunities, political influence and power, which shape access and exposure to the social determinants of health (Graham, 2004, pp. 107–108). As such, the social determinants of health are not to be conflated with the social determinants of health inequity (Baum, 2016). A case in point is observed in many Western high-income countries where both living standards and population health have significantly improved over the past 50 years. Yet, at the same time, health inequities have persisted and even increased in some cases (Graham, 2004; Mackenbach, 2012; Mackenbach et al., 2015). Nonetheless, this confusion appears to often be the case in health impact assessments which struggle to include macro-economic policy as a determinant (Buse et al., 2019; Povall et al., 2013).

Despite the honourable intention of tackling the twin challenges of reducing ill health at a population level and diminishing social inequities in health, the blurring between the two perpetuates the assumption that social inequities in health can be reduced by policies focusing only on the social determinants of health. This tends to give prominence to population health concerns rather than equity in HiAP-inspired policymaking (Graham, 2004; Kvåle et al., 2020; van Eyk et al., 2017) and is made even more likely given the difficulties in "selling" the re-distribution requirements that social equity policies demand.

This shortcoming is partly due to (or justified by) the assumption that action on the SDH will "trickle down"; overall improvements in SDH are expected to reduce social inequities in health over time (van Eyk et al., 2017). According to this logic, for instance, policies focused on reducing smoking prevalence at a population level should in turn reduce social inequities in smoking because the prevalence of smoking is highest among lower SES-groups. However, this logic constitutes what we would define as a health drift: a displacement where the intention of HiAP to address social inequity in health translates as more limited PHPs addressing only intermediary SDH, if not just the risk factor itself (Graham, 2009).

One such example is the Scottish tobacco control policy *Creating a Tobacco-Free Generation: A Tobacco Control Strategy for Scotland*, which sets itself apart from other countries' tobacco control policies by having a distinct focus on inequities (Healthier Scotland, 2013). This comprehensive and ambitious policy aims to reduce smoking prevalence to 5% or less by the year 2034. Moreover, it distinguishes itself from those of many countries because it aims specifically to reduce stark social inequities in smoking in Scotland.

However, rather than focusing on the social determinants of health inequities in the policy, smoking is considered to be a crucial contributing cause of health inequities. As phrased in the document:

> the patterns of smoking prevalence rates [...] are a very direct cause of Scotland's continuing health inequalities. It therefore follows that reducing smoking prevalence rates in the most deprived communities will make a decisive contribution to reducing Scotland's health inequalities. (Healthier Scotland 2013, p. 7)

Although underlying environmental and living conditions (e.g., built environment, income, education and employment) are discussed as determinants of inequalities in the policy, efforts to address these underlying factors are delegated to the Scottish Government's Ministerial Task Force on Health Inequalities. The remainder of the policy elucidates how to reduce smoking prevalence by: (1) preventing smoking initiation in youth; (2) protecting the population from second-hand smoke, especially children; and (3) offering more cessation services to help those who are smoking to quit (Healthier Scotland, 2013). As such, the policy may primarily be categorized as a behavioural-type public health policy (PHP) focusing largely on the reduction of smoking as a behaviour rather than the social conditions that lead to smoking inequities (e.g., poverty). This is important because, while tobacco control policies have been immensely productive in reducing the population prevalence of smoking during the last 30 years, evidence indicates that they may have simultaneously aggravated social inequities in smoking (Corsi et al., 2014; Frohlich & Potvin, 2008; Smith et al., 2009). As such, the use of similar approaches in tobacco control may no longer be a feasible option if the reduction in social inequities in smoking is the goal.

The tobacco control example is not unique. For example, Thomson et al. (2018) have shown how some PHPs that may be efficient in improving overall population health either have no differential health effects or may even increase inequities by disproportionately benefitting more advantaged groups. Lorenc et al. (2013) also caution against such intervention-generated inequities. They find that downstream policies often risk producing differential effects by benefitting higher SES-groups the most. In Canada, for instance, smoking prevalence among women with a university education decreased from 45% in 1950 to 8% in 2011. In contrast, prevalence of smoking in women with less than a high school education only decreased from 40 to 33% (Corsi et al., 2014. See Manuel et al. (2020) for projections to 2041). In concrete terms, the most socio-economically disadvantaged Canadians have benefitted the least from these PHPs (Frohlich & Potvin, 2008).

This critique is not restricted to PHPs such as tobacco regulation. When HiAP sets out to address working and living conditions, based on a social model of health, this does not necessarily entail a redistribution of these factors and thus would not necessarily improve health equity (Baum et al., 2017; Fisher et al., 2017; Graham, 2004). For instance, a study by Chaufan et al. (2014) highlights a blind spot in public health with regard to the drivers of SDH. Chaufan and colleagues argue that environmental changes to the built environment are often suggested as an SDH approach to improve health equity without considering the drivers of inequity such as poverty. Instead, environmental changes are proposed to facilitate behavioural changes (i.e., to make neighbourhoods safer to walk or bike in and increase access to healthy foods). Such HiAP policies thus fall victim to a similar health drift: they reduce complex issues of health equity to focus primarily on health behaviour. A similar critique can be found in a study by Holt et al. (2017) in which the authors found that environmental changes to the school environment to improve children's level of physical activity and dietary choices (in order to improve their cognitive ability and learning outcomes) may compromise action on the broader SDH.

In sum, the consequence of the dual aim of promoting both population health and health equity is that the intentionality of HiAP is not always clear. In some examples of HiAP, either the policies have sought outcomes other than reductions in social inequities in health, and/or could potentially cause unintentional concentrations of vulnerabilities and increase inequities in health (Baum et al., 2017; Frohlich & Potvin, 2008; van Eyk et al., 2017). For a policy framework to efficiently address social inequities in health, it needs to specifically apply an equity lens, be prepared to confront the issue of inequities as being unfair and mutable and be willing to consider redistributive policy options. This involves an explicit focus on the drivers of inequity rather than merely the health behaviours of the disadvantaged.

3.2 Ambiguous Directionality: The Contribution of Non-health Sectors to Health

A second criticism of HiAP concerns how it is interchangeably considered to place health as the main intersectoral objective (Freiler et al., 2013; Greer & Lillvis, 2014; Wismar et al., 2013) and to entail a "networking strategy" that advances broader societal goals such as sustainability and equity, as well as health (Kickbusch, 2010; Kickbusch & Buckett, 2010; Kranzler et al., 2013; Rudolph et al., 2013). This ambiguity involves a question of how HiAP constructs the role and contribution of non-health sectors. Specifically, should non-health sectors integrate health (equity) objectives as part of their sectoral mission and core services or could the core services of non-health sectors be health promoting in their own right? This distinction is crucially important as it brings attention to the sectoral interests involved and, in doing so, an inherent problem of existing HiAP; which is to ensure legitimacy and to create motivation among non-health sectors to engage in intersectoral collaboration with the health sector (Degeling, 1995; Holt, Carey, et al., 2018; Khayatzadeh-Mahani et al., 2019).

According to the definition of HiAP, its aim is to make health (equity) concerns a *shared* objective across government sectors. As such, HiAP represents "a continuation of the imperative of health" whereby health is sanctioned as one of the most important policy issues for governments to address (Carey & Crammond, 2014, p. 500). For instance, Wismar and colleagues (2013, p. 2) argue that "we need to better understand how diverse actors such as government officials, private industry and citizens may internalize health as an important objective, as we all have internalized evidence, efficiency, integrity, anti-discrimination and many other values". Kickbusch et al. (2014, p. 186) describe how HiAP "… implies challenging nearly every societal actor, sector, and institution at all levels of governance to 'think health' and to contribute to the circumstances in which people can be healthy". At least two problems follow from this health imperative.

First, regarding policy content, most SDH are characterized by the fact that they lie outside the health sector. That is, SDH involve the circumstances in which people are born, grow, live, work and age, as it is commonly phrased, and the unequal distribution of these determinants is seen as the driver of health inequity (Graham, 2004; Irwin & Scali, 2010). De Leeuw (2017) lists the most commonly identified sectors as: education, housing and urban planning, transport and mobility, social protection and welfare support systems, as well as energy and sustainable development. As such, the SDH belong to non-health sector domains. This is generally accepted as a fact in the public health community and is the main argument for introducing HiAP. However, it follows that non-health sectors' main contribution to addressing the unequal distribution of SDH must lie within their sectoral mission and core service provision. That is, targeting the social determinants of health inequity primarily concerns (coordinated) sectoral policy and action by non-health sectors such as providing free, good quality education, proper working conditions, employment opportunities and a minimum income, among others. Thus, the promotion of health itself is not the objective, and the health sector would need to emphasize the importance of resource redistribution in other sectors in order to reach both their own equity goals, as well as the health sector's objective of reducing social inequity in health (Lynch, 2017).

HiAP is conceptually flawed if the assumption being made is that making health (rather than equity), the objective of non-health sectors will significantly reduce social inequities in health. This reduces the role of non-health sectors in HiAP to be implementers of health policy and, thus, neglects their main sectoral contribution to (health) equity. By contrast, many public policies with (intended or unintended) health effects are not based on a health rationale (de Leeuw, 2017; Storm et al., 2016).

This leads to the second problem of confused directionality: the motivation of non-health sectors to engage in intersectoral collaboration. Health (equity) is often not effective as a "collaboration magnet" to engage non-health sectors (Khayatzadeh-Mahani et al., 2019). At times it may be easy to frame a win–win argument regarding the interrelations and shared interests between sectors, one example being the interrelationships between early child development, education and social inequities in health (Diderichsen et al., 2012; Hahn et al., 2016; Maggi et al., 2010). Another example used by advocates of a HiAP approach is the shared interest across government in reducing ever-expanding health expenditures (Baum et al., 2017; Baum, Ollila, et al., 2013). As described by Cairney et al. in Chapter 11 (2022), policymakers may find it easy to show support to a vague solution to an unclear problem like health inequity before they assign meaning to it (also see Holt, Rod, et al., 2018). It becomes a much greater challenge, however, when government actors need to resolve ambiguity and agree on specific policy designs and instruments, when overall shared aims are to be operationalized and prioritized in the development and implementation of specific policies (Brunsson, 2002; Carey & Crammond, 2014; Holt, Carey, et al., 2018). Then the vague agreement is confronted with the reality of complex policy environments with path dependencies of existing policies, sectoral logics, and various dominant frames, and all potential solutions may be divisive or compete with other government priorities. Non-health sectors may consider the HiAP aim of reducing social inequities in health to be peripheral to, if not incompatible with, their own equity-related objectives. Smith and Weinstock (2019), for instance, argue that intersectoral strategies for health equity by their very nature risk limiting the motivation of non-health sectors to engage in intersectoral collaboration because these strategies take as their starting point the privileging of *health* equity, over equity for other social goods (Smith & Weinstock, 2019). Similarly, de Leeuw (2017) and Holt (2018) find that starting with a *health* argument may sometimes be counterproductive to the aim of engaging non-health sectors in intersectoral collaboration. Lynch (2017, p. 656) even warns that the framing of social inequity as a problem of health tends to medicalize the problem of inequity, "making it seem less amenable to structural solutions" while implying health imperialism. The problem arises when HiAP supporters collapse complex issues of social disadvantage and inequity into matters of health and advocate health-centric solutions. This type of approach is unlikely to be welcomed by those working in the non-health sectors (Carey & Crammond, 2014). HiAP's tendency to solely promote the integration of health (equity) concerns across government, together with the encouragement for the health sector to take a leadership role (Marmot, 2010), is, therefore, most likely to limit HiAP's ability to create a coordinated approach to addressing the drivers of health inequity (Khayatzadeh-Mahani et al., 2019; Smith, 2013).

Acknowledging this challenge, several scholars have argued for a "win–win" approach (Freiler et al., 2013; Molnar et al., 2016), synergy (Ollila et al., 2013), or for HiAP supporters to use strategic framing or "speak the same language" as collaborating sectors (Hall & Jacobson, 2018; WHO, 2015; Storm et al., 2016; Molnar et al., 2016; Freiler et al., 2013). While this has proven successful in some cases, we caution that a win–win approach risks maintaining the imperative of health if other sectors are treated as instrumental to the aim of improving health (equity) only. In siloed systems (reflecting a bureaucratic logic of specialization), the health sector would find it challenging to legitimately engage non-health sectors in intersectoral policymaking on matters that lie within non-health sectors' own domains, if it is not (at least rhetorically) a matter of health. That is, if policy changes within non-health sectors are sectoral (e.g., better and more equitable education), the health sector would generally not have a legitimate seat at the table. Therefore, HiAP involves a dynamic which tends to maintain the health imperative and, thus, reproduce the challenge of intersectoral engagement, which HiAP is intended to overcome.

To sum up our critiques of the intentionality and directionality of HiAP, we are arguing that the opportunities, as well as the aim of establishing intersectoral engagement and collaboration, are quintessentially different when promoting population health from reducing social inequities in health. For public policy to effectively reduce social inequities in health, it should focus desired change away from any one health issue in isolation, towards the drivers of inequities in the same. Moreover, the health imperative involved with a HiAP approach may discourage non-health sectors from engaging substantially in intersectoral policymaking beyond peripheral concerns. While, theoretically, the main contribution of non-health sectors to health equity lies within their sectoral domains, the ability of the health sector to facilitate intersectoral policymaking is largely dependent on the legitimacy derived from focusing on health.

Building on Julia Lynch (2017), we suggest that public health would benefit from changing its intersectoral advocacy to ensure equity within the provision of non-health sector's core missions and services, rather than framing it as a health inequity problem (Lynch, 2017). Not only would this hold more potential for targeting the drivers of social inequities (in health), but it would also permit non-health sectors to take leadership of their own equity-related policies and objectives. This would mean less direct policy instruction from the health sector to non-health sectors (which is likely to be met with limited success) and place more emphasis on the connections between sectoral domains. While acknowledging the tremendous task of advocating for social equity in a neo-liberal era, we believe that such an approach holds greater promise in terms of ensuring the creation of public policies that address social equity. As Lynch (2017) argues, health inequity may be an appealing problem frame that makes certain inequality issues more palatable in a neo-liberal policy paradigm than re-distribution policy. However, this framing underscores the inherent complexity: dealing with a wicked problem with multiple interacting, unclear, and distal causes and making the problem seem unamenable to policy intervention and thus making it difficult to act. In contrast, sectoral equity policies have the benefit of being relatively simple to imagine and can be implemented by a much smaller number of actors within one or only a few policy sectors.

4   TOWARDS A FRAMEWORK FOCUSED ON THE REDUCTION OF SOCIAL INEQUITIES

We propose the capability approach (CA) as a policy framework to guide thinking about how policies from all sectors can increase people's capabilities as an intersectoral goal, rather than health. The capability approach is an explanatory theory of well-being and a normative theory of justice that emerged as a response to the standard limitations to distributional theory (such as utilitarianism and other welfare theories) (Sen, 1992). Over the last 10–15 years, this approach has been proposed as being potentially important for public health action concerned with the reduction of social inequities in health. The work of the WHO Commission on Social Determinants of Health (CSDH, 2008) and the writings of experts like Jennifer Ruger (2010) have emphasized the importance of considering distributive justice from a capability standpoint in order to effectively address inequities in health (Ruger, 2004). More importantly, for the sake of our argument, the capability approach helps us re-frame the question of "equity of what?" by steering the answer away from equity in health to equity in capabilities.

The core characteristic of the capability approach is its focus on what people are effectively able to do and be; that is, on their capabilities (Robeyns, 2005). Individuals' opportunities to undertake the actions and activities that they want to engage in are what matter. These actions and activities ("doings") together with the "beings", or what Sen calls "functionings", constitute a valuable life. Functionings include, but are not limited to, being healthy, being active as a community member, working, resting, being literate, etc. The distinction between realizable and realized functionings is crucial to the capability approach. "A functioning is an achievement, whereas a capability is the ability to achieve" (Sen, 1987, p. 36). Sen puts much emphasis on the distinction between functionings and capabilities because he believes that well-being should not only include realized functionings but that the ability to choose from a set of alternative functionings is a freedom sui generis (Sen, 1999).

Here Sen puts great emphasis on freedom. Freedom is important to equity issues for Sen for at least two different reasons. First, more freedom gives people more opportunities to pursue their objectives. It helps, for example, in their ability to decide to live as they would like and to promote the ends that they may want to advance (in some public health jargon, this could be equivocated with empowerment). This aspect of freedom is concerned with people's ability to achieve what they value, no matter what the process is through which that achievement comes about (Sen, 2009). Second, we may attach importance to the process of choice itself. We may, for example, want to make sure that people are not being forced to do certain things, take on certain health or social practices, or not able to behave in the way they wish, because of specific constraints.

The focus of the capability approach is not just on what a person ends up doing (or achieving), but also whether he or she chooses freely to make use of that opportunity and what their overall options are. The focus is therefore on the ability of people to choose to live different kinds of lives within their reach, rather than confining attention only to what may be described as the culmination—or aftermath—of choice. In this sense, freedom is both structured (having collective/shared aspects) and individual. It is this inequity in capabilities, understood as an inequity in choice, that Sen argues is at the core of inequity in society.

Consequently, and in relation to the social determinants of health inequities, HiAP considerations of public policies and programmes based on the CA would include, on the structural side, not only the quality and quantity of available resources, or the realized doings and beings on the agency side, but also, the range of capabilities available to people. As Smith and Seward note, an "individual's capabilities emerge from the combination and interaction of individual-level capacities and the individual's relative position vis-à-vis social structures that provide reasons and resources for particular behaviors" (2009, p. 213). People's ability to use resources will determine the range of options for health practices by shaping their capabilities. In other words, we must consider the "capability sets" from which individuals can draw (Sen, 1992) in order to understand how inequities in health practices come about.

As such, health equity policy discussions must grapple with the larger issues of fairness and justice in social arrangements, including economic allocations, paying appropriate attention to the role of health in human life and freedom. Fundamentally, health equity is not just about the distribution of health (Sen, 1992). Rather, addressing health inequity is about the distribution of a much wider array of resources.

5 Conclusion

To conclude, we suggest that the capability approach may function as a meta-framework for addressing social inequities (in health) when considering HiAP. The CA helps us avoid the health drift of confused intentionality as it demands us to focus on how each sector can promote equity in capabilities within their sectoral domains. As such, it helps us to value the contribution of each sector in reducing social inequities and thus to avoid the problem of ambiguous directionality. While the CA does not prescribe the most efficient governance structures to be used to ensure intersectoral collaboration, it involves understanding sectoral missions in context. Focusing on how each sector can promote capabilities within their sectoral domains may help reduce the complexity of intersectoral policymaking to address the social determinants of health inequity. We propose that a CA inspired approach to intersectoral policymaking would tend to focus more on the connections between sectoral domains rather than attempting to direct policy action of non-health sectors.

Insisting on an equity lens does represent an enormous and difficult task in a neo-liberal era. However, we argue, the solution to this is not found in an intersectoral "fix" like HiAP. Rather, what is required is the mobilization of multiple stakeholders to establish a social movement and, in turn, public pressure for change.

Acknowledgements We would like to acknowledge the significant contributions made by Dr. Luke Craven and Dr. Josée Lapalme in helping to develop the original idea behind this paper and in discussing several drafts of the manuscript. The idea for this paper was first conceived at the 2017 workshop: "Public management and policy implementation for public health policy – new directions for research and practice" organized by Gemma Carey and colleagues, and hosted by the Center for Public Service Research at the University of New South Wales, Canberra, Australia.

References

Bacchi, C. L. (2009). *Analysing policy: What's the problem represented to be?* Pearson.

Baum, F. (2016). *The new public health* (4th ed.). Oxford University Press.

Baum, F., Delany-Crowe, T., MacDougall, C., Lawless, A., van Eyk, H., & Williams, C. (2017). Ideas, actors and institutions: Lessons from South Australian Health in All Policies on what encourages other sectors' involvement. *BMC Public Health, 17*(1), 811. https://doi.org/10.1186/s12889-017-4821-7

Baum, F., Lawless, A., Delany, T., Macdougall, C., Williams, C., Broderick, D., Wildgoose, D., Harris, E., McDermott, D., Kickbusch, I., Popay, J., & Marmot, M. (2014). Evaluation of Health in All Policies: Concept, theory and application. *Health Promotion International, 29*(Suppl 1), i130–142.

Baum, F., Lawless, A., & Williams, C. (2013). Health in All Policies from international ideas to local implementation: Policies, systems, and organizations. In C. Clavier & E. de Leeuw (Eds.), *Health promotion and the policy process* (pp. 188–217). Oxford University Press.

Baum, F., Ollila, E., & Peña, S. (2013). History of HiAP. In K. Leppo, E. Ollila, S. Peña, M. Wismar, & S. Cook (Eds.), *Health in All Policies: Seizing opportunities, implementing policies* (pp. 25–42). Ministry of Social Affairs and Health.

Bettcher, D., & Silva, V. L. d. C. e. (2013). Tobacco or health. In K. Leppo, E. Ollila, S. Peña, M. Wismar, & S. Cook (Eds.), *Health in All Policies: Seizing opportunities, implementing policies* (pp. 203–224). Ministry of Social Affairs and Health.

Brunsson, N. (2002). *The organization of hypocrisy: Talk, decisions and actions in organizations* (2nd ed.). Abstrakt forlag AS 2002.

Buse, C. G., Lai, V., Cornish, K., & Parkes, M. W. (2019). Towards environmental health equity in health impact assessment: Innovations and opportunities. *International Journal of Public Health, 64*(1), 15–26.

Cairney, P., Mitchell, H., & St Denny, E. (2022). Addressing the expectations gap in preventative public health and 'Health in All Policies': How can policy theory help? In P. Fafard, A. Cassola, & E. De Leeuw (Eds.), *Integrating science and politics for public health*. Palgrave Springer.

Carey, G., & Crammond, B. (2014). Help or hindrance? Social policy and the 'social determinants of health.' *Australian Journal of Social Issues, 49*(4), 489–507.

Carey, G., Crammond, B., & Keast, R. (2014). Creating change in government to address the social determinants of health: How can efforts be improved? *BMC Public Health, 14*, 1087.

Chaufan, C., Yeh, J., Ross, L., & Fox, P. (2014). You can't walk or bike yourself out of the health effects of poverty: Active school transport, child obesity, and blind spots in the public health literature. *Critical Public Health, 25*(1), 32–47.

Clavier, C., & de Leeuw, E. (2013). Framing public policy in health promotion: Ubiquitous yet elusive. In C. Clavier & E. de Leeuw (Eds.), *Health promotion and the policy process* (pp. 1–22). Oxford University Press.

CSDH, Commission on Social Determinants of Health. (2008). *Closing the gap in a generation: Health equity through action on the social determinants of health*. World Health Organization.

Corsi, D. J., Boyle, M. H., Lear, S. A., Chow, C. K., Teo, K. K., & Subramanian, S. V. (2014). Trends in smoking in Canada from 1950 to 2011: Progression of the tobacco epidemic according to socioeconomic status and geography. *Cancer Causes and Control, 25*(1), 45–57. https://doi.org/10.1007/s10552-013-0307-9

de Leeuw, E. (2015). Intersectoral action, policy and governance in European healthy cities. *Public Health Panorama, 1*(2), 175–182.

de Leeuw, E. (2017). Engagement of sectors other than health in integrated health governance, policy, and action. *Annual Review of Public Health, 38*(1), 329–349.

de Leeuw, E., & Clavier, C. (2011). Healthy public in all policies. *Health Promotion International, 26*(suppl 2), ii237–ii244.

de Leeuw, E., Clavier, C., & Breton, E. (2014). Health policy—why research it and how: Health political science. *Health Research Policy and Systems, 12*(1), 55.

de Leeuw, E., Keizer, M., & Hoeijmakers, M. (2013). Health policy networks: Connecting the disconnected. In C. Clavier & E. de Leeuw (Eds.), *Health promotion and the policy process* (pp. 154–173). Oxford University Press.

de Leeuw, E., & Peters, D. (2015). Nine questions to guide development and implementation of Health in All Policies. *Health Promotion International, 30*(4), 987–997. https://doi.org/10.1093/heapro/dau034

Degeling, P. (1995). The significance of 'sectors' in calls for urban public health intersectoralism: An Australian perspective. *Policy & Politics, 23*(4), 289–301 (213).

den Broeder, L., Scheepers, E., Wendel-Vos, W., & Schuit, J. (2015). Health in All Policies? The case of policies to promote bicycle use in the Netherlands. *Journal of Public Health Policy, 36*(2), 194–211.

Diderichsen, F., Andersen, I., Manuel, C., Andersen, A.-M. N., Bach, E., Baads-gaard, M., Brønnum-Hansen, H., Hansen, F. K., Jeune, B., Jørgensen, T., & Søgaard, J. (2012). Health Inequality—Determinants and policies. *Scandinavian Journal of Public Health, 40*(suppl 8), 12–105.

Fafard, P., Cassola, A., & Weldon, I. (2022). Political science in, of, and with public health: Implications for the role of evidence. In P. Fafard, A. Cassola, & E. de Leeuw (Eds.), *Integrating science and politics for public health*. Palgrave Springer.

Fisher, M., Baum, F. E., MacDougall, C., Newman, L., McDermott, D., & Phillips, C. (2017). Intersectoral action on SDH and equity in Australian health policy. *Health Promotion International, 32*(6), 953–963.

Freiler, A., Muntaner, C., Shankardass, K., Mah, C. L., Molnar, A., Renahy, E., & O'Campo, P. (2013). Glossary for the implementation of Health in All Policies (HiAP). *Journal of Epidemiology and Community Health, 67*(12), 1068–1072. https://doi.org/10.1136/jech-2013-202731

Frohlich, K. L., & Potvin, L. (2008). The inequality paradox: The population approach and vulnerable populations. *American Journal of Public Health, 98*(2), 216–221.

Graham, H. (2004). Social determinants and their unequal distribution: Clarifying policy understandings. *Milbank Quarterly, 82*(1), 101–124.

Graham, H. (2009). Health inequalities, social determinants and public health policy. *Policy & Politics, 37*(4), 463–479.

Greer, S. L., & Lillvis, D. F. (2014). Beyond leadership: Political strategies for coordination in health policies. *Health Policy, 116*(1), 12–17. https://doi.org/10.1016/j.healthpol.2014.01.019

Hahn, R. A., Barnett, W. S., Knopf, J. A., Truman, B. I., Johnson, R. L., Fielding, J. E., Muntaner, C., Jones, C. P., Fullilove, M. T., Hunt, P. C., &

Community Preventive Services Task Force. (2016). Early childhood education to promote health equity: A community guide systematic review. *Journal of Public Health Management and Practice, 22*(5), E1–E8. https://doi.org/10.1097/PHH.0000000000000378

Hall, R. L., & Jacobson, P. D. (2018). Examining whether the health-in-all-policies approach promotes health equity. *Health Affairs, 37*(3), 364–370. https://doi.org/10.1377/hlthaff.2017.1292

Hancock, T. (1985). Beyond health care: From public health policy to healthy public policy. *Canadian Journal of Public Health, Revue Canadienne De Sante Publique, 76*(Suppl 1), 9–11.

Healthier Scotland, The Scottish Government. (2013). *Creating a Tobacco-Free Generation: A Tobacco Control Strategy for Scotland.* Edinburgh.

Holt, D. H. (2018). Rethinking the theory of change for Health in All Policies; Comment on "Health promotion at local level in Norway: The use of public health coordinators and health overviews to promote fair distribution among social groups." *International Journal of Health Policy and Management, 7*(12), 1161–1164.

Holt, D. H., Carey, G., & Rod, M. H. (2018). Time to dismiss the idea of a structural fix within government? An analysis of intersectoral action for health in Danish municipalities. *Scandinavian Journal of Public Health, 46*(suppl 22), 48–57. https://doi.org/10.1177/1403494818765705

Holt, D. H., Frohlich, K. L., Tjørnhøj-Thomsen, T., Clavier, C. (2017). Intersectoriality in Danish municipalities: Corrupting the social determinants of health? *Health Promotion International, 32*(5), 881–890. https://doi.org/10.1093/heapro/daw020

Holt, D. H., Rod, M. H., Waldorff, S. B., & Tjørnhøj-Thomsen, T. (2018). Elusive implementation: An ethnographic study of intersectoral policymaking for health. *BMC Health Services Research, 18*(1), 54. https://doi.org/10.1186/s12913-018-2864-9

Irwin, A., & Scali, E. (2010). *Action on the Social Determinants of Health: Learning from previous experiences* (Social Determinants of Health Discussion Paper 1 (Debates)). World Health Organization.

Khayatzadeh-Mahani, A., Labonte, R., Ruckert, A., & de Leeuw, E. (2019). Using sustainability as a collaboration magnet to encourage multi-sector collaborations for health. *Global Health Promotion, 26*(1), 100–104. https://doi.org/10.1177/1757975916683387

Kickbusch, I. (2010). Health in all policies: Where to from here? *Health Promotion International, 25*(3), 261–264. https://doi.org/10.1093/heapro/daq055

Kickbusch, I. (2013). Health in all policies. *BMJ (Clinical research ed.), 347*(f4283). https://doi.org/10.1136/bmj.f4283

Kickbusch, I., & Buckett, K. (2010). *Implementing health in all policies: Adelaide 2010.* Government of South Australia.

Kickbusch, I., Williams, C., & Lawless, A. (2014). Making the most of open windows: Establishing health in all policies in south Australia. *International Journal of Health Services, 44*(1), 185–194. https://doi.org/10.2190/HS.44.1.k

Kranzler, Y., Davidovich, N., Fleischman, Y., Grotto, I., Moran, D. S., & Weinstein, R. (2013). A health in all policies approach to promote active, healthy lifestyle in Israel. *Israel Journal of Health Policy Research, 2*(1), 16. https://doi.org/10.1186/2045-4015-2-16

Kvåle, G., Kiland, C., & Torjesen, D. O. (2020). Public health policy to tackle social health inequalities: A balancing act between competing institutional logics. In P. Nugus, C. Rodriguez, J.-L. Denis, & D. Chênevert (Eds.), *Transitions and boundaries in the coordination and reform of health services: Building knowledge, strategy and leadership* (pp. 149–165). Springer International Publishing.

Lorenc, T., Petticrew, M., Welch, V., & Tugwell, P. (2013). What types of interventions generate inequalities? Evidence from systematic reviews. *Journal of Epidemiology and Community Health, 67*(2), 190–193. https://doi.org/10.1136/jech-2012-201257

Lynch, J. (2017). Reframing inequality? The health inequalities turn as a dangerous frame shift. *Journal of Public Health, 39*(4), 653–660. https://doi.org/10.1093/pubmed/fdw140

Mackenbach, J. P. (2012). The persistence of health inequalities in modern welfare states: The explanation of a paradox. *Social Science and Medicine, 75*(4), 761–769.

Mackenbach, J. P., Kulhánová, I., Menvielle, G., Bopp, M., Borrell, C., Costa, G., Deboosere, P., Esnaola, S., Kalediene, R., Kovacs, K., Leinsalu, M., Martikainen, P., Regidor, E., Rodriguez-Sanz, M., Strand, B. H., Hoffmann, R., Eikemo, T. A., Östergren, O., & Lundberg, O. (2015). Trends in inequalities in premature mortality: A study of 3.2 million deaths in 13 European countries. *Journal of Epidemiology and Community Health, 69*(3), 207–217. https://doi.org/10.1136/jech-2014-204319

Maggi, S., Irwin, L. J., Siddiqi, A., & Hertzman, C. (2010). The social determinants of early child development: An overview. *Journal of Paediatrics and Child Health, 46*(11), 627–635. https://doi.org/10.1111/j.1440-1754.2010.01817.x

Manuel, D. G., Wilton, A. S., Bennett, C., Dass, A. R., Laporte, A., & Holford, T. R. (2020, November 18). *Health Reports. Smoking patterns based on birth-cohort-specific histories from 1965 to 2013, with projections to 2041.* Retrieved August 31, 2021, from https://www150.statcan.gc.ca/n1/pub/82-003-x/2020011/article/00002-eng.htm

Marmot, M. (2010). *Fair society, healthy lives: The Marmot Review*. Strategic Review of Health Inequalities in England post-2010.

Marmot, M., & Allen, J. (2013). Prioritizing health equity. In K. Leppo, E. Ollila, S. Peña, M. Wismar, & S. Cook (Eds.), *Health in All Policies: Seizing opportunities, implementing policies* (pp. 63–80). Ministry of Social Affairs and Health.

McQueen, D., Wismar, M., Lin, V., Jones, C. M., & Davies, M. (2012). *Intersectoral Governance for Health in All Policies: Structures, actions and experiences*. World Health Organization on behalf of the European Observatory on Health Systems and Policies.

Milio, N. (1981). *Promoting health through public policy*. FA Davis Company.

Molnar, A., Renahy, E., O'Campo, P., Muntaner, C., Freiler, A., & Shankardass, K. (2016). Using win-win strategies to implement health in all policies: A cross-case analysis. *PloS One, 11*(2), e0147003.

Ollila, E. (2011). Health in all policies: From rhetoric to action. *Scandinavian Journal of Public Health, 39*(6), 11–18. https://doi.org/10.1177/140349 4810379895

Ollila, E., Baum, F., & Peña, S. (2013). Introduction to Health in All Policies and the analytical framework of the book. In K. Leppo, E. Ollila, S. Peña, M. Wismar, & S. Cook (Eds.), *Health in All Policies: Seizing opportunities, implementing policies* (pp. 3–23). Ministry of Social Affairs and Health.

Oneka, G., Vahid Shahidi, F., Muntaner, C., Bayoumi, A. M., Mahabir, D. F., Freiler, A., O'Campo, P., & Shankardass, K. (2017). A glossary of terms for understanding political aspects in the implementation of Health in All Policies (HiAP). *Journal of Epidemiology and Community Health, 71*(8), 835–838. https://doi.org/10.1136/jech-2017-208979

Povall, S. L., Haigh, F. A., Abrahams, D., & Scott-Samuel, A. (2013). Health equity impact assessment. *Health Promotion International, 29*(4), 621–633. https://doi.org/10.1093/heapro/dat012

Rashad, H., & Khadr, Z. (2014). Measurement of health equity as a driver for impacting policies. *Health Promotion International, 29*(suppl_1), i68–i82. https://doi.org/10.1093/heapro/dau045

Robeyns, I. (2005). The capability approach: A theoretical survey. *Journal of Human Development, 6*(1), 93–114.

Rudolph, L., Caplan, J., Mitchell, C., Ben-Moshe, K., & Dillon, L. (2013). *Health in all policies: Improving health through intersectoral collaboration* (Discussion Paper). Institute of Medicine of the National Academies.

Ruger, J. P. (2004). Ethics of the social determinants of health. *The Lancet, 364*, 1092–1097.

Ruger, J. P. (2010). Health capability: Conceptualization and operationalization. *American Journal of Public Health, 100*(1), 41–49.

Sen, A. (1987). The standard of living. In G. Hawthorn (Ed.), *The Standard of Living*. Cambridge University Press.

Sen, A. (1992). *Inequality re-examined*. Russell Sage Foundation.

Sen, A. (1999). *Development as freedom*. Random Books.

Sen, A. (2009). *The idea of justice*. The Belknap Press.

Smith, K. (2013). Institutional filters: The translation and re-circulation of ideas about health inequalities within policy. *Policy & Politics, 41*(1), 81–100. https://doi.org/10.1332/030557312X655413

Smith, M. J., & Weinstock, D. (2019). Reducing health inequities through inter-sectoral action: Balancing equity in health with equity for other social goods. *International Journal of Health Policy and Management, 8*(1), 1–3.

Smith, M. L., & Seward, C. (2009). The relational ontology of Amartya Sen's capability approach: Incorporating social and individual causes. *Journal of Human Development and Capabilities, 10*(2), 213–235. https://doi.org/10.1080/19452820902940927

Smith, P., Frank, J., & Mustard, C. (2009). Trends in educational inequalities in smoking and physical activity in Canada: 1974 2005. *Journal of Epidemiology & Community Health, 63*, 317–323.

Storm, I., den Hertog, F., van Oers, H., & Schuit, A. J. (2016). How to improve collaboration between the public health sector and other policy sectors to reduce health inequalities?—A study in sixteen municipalities in the Netherlands. *International Journal for Equity in Health, 15*(1), 97. https://doi.org/10.1186/s12939-016-0384-y

Ståhl, T. (2018). Health in All Policies: From rhetoric to implementation and evaluation—The Finnish experience. *Scandinavian Journal of Public Health, 46*(suppl 20), 38–46. https://doi.org/10.1177/1403494817743895

Thomson, K., Hillier-Brown, F., Todd, A., McNamara, C., Huijts, T., & Bambra, C. (2018). The effects of public health policies on health inequalities in high-income countries: An umbrella review. *BMC Public Health, 18*(1), 869. https://doi.org/10.1186/s12889-018-5677-1

van Eyk, H., Harris, E., Baum, F., Delany-Crowe, T., Lawless, A., & MacDougall, C. (2017). Health in All Policies in South Australia—Did it promote and enact an equity perspective? *International Journal of Environmental Research and Public Health, 14*(11), 1288.

Wismar, M., McQueen, D., Lin, V., Jones, C. M., & Davies, M. (2013). Rethinking the politics and implementation of health in all policies. *Israel Journal of Health Policy Research, 2*(1), 17. https://doi.org/10.1186/2045-4015-2-17

WHO, World Health Organization. (2013, June 10–14). *The Helsinki Statement on Health in All Policies*. The 8th Global Conference on Health Promotion.

WHO, World Health Organization. (2015). *Health in All Policies: Training manual*.

WHO, World Health Organization, Canadian Public Health Association, & Health Canada. (1986). The Ottawa charter for health promotion. *Health Promotion, 1*, i–v. Retrieved September 7, 2021, from http://www.who.int/healthpromotion/conferences/previous/ottawa/en/

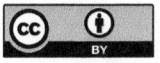

Mechanisms to Bridge the Gap Between Science and Politics in Evidence-Informed Policymaking: Mapping the Landscape

Adèle Cassola, Patrick Fafard, Michèle Palkovits, and Steven J. Hoffman

1 INTRODUCTION

Efforts to improve the link between public health policy and scientific evidence are pervasive. The literature on evidence-based and evidence-informed policymaking has proliferated in recent decades, often reflecting

A. Cassola (✉) · M. Palkovits
Global Strategy Lab, York University, Toronto, ON, Canada
e-mail: adele.cassola@globalstrategylab.org

P. Fafard
Global Strategy Lab; Faculty of Social Sciences, Faculty of Medicine, Ottawa, ON, Canada

S. J. Hoffman
Global Strategy Lab; Global Health, Law, and Political Science, York University, Toronto, ON, Canada

© The Author(s) 2022
P. Fafard et al. (eds.), *Integrating Science and Politics for Public Health*,
Palgrave Studies in Public Health Policy Research,
https://doi.org/10.1007/978-3-030-98985-9_13

the idea that policy should "follow" evidence. However, criticisms during the COVID-19 pandemic (among other examples) that politicians did not base their decisions on scientific advice and data demonstrated that the relationship between evidence and policy is not straightforward. In particular, unresolved tensions remain between the importance of basing policy decisions on the best available scientific evidence and the need for elected decision-makers to balance competing goals, interests, values, and evidentiary sources in representative democracies. This chapter refers to this set of tensions as the "science-politics" gap.

1.1   Understanding the Gap Between Science and Politics in Public Health Policymaking

Three key strands of literature examine the gap between science and politics in public health policymaking from different (but not mutually exclusive) viewpoints. The "two communities"[1] perspective proceeds from the observation that "[t]here is a considerable gap between what research shows is effective and the policies that are enacted and enforced" (e.g., Brownson et al., 2009, p. 1576; Oxman et al., 2009). The literature identifies multiple potential barriers to the effective use of scientific evidence in policy processes, including a lack of scientific evidence that is accessible, relevant, or known to policymakers; a lack of capacity among policymakers to evaluate existing evidence; inadequate understanding of or interaction with the policy process by researchers; the different incentives and logics driving policymakers and scientists; a lack of political will or value attached to evidence-informed policymaking; the complexity and diffuseness of the policymaking process; and decision-makers' deference to interest group pressures or commitment to ideological positions that are not supported by the evidence base (Bonell et al., 2018; Brownson, 2011; Brownson et al., 2009; Choi, 2005; Pantoja et al., 2018). Although the "two communities" literature often acknowledges the diverse priorities and evidentiary sources that influence decision-makers, proponents of this perspective typically hold that the policy process would produce more health-promoting outcomes if it had a stronger foundation in scientific knowledge—particularly knowledge contained in rigorous evidence reviews or syntheses (such as systematic reviews of randomized control

---

[1] See Caplan (1979).

trials) (e.g., Anderson et al., 2005; Fielding & Briss, 2006; Oxman et al., 2009). In sum, the "gap" from this perspective is between the body of evidence that scientists have accumulated on the one hand and policymakers' use of that evidence on the other.

The "politics of evidence" strand of literature problematizes the question of what constitutes "evidence." This perspective challenges the idea of scientific evidence as objective and apolitical and points out that knowledge creation, analysis, interpretation, and utilization are all value-based processes that are influenced by, and reinforce, existing power structures (Cairney, 2016; Jasanoff, 2004; Stewart & Smith, 2015). Choices about how to frame research questions, which methods to use, what data to draw on, and how to evaluate success are all driven by researchers' and funders' priorities and worldviews. This perspective cautions against a belief in the "primacy and purity of scientific evidence" (Greer et al., 2017, p. 41), which can manifest in excessive trust in technical expertise and evidentiary hierarchies, limit debate about ethics and values, and prevent practical and experience-based knowledge from being considered in policy decisions (Corburn, 2007; Russell et al., 2008). Moreover, a focus on measuring problems and effects shifts attention to those issues and solutions that lend themselves to quantification, while populations or crises that are more difficult to research remain invisible and unaddressed (Corburn, 2007; Parkhurst, 2017; Russell et al., 2008). Here, the "gap" refers to understandings of what constitutes evidence between a technocratic or expert-oriented view and a more socially embedded conception.

The "policy complexity" strand of literature focuses on the nature of the policymaking process and the role of politics and evidence within it. Similar to the literature on the social construction of evidence, this perspective starts with the assumption that the production of evidence and its use in policymaking are fundamentally political (Cairney, 2016; Fafard, 2015; Hawkins & Parkhurst, 2016). The policymaking process is value-laden, involves multiple levels and actors, and is shaped by ideological, economic, financial, and temporal considerations; even when policymakers are aware of the evidence and wish to base their decisions on it, doing so may not be politically or financially feasible (Cairney, 2016; Cairney & Oliver, 2017; de Leeuw et al., 2014; K. Smith, 2013). Amid the complexity of the policy environment and the incomplete and contested nature of scientific evidence, the latter constitutes an important source of information but cannot yield certainty to decision-makers

(Fafard, 2015; French, 2018; Stewart & Smith, 2015). From this perspective, the "gap" refers to the difference between how some proponents of evidence-informed policy perceive the use of evidence by policymakers, and the complex, diffuse, and intrinsically political way in which it unfolds in practice.

1.2   Bridging the Gap Between Science and Politics in Public Health Policymaking

Although these three perspectives highlight different aspects of the science-politics gap, they share much potential common ground. For example, few would argue the extreme view that "politics is so pathological that no decision is based on an appeal to scientific evidence if it gets in the way of politicians seeking election, or so messy that the evidence gets lost somewhere in the political process" (Cairney, 2016, p. 2). Similarly, most would agree that the value-laden and political nature of evidence does not imply that facts are marginal or irrelevant to policymaking (Jasanoff, 2004; Latour, 2004). Consequently, there is a growing effort to bring insights on the nature of evidence and policymaking together with insights regarding robust scientific knowledge, with the goal of improving both the technical and democratic legitimacy of decision-making processes. These efforts ultimately aim to create systems of evidence utilization that reduce "issue bias" (the sidelining of social values and concerns through the prioritization of technical evidence) and "technical bias" (the use of evidence in ways that are not scientifically valid) (Parkhurst, 2017, pp. 7–8). Although numerous mechanisms have been proposed to achieve this goal, the field lacks a comprehensive conceptual overview of these mechanisms' objectives and potential contributions to the evidence-informed policymaking process. Proceeding from the perspective that the tensions between technical and political considerations can, and should, be reconciled, this chapter presents an inventory of relevant mechanisms, describes salient design considerations and trade-offs, and proposes a typology informed by key dimensions of variation.

2   METHODS

Using the above-mentioned tensions and debates as a starting point, we synthesized the literature on mechanisms that have been proposed to bring scientific evidence into public health policymaking in democratically and technically robust ways. We focused on two questions (Fafard & Cassola, 2020):

1. Which mechanisms have been proposed to produce and evaluate evidence in more participatory ways?
2. Which mechanisms have been proposed to enhance the integration of robust scientific evidence into the decision-making processes of institutions of representative democracy?

We focused on conceptual and empirical studies in public health and related fields (such as healthcare and environmental health) that specifically discussed tools to reconcile political and scientific considerations in evidence-informed policymaking. We identified sources through (1) our previous knowledge of the literature; (2) an iterative search of databases[2] covering public health and similar topic areas using search terms related to evidence-informed policymaking, bridging the science-politics gap, and specific types of mechanisms; and (3) forward-searching from article bibliographies. Where available, we prioritized review articles, overviews of multiple empirical cases, seminal and highly-cited articles, and articles that directly discussed the relevant mechanisms as bridges between scientific and political considerations in policymaking. We included articles that discussed mechanisms generally (not specifically in relation to public health or related fields) when they provided foundational information.

When reviewing sources, we listed the mechanisms they mentioned and extracted information about their goals, theories of impact, and operation.[3] We grouped the mechanisms into broad categories based on their objectives as they relate to the science-politics gap. We stopped reviewing articles at the point of saturation, when new sources did not yield substantially new types of mechanisms or information in these categories. We then synthesized salient themes and categorizations to develop a conceptual typology of mechanisms. In summarizing a vast and dispersed literature that lacks terminological or conceptual coherence, we employ the term

---

[2] Including ProQuest, ScienceDirect, EMBASE, MEDLINE, PsycInfo, Scholars Portal, Ingenta Connect, and Wiley Online.

[3] It was outside the scope of the chapter to evaluate mechanisms' effectiveness in achieving their goals.

"typology" to describe an organizational tool that helps to situate mechanisms in relation to one another and the field overall by identifying key dimensions of variation (Bailey, 1994; Collier et al., 2011).

3   MAPPING THE LANDSCAPE

We identified five broad categories of mechanisms that have been proposed in the literature to bridge the science-politics gap in public health and related fields: (1) co-production of evidence; (2) public deliberation of evidence; (3) knowledge mobilization[4]; (4) expert advisory bodies and roles; and (5) policy experimentation and evaluation (Table 1).[5] These categories were chosen because we identified considerable consistency in the literature regarding the objectives within them. At the same time, the categories often overlap, and mechanisms are sometimes differentially categorized and defined in the literature. For example, the *integrated knowledge translation* mechanism that we categorized under "knowledge mobilization" is sometimes discussed as a form of "co-production of evidence." Similarly, *citizens' juries* and *participatory Health Impact Assessments (HIAs) and Health Technology Assessments (HTAs)* may fall within either (or both) the co-production and deliberation categories of mechanisms discussed in this chapter, depending on the purpose and design of the process. Consequently, although we place them into discrete categories for the sake of analytical clarity, these mechanisms might in practice be considered to exist along a continuum. This section describes the objectives of each category of mechanisms, highlights examples, and describes challenges and design considerations associated with their use.

---

[4] In this chapter, we consider the term "knowledge mobilisation" to be interchangeable with another term that is often used to discuss this category of mechanisms—"knowledge translation and exchange."

[5] This chapter focuses on specific mechanisms that have been operationalized and implemented to address the science-politics gap. In a related approach, de Leeuw et al. (2008) identified seven categories of theories that address the integration of research, policy, and practice, which they term *institutional re-design, blurring the boundaries, utilitarian evidence, conduits, alternative evidence, narratives,* and *resonance.* The categories of mechanisms discussed in this chapter can all be seen as attempts at *institutional re-design* (i.e., devising institutional arrangements and channels of interaction that bridge the science-politics gap), although the mechanisms themselves variously target the structural and communicative concerns represented by the other six categories of theories.

Table 1 Mechanisms identified in the literature to bridge the gap between science and politics in public health policymaking

Category	Purpose	Theory of impact	Examples	Key design considerations and trade-offs
(1) Co-production of evidence	Address the socially embedded nature of evidence production by creating knowledge together with affected populations and/or knowledge users	Combining scientific expertise with the lay knowledge of service users and affected populations (and in some cases, the practical knowledge of policymakers and practitioners) will result in more contextually robust, relevant, and publicly acceptable knowledge for decision-making	• Community-based participatory research • Participatory health impact assessments • Participatory health technology assessments • Evidence-based activism	Timelines, goals, and epistemological views of participants may conflict. Decisions about who participates, at what stage, and with what decision-making power may be contested. Trade-offs may arise between scientific rigor on the one hand, and community relevance and legitimacy on the other.
(2) Public deliberation of evidence	Integrate public knowledge, values, and debate into evidence interpretation and decision-making processes	Holding informed and facilitated dialogues among researchers, policymakers, and/or members of the public will increase the likelihood that a diversity of values and considerations is accounted for in decision-making, thus enhancing democratic legitimacy	• Citizens' juries • Participatory budgeting • Consensus conferences • Deliberative polling • Stakeholder dialogues and roundtables	Trade-offs exist among size, representativeness, and deliberation quality. A priori decisions about process design (such as question and evidence selection) influence outcomes. A lack of participant authority or decision-maker accountability can lead to cynicism and disengagement.

(continued)

Table 1 (continued)

Category	Purpose	Theory of impact	Examples	Key design considerations and trade-offs
(3) Knowledge mobilization	Ensure that the appropriate policymakers have timely access to relevant and robust scientific evidence in an effective format	Enhancing the accessibility and relevance of scientific findings, and policymakers' ability to interpret them, will increase the use of robust scientific evidence in policymaking	• Knowledge platforms • Knowledge brokers and intermediaries • Integrated knowledge translation • Knowledge translation networks	Mismatches may arise between the nature and timelines of the scientific process in contrast to knowledge users' expectations and timeframes. Early and ongoing collaboration can enhance relevance and uptake and intermediary. platforms can provide resources and credibility Researchers must understand the complexity of the policy process.

Category	Purpose	Theory of impact	Examples	Key design considerations and trade-offs
(4) Expert advisory bodies and roles	Improve the technical quality, reliability, and relevance of scientific evidence available to inform decision-making	Establishing formal entities or roles composed of scientific experts who oversee or advise on the use of evidence in government decision-making will enhance the scientific basis and technical legitimacy of policy decisions	• Scientific advisory committees/panels • Scientific oversight and advisory roles • Organizations that systematically review or synthesize evidence for policy use • International evidentiary bodies	Elements of effective design include quality (soundness), relevance (applicability), and legitimacy (fairness, inclusivity, impartiality), but trade-offs may arise. The transparency that contributes to legitimacy may conflict with the privacy that can enhance quality. The participation of policymakers that can enhance relevance may conflict with the independence that can increase legitimacy.

(continued)

Table 1 (continued)

Category	Purpose	Theory of impact	Examples	Key design considerations and trade-offs
(5) Policy experimentation and evaluation	Determine the applied effectiveness and context-specific viability of policy interventions, as and after they are implemented	Evaluating new or amended policies or programs after a limited rollout under experimental conditions or over long time periods will generate contextual evidence of effectiveness to inform decisions about whether (and how) the policy or program should be implemented more widely	• Policy experiments • Pilot evaluations • Long-term impact evaluations • Design experiments • Policy innovation labs	The degree of integration or independence from government involves trade-offs between influencing policy and challenging the status quo. High degrees of experimental control can undermine generalizability. Expert-led technocratic experiments may have less policy influence than those that involve a broader set of societal actors.

3.1 Co-production of Evidence

Concern about excessive reverence toward technical and expert knowledge in policymaking has produced efforts to account for the social embeddedness of science and technology by increasing involvement of practitioners, patients, and/or affected communities in negotiating research priorities and generating evidence (Corburn, 2007; Rabeharisoa et al., 2014; Williams et al., 2020).[6] Co-productive research may be motivated by the normative goal of democratizing evidence production as an end in itself, as well as the practical goals of improving research quality, relevance, impact, and perceived legitimacy by integrating experience-based expertise (Corburn, 2007; Oliver et al., 2019; Williams et al., 2020).

Although it shares similarities with broader collaborative or participatory approaches to research, co-production is traditionally concerned with redistributing some of the power to frame and produce evidence from researchers and experts to affected communities and service users (Corburn, 2007; Williams et al., 2020). For example, *community-based participatory research (CBPR)* involves the structured participation of community members and organizations in research, recognizing them as experts in their own right and often including a capacity-building element (Jull et al., 2017; Viswanathan et al., 2004). Community participants in CBPR are viewed as equal partners rather than subjects, share in decision-making power and project ownership, and are ideally involved at all stages of the research process, including identifying research priorities and interpreting findings (Cashman et al., 2008; Jull et al., 2017; Richardson, 2014; Viswanathan et al., 2004). In a similar approach, patients' organizations involved in *evidence-based activism* "articulate credentialed knowledge with 'experiential knowledge'" in an effort to reshape dominant understandings of areas of concern and raise their political salience (Rabeharisoa et al., 2014, p. 115).

Similar principles have been integrated into processes like *participatory HIAs* and *HTAs*, which consider experience-based knowledge alongside

---

[6] The term 'co-production' is sometimes also used to refer to processes in which researchers and knowledge end-users (such as policymakers) collaborate at different stages of the research process. This is frequently termed *integrated knowledge translation (iKT)* and is discussed in more detail below (see Knowledge Mobilisation).

technical expertise in health-related decisions. HIAs often combine quantitative assessments of effectiveness and efficiency with residents' local knowledge to generate a more representative picture of the potential health impacts and underlying values of policy alternatives, encourage more transparent, accountable, equitable, and responsive policymaking, and increase community influence on policy decisions (Bhatia & Corburn, 2011; Den Broeder et al., 2017; Haigh et al., 2012; Harris-Roxas et al., 2012; Wright et al., 2005). Members of the affected community may be involved in developing the goals, questions, measures, and policy alternatives under review and can also identify gaps in knowledge that technical experts then work to address (Bhatia & Corburn, 2011). Patients' experiences and the public's views may also be included in HTAs, in combination with evaluations of technical and cost effectiveness, to incorporate more comprehensive knowledge and values into decisions about the use of these technologies (Abelson et al., 2007; Gagnon et al., 2011). This may involve participation in the "prioritization, scoping, evidence assessment, and dissemination of HTA findings" (Gagnon et al., 2011, p. 35), thus potentially spanning the co-production, deliberative, and knowledge mobilization categories of mechanisms discussed in this chapter.

There are several considerations and trade-offs associated with the selection and design of co-productive mechanisms. Because co-production involves prolonged engagement between experts and affected groups, it is time- and resource-intensive, raises complex research ethics considerations, involves potential costs to researchers and participants, and requires facilitation, relationship-building, and brokering skills (Cashman et al., 2008; Nyström et al., 2018; Oliver et al., 2019; E. Smith et al., 2008). The timelines, goals, and epistemological outlooks of traditional knowledge producers and their partners do not always align; for example, trade-offs may arise between the time required to effectively engage with communities and the desire for co-produced knowledge to influence time-sensitive policy processes (Cashman et al., 2008; Nyström et al., 2018; Wright et al., 2005). Careful attention to design is also required to ensure that co-production processes fulfill their objective of knowledge co-creation among technical and experiential experts, including in decisions regarding who participates, to what end, at what stage, and with what level of decision-making power (E. Smith et al., 2008; Wright et al., 2005). For example, involving community partners in decisions about research design and priorities can help increase equity and relevance at the outset of the research process (E. Smith et al., 2008; Williams et al., 2020). At the same time, considerations about who is included among the "affected community" or "service users" can be contested and will influence the representativeness and reliability of the knowledge produced through these mechanisms (Den Broeder et al., 2017; Oliver et al., 2019; E. Smith et al., 2008; Wright et al., 2005).

3.2 Public Deliberation of Evidence

Deliberative approaches involve structured fora that aim to integrate diverse knowledge and values into the evaluation of evidence, increase decision-makers' access to timely, relevant, and contextualized evidence interpretation, and enhance the public legitimacy of decisions (Boyko et al., 2012; Degeling et al., 2015; Fung, 2003; Lavis et al., 2014). Although a variety of deliberative approaches exists with different aims and designs (Fung, 2003), these mechanisms share roots in a long tradition of deliberative democracy in which including public stakeholders in dialogic decision-making spaces is considered important for democratic legitimacy and, indeed, a democratic ideal in itself (e.g., Cohen, 1997; Fafard, 2009).

Deliberative mechanisms typically bring participants up to date on the appropriate evidence base and possible interventions and enable them "to explore value-laden problems from a variety of perspectives and then work through the trade-offs of potential solutions" (Boyko et al., 2012, p. 1943). In *deliberative polling*, a random sample of several hundred members of the public is recruited for a deliberative dialogue that usually takes place over the course of a few days (Abelson et al., 2003; Fishkin et al., 2000; Maxwell et al., 2002). Participants receive background information about the issue at hand, take part in moderated discussions with other participants, and hear from expert panels representing diverse perspectives (Fishkin et al., 2000; Johnson, 2009). Participants' views are polled before and after deliberation, with the goal of measuring the change in opinions following education and deliberation—and ultimately of "expos[ing] [policymakers] to what a more informed state of public opinion would be like" (Fishkin et al., 2000, p. 664; Johnson, 2009).

In a slightly different approach, *citizens' juries* aim to ensure that public concerns and values guide the interpretation and use of evidence by assembling a small group of lay members of the public (often randomly selected), educating them about a policy issue, providing time for structured deliberation, and having them produce a decision or recommendation (Degeling et al., 2017; G. Smith & Wales, 2000; Street et al., 2014). The proceedings are moderated by trained facilitators, and participants typically hear from witnesses who represent a range of areas of expertise and relevant interests (G. Smith & Wales, 2000). Decisions are often reached through consensus, and in some cases, decision-makers may be required to respond to or adopt the jury's recommendations (Ritter et al., 2018; G. Smith & Wales, 2000; Street et al., 2014).

Deliberative decision-making can also be used to address equity for populations facing conditions of marginalization. *Participatory budgeting* processes involve sequential deliberative meetings during which a jurisdiction's residents participate equally alongside government representatives and other organizations to develop and vote on proposals for allocating public funds (Hagelskamp et al., 2018; Johnson, 2009; Wampler, 2007). Because this process usually enables the voting public to initiate the spending proposals that are put on the ballot, it can "raise awareness of community needs that may be forgotten or invisible under politics-as-usual" (Hagelskamp et al., 2018, p. 769), and although not a panacea, such processes may have a "moderate capacity to challenge social and political exclusion while promoting social justice" (Wampler, 2007, p. 45). Well-designed processes can also encourage more active citizenship and increased decision-making transparency, accountability, and legitimacy (Wampler, 2007).

Other deliberative mechanisms, such as *stakeholder dialogues and roundtables*, bring together representatives of groups that are identified as key stakeholders on different sides of a policy issue for structured meetings; these meetings provide opportunities for engagement that might not otherwise occur in traditional decision-making processes (Cuppen, 2012; Johnson, 2009). The goal is not necessarily to reach consensus, but rather to facilitate learning about the nature of the issue and potential policy responses through deliberation and synthesis of stakeholders' divergent expertise, values, and perspectives (Cuppen, 2012).

Despite these mechanisms' promise for broadening participation in evidence deliberation and interpretation, several design considerations and trade-offs exist. First, as with co-production, complex questions can arise regarding the affected population or stakeholder groups from which participants are drawn (Cuppen, 2012; G. Smith & Wales, 2000). In the case of open processes like participatory budgeting, citizens may face material, trust, interest-based, or other barriers to participating

(Ganuza & Francés, 2012; Hagelskamp et al., 2018). In processes like citizens' juries, assembling a small group can enhance the quality of deliberations, but may also hinder the recruitment of a geographically, demographically, and politically representative sample (Abelson et al., 2003; Boyko et al., 2012; G. Smith & Wales, 2000; Street et al., 2014). Second, although the equality of participants is a key tenet of deliberative dialogues, tacit beliefs or assumptions may lead to certain voices being devalued or excluded (Milewa, 2006). Third, decisions made prior to the proceedings—such as in the case of citizens' juries, the formulation of the question and the selection of witnesses and evidence—critically influence the outcomes of deliberative processes (Abelson et al., 2003; G. Smith & Wales, 2000). Fourth, when they do not include decision-making power for public participants, deliberative models may be perceived as tokenistic, unaccountable, or intended to legitimize foregone decisions and can lead to cynicism and disengagement (Abelson et al., 2003; Fung, 2015; Safaei, 2015). Finally, deliberative processes can be resource-intensive to implement (Boyko et al., 2012).

3.3   Knowledge Mobilization (KM)

One of the most common strategies discussed in the research literature to enhance the use of scientific evidence in public health decisions involves making existing knowledge more accessible and relevant to policymakers. This approach typically focuses on how the research community can increase the policy impact of empirical evidence (and particularly sources like systematic reviews and other evidence syntheses) by addressing policy-relevant questions and transferring research knowledge to decision-makers more effectively (e.g., Catallo et al., 2014; Grimshaw et al., 2012; Mitton et al., 2007).

KM mechanisms typically promote the tailoring of evidence for the relevant audience and increased interaction among knowledge creators and users. For example, *knowledge brokering* efforts aim to ensure that existing research evidence is effectively packaged (through briefs, summaries, reports, etc.) and actively shared (through dialogues, work-shops, briefings, etc.) to increase its demand and use by policymakers (Catallo et al., 2014; Ward et al., 2009). *Knowledge platforms* employ tools such as evidence briefs and policy dialogues to support the evidence-informed policy process and often involve partnerships among researchers and a range of knowledge users (El-Jardali et al., 2014; Partridge et al.,

2020). Some platforms, such as the Cochrane and Campbell Collaborations, are dedicated to increasing access to high-quality and reliable evidence syntheses.

With increased recognition of the complexity of the policy process and the need for more active engagement with decision-makers, a focus on *integrated knowledge translation (iKT)* has emerged. This strategy resembles co-production in that it involves collaboration between researchers and knowledge users (often policymakers) throughout the research and dissemination process (Jull et al., 2017; Kothari & Wathen, 2013; Lawrence et al., 2019; Nguyen et al., 2020). Like co-production models, iKT is based on a recognition that researchers and knowledge users have complementary expertise in producing relevant and grounded policy research (Jull et al., 2017). However, iKT processes are typically motivated by the goals of increasing research relevance and utilization and are usually less concerned with addressing issues of social embeddedness or power dynamics (Jull et al., 2017; Lawrence et al., 2019; Nguyen et al., 2020; Williams et al., 2020).

Like co-production and deliberative mechanisms, all KM strategies require extensive time and resource investments to build the relationships and trust that underpin their success (Lawrence et al., 2019; Mitton et al., 2007; Nguyen et al., 2020; Oliver et al., 2019). Because successful KM requires researchers to have time, resources, skills, and credibility, the presence of intermediary organizations, platforms, or structures dedicated to this work may facilitate successful efforts (Edwards et al., 2019; Grimshaw et al., 2012). The effectiveness of KM processes can be jeopardized by mismatches between the nature and timelines of the scientific process in contrast to knowledge users' expectations and timeframes, but early, phased, and ongoing collaboration can increase mutual understanding, enhance the relevance of research questions, and ultimately improve research uptake (Edwards et al., 2019; Kothari & Wathen, 2013; Lawrence et al., 2019; Mitton et al., 2007; Ward et al., 2009). Effective KM for public health policy also requires a robust understanding of the complexity of the policymaking process by those looking to improve evidence uptake (Fafard & Hoffman, 2020; Mitton et al., 2007; Oliver & Cairney, 2019).

3.4 Expert Advisory Bodies and Roles

Another set of mechanisms aims to provide timely and appropriate scientific expertise to policymakers by establishing formal entities or roles with a mandate to inform policy decisions through high-quality, relevant, and legitimate scientific evidence (Hoffman et al., 2018; Parkhurst, 2017). For example, *scientific advisory committees* are typically established to inform policy decisions "with the best available research evidence such that positive impact is maximized and negative (often unintended) consequences are minimized" (Hoffman et al., 2018, p. 2). Expert advisory bodies may be: ad hoc or permanent; statutorily mandated or voluntarily commissioned; designed to address broad science policy or more bounded issues; targeted at audiences internal or external to the institution that established them; and embedded within the government or at arm's length (Groux et al., 2018; OECD, 2015). As discussed in Chapter 9 (Hawkins & Oliver, 2022) of this book, *parliamentary committees* are another mechanism through which a range of evidence, including expert testimony, can be synthesized in order to support the scrutiny and development of policy action (Earwicker, 2012).

In some cases, individual officials exercise a similar mandate. *Scientific oversight/advisory roles*, such as Chief Science Advisors, are positioned "as broker[s] and expert navigator[s] between the government and the scientific community" and aim to ensure that policymakers interpret and use technical evidence in appropriate ways (OECD, 2015, p. 15; Parkhurst, 2017). In some cases, an individual official has multiple roles of which scientific oversight or advice is but one, as is the case with Chief Medical Officers in several Westminster countries and the Surgeon General in the United States (Fafard et al., 2018; MacAulay et al., 2021; Sheard & Donaldson, 2006; Stobbe, 2014).

The transnational nature of many contemporary scientific problems has also given rise to the establishment of *international advisory or evidentiary bodies*. For example, the World Health Organization (WHO) regularly convenes expert advisory panels and committees to provide technical guidance in specific areas (Gopinathan et al., 2018; WHO, 2021). Another mechanism that aims to institutionalize governments' access to expertise involves formal *organizations with a mandate to review and/or synthesize evidence to inform policy* (Parkhurst, 2017). For instance, the National Institute for Health and Care Excellence (NICE) in the

UK combines rigorous technical analyses of the effectiveness and efficiency of healthcare interventions with considerations of social and ethical values to inform the National Health Service and other health decision-makers (NICE, 2019; Parkhurst, 2017; Rawlins, 2015). Although the above-mentioned mechanisms aim to better ground public health policy decisions in technical evidence and expertise, these decisions nonetheless continue to require reconciliation of different values, interests, and goals—that is, they remain inherently political in nature (Gelijns et al., 2005; Lee, 2020).

The effectiveness of scientific advisory bodies may be thought of as a function of the quality (scientific soundness), relevance (applicability to the question at hand), and legitimacy (procedural fairness, inclusiveness, and impartiality) of their advice (Hoffman et al., 2018). The way in which these bodies are designed can influence perceptions of quality, relevance, and legitimacy. For example, perceptions of legitimacy may be influenced by the transparency of the advisory body's composition and processes, the representation of a diversity of experts, and the experts' degree of independence from the entities that convene the body, those that will use its advice, and those with which its expert members are affiliated (Behdinan et al., 2018; Gopinathan et al., 2018; Groux et al., 2018; Rowe et al., 2013). At the same time, design trade-offs exist (Gopinathan et al., 2018). For example, although transparent proceedings are critical to enhance legitimacy, closed-door discussions may be important for high-quality deliberations (Gopinathan et al., 2018). Additionally, although representation within advisory bodies is important to reduce bias and increase relevance, achieving this may prove challenging in specialized technical areas, within short timelines, or when strict conflict-of-interest exclusions reduce the pool of potential experts (Behdinan et al., 2018; Gopinathan et al., 2018). And although including policymakers and other end users in the proceedings can increase relevance, doing so may also cast doubt on the quality and legitimacy of the resulting advice (Andresen et al., 2018; Gopinathan et al., 2018).

3.5   Policy Experimentation and Evaluation

Once policymakers have considered different inputs into the policy process and proposed a path forward, policy experimentation and evaluation can generate additional knowledge of how a policy performs in context (Campbell, 1998; McFadgen & Huitema, 2018; Pearce &

Raman, 2014; Sanderson, 2002, 2009). This category of mechanisms seeks to address the inadequacy of a priori evidence for determining what will happen in practice, by helping policymakers to evaluate their proposed policies through pragmatic knowledge gained "in the experience of delivery" (Sanderson, 2009, p. 711).

Policy pilots and *policy experiments* typically aim to evaluate a limited rollout of a policy or program, often using randomized control trials or quasi-experimental methods, based on the assumption that the strong internal validity of such methods will lead to high-quality evidence that may be convincing to policymakers (Ettelt et al., 2015a, 2015b). Policy experiments can take different forms, including "technocratic" experiments led by scientific experts who proceed independently and present their results to policymakers; "boundary" experiments developed collaboratively among governmental and non-governmental actors that integrate "multiple knowledge systems" and "multiple value perspectives" in assessing solutions; and "advocacy" experiments led by policymakers in consultation with traditional interests who agree on the underlying framing of the problem at hand (McFadgen & Huitema, 2018, pp. 166–167).

Although experimental or quasi-experimental methods may be most suitable where there is considerable uncertainty regarding policy effects, *observational policy evaluations* are also useful for generating evidence of policy impact, particularly in cases characterized by less uncertainty, on questions that are not appropriately answered through experimentation, and to track policy outcomes during longer-term implementation processes (Petticrew, 2013; Sanderson, 2002, 2009). *Policy innovation labs* use a range of methodologies, including experimental methods, advanced data analytics, and/or user-centered design techniques (which often include ethnographic or participatory approaches) to foster new approaches to generate, test, and evaluate solutions to complex policy and service delivery problems (McGann et al., 2018; Olejniczak et al., 2020).

As is the case with other categories of mechanisms, the time horizons of policy experiments, pilots, and evaluations may not line up with those of policymaking, particularly when they aim to assess how policies address complex problems (Pearce & Raman, 2014; Sanderson, 2002). The degree of integration or independence from government of a policy lab, evaluation, or experiment may also involve trade-offs between policymaking influence and ability to challenge the status quo (McGann et al., 2018). Mechanisms that rely on experimental methods also face specific challenges. Although policy experiments can determine with some credibility the effectiveness of a policy in a specific social context, their conclusions are usually limited to a narrow selection of measurable outputs, and the high degree of experimental control can undermine the generalizability of the findings (Jensen, 2020; Sanderson, 2002). Some experiment designs may also be more influential on policymaking than others. For example, one analysis showed that expert-led technocratic experiments were considered by policymakers to have lower credibility, salience, and legitimacy compared to boundary and advocacy experiments, demonstrating that "when a broad set of actors contribute contextual, practical knowledge, this place-based knowledge improves credibility over scientifically defensible knowledge alone" (McFadgen & Huitema, 2018, p. 176).

4   Toward a Typology

Our analysis of mechanisms that have been proposed to bridge the science-politics gap identified several key dimensions of variation (Table 2) that represent a set of considerations for thinking through the selection and design of different mechanisms (Fig. 1). Although some of these dimensions differentiate categories of mechanisms (e.g., co-production and expert advisory bodies typically address different types of bias), others vary across mechanisms within the same category (e.g., different types of deliberative mechanisms may involve different actors or loci of authority).

4.1   Type of Bias Addressed

As discussed above, Parkhurst (2017) identifies two sources of bias relevant to evidence-informed policymaking: "issue bias" and "technical bias." The categories of mechanisms discussed here are typically oriented more strongly to addressing one or the other of these biases. For example, expert advisory bodies are established to reduce technical bias in policymaking by institutionalizing scientific expertise, while many deliberative mechanisms aim to reduce issue bias by fostering public debate of the evidence on value-laden issues. Because mechanisms that address one type of bias may fall short on considerations of another (such as when expert advisory bodies are critiqued as too technocratic or co-produced evidence is considered insufficiently scientific), mechanisms from different

Table 2 Proposed typology of mechanisms to bridge the gap between science and politics in public health policymaking

	Dimension	*Options*
Mechanism selection	Type of bias addressed[a]	Technical bias Issue bias
	Phase of the evidence-policy process[b]	Defining policy problems and priorities Generating evidence Evaluating evidence Inputting evidence into formal decision-making processes Evaluating policy outputs
	Relevant policy concerns	Uncertainty regarding outcomes Equity/social justice concerns Contested value-based issues "Hybrid" technical and value-based issues[c] Highly technical issues
Mechanism design	Actors and institutions involved	Researchers Technical experts Practitioners Policy/decision-makers Naïve publics[d] Affected publics[d] Partisan publics[d]
	Locus of authority	Traditional knowledge creators (experts/researchers) Traditional knowledge users (policy/decision-makers) Participating publics Shared
	Relationship with government actors	Independent Intermediated In partnership Integrated

[a]See Parkhurst (2017)
[b]Loosely adapted from de Leeuw and Peters (2014)
[c]See Degeling et al. (2015, 2017)
[d]See Degeling et al. (2015)

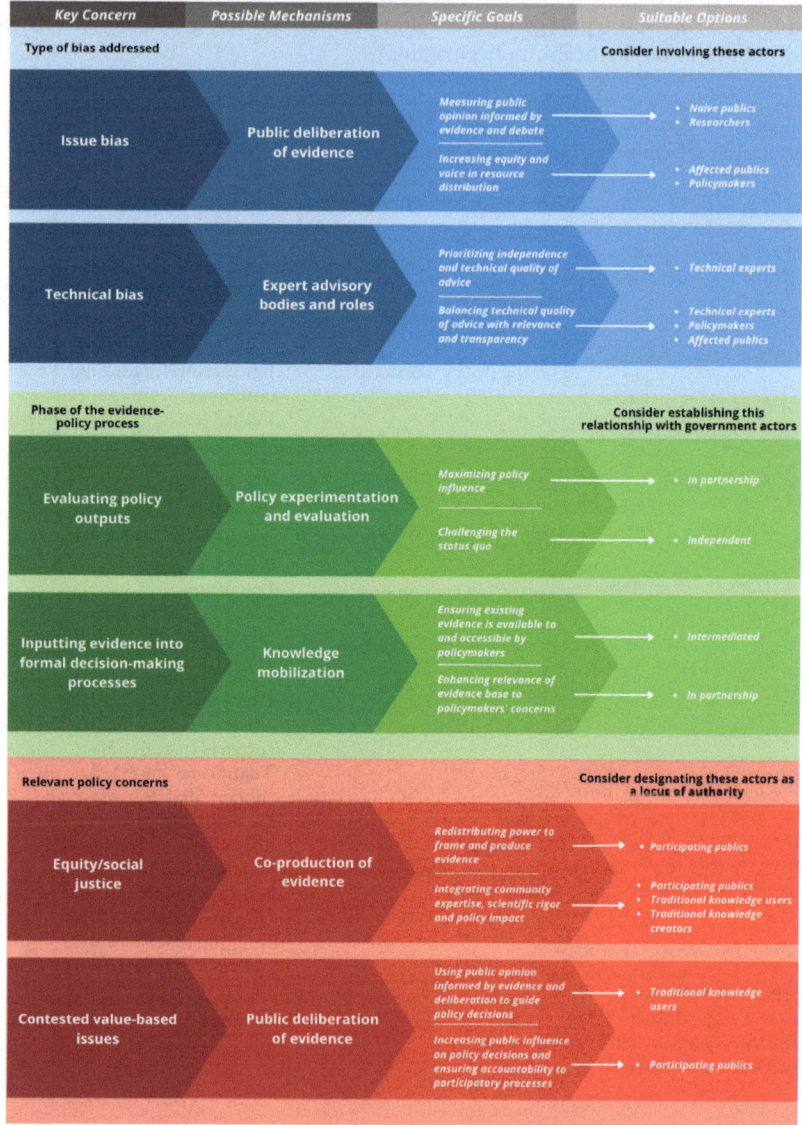

Fig. 1 Examples of typology dimensions in relation to mechanism selection and design[7]

[7] This figure is illustrative of different decision processes that the typology in Table 2 can help to facilitate. It is not a comprehensive list of all possible mechanisms, goals, or suitable options associated with addressing each concern.

categories may be combined to strengthen evidence-informed policy processes. For example, the mandate of NICE involves reducing technical bias in health decision-making through the rigorous and systematic review of evidence; however, the organization's Citizens Council, solicitation of commentary from pluralistic stakeholders on guidelines, and other participatory efforts are examples of strategies to reduce issue bias (Parkhurst, 2017; Rawlins, 2015).

4.2   Phase of the Evidence-Policy Process

Although policymaking is complex and cannot be neatly divided into sequential steps, each of the mechanisms reviewed in this chapter can be thought of as contributing to a different phase of the evidence-informed policymaking process, broadly conceived. For example, co-productive mechanisms such as CBPR can help to *define or redefine a problem* by marshaling locally-*generated evidence* that has traditionally not been part of the policy conversation. Deliberative mechanisms such as citizens' juries are often designed to *evaluate evidence* about a policy issue through a mediated dialogue among informed participants. Traditional KM mechanisms focus on *inputting existing evidence into formal decision-making processes*, while iKT may also span *problem definition* and *evidence generation*. Expert advisory bodies typically *evaluate evidence* and have channels for *inputting evidence into the decision-making processes*. Finally, policy experimentation and evaluation mechanisms typically focus on *evaluating policy outputs* to *generate evidence* that informs future decision-making (although policy innovation labs sometimes contribute more broadly across the evidence-policy process).

4.3   Relevant Policy Concerns

Within and across categories, different mechanisms may also be appropriate for addressing different policy concerns. For example, citizens' juries have been identified as useful for deliberating policy questions involving difficult value judgments that may benefit from the integration of expert and experience-based knowledge (Degeling et al., 2017). SACs may be most appropriate for highly technical questions—although principles of open deliberation, transparency, accountability, and contestability should still apply (Andresen et al., 2018; OECD, 2015; Parkhurst, 2017). Co-production mechanisms like CBPR (which broadens the locus of authority on problem definition and evidence generation) and participatory budgeting (which expands decision-making and voice on resource allocation issues) may be most appropriate where the concern is to increase equity and social justice in policymaking. Finally, where the policy concern involves a high level of uncertainty regarding policy outcomes, experimental policy pilots may be the most appropriate mechanism.

4.4   Actors and Institutions Involved

Considerable variation exists across and within mechanisms regarding the actors and institutions involved. Expert bodies such as SACs are typically composed of purposively selected professionals with specialized and in-depth technical knowledge of a particular subject. Traditional KM approaches often rely on self-selected researchers or research platforms that attempt to transfer their knowledge to relevant decision-makers, although knowledge users may also be directly and formally involved in knowledge platforms and iKT processes. As discussed above, policy experiments can also be led by different constellations of actors, including scientific experts, governmental entities, and groups with affected interests (McFadgen & Huitema, 2018). Among mechanisms that involve public participation, a key distinction involves the type of "public" that participates. Degeling and co-authors (2015, p. 117) identify three categories: (1) citizens or naïve publics, who are construed as "a subject of education, and then, potentially as decision maker"; (2) affected consumers, who are seen as "the authentic expert[s]" about the issue at hand; and (3) partisan publics, who represent interest groups and affected organizations. For example, stakeholder roundtables typically bring together purposively selected members of partisan publics while deliberative polling typically involves randomly selected members of the naïve public.

4.5   Locus of Authority

Mechanisms also vary in the level of authority or decision-making power allocated to different actors. One consideration involves the degree to which the input of different parties is considered binding or advisory. For instance, the recommendations of expert advisory bodies carry authority but are, as the name suggests, typically non-binding, while the findings of citizens' juries are occasionally designed to be binding on decision-makers or to require a formal response. Another consideration for mechanisms that involve evidence creation and deliberation concerns the degree of control at different stages of the process, such as defining the policy problem and deciding how to frame results. As discussed above, the ways in which considerations about authority are addressed in mechanisms' design have implications for, and raise trade-offs among, the perceived legitimacy, quality, and relevance of the resulting processes. For example, trade-offs may arise in co-production processes when it comes to balancing scientific rigor (implying a measure of control for researchers) with relevance and legitimacy (implying a measure of control for members of affected communities).

4.6   Relationship with Government Actors and Institutions

Finally, variation exists both across and within categories of mechanisms regarding their relationship with government entities. At a local level, for example, CBPR initiatives may emerge *independently* through research institutions or civil society or may be undertaken *in partnership* with planners and policymakers. Citizens' juries can similarly take place as independent research exercises or in partnership with decision-makers; if designed independently from government actors, they are likely to require an *intermediary* such as a knowledge broker to influence the policy process (Degeling et al., 2017). Policy experiments may emerge independently from, in partnership with, or at the behest of government actors and may be characterized by different levels of government funding and oversight (McFadgen & Huitema, 2018; McGann et al., 2018). Expert advisory committees may be *integrated* within the structures of government or exist at arm's length (Groux et al., 2018; OECD, 2015).

5   DISCUSSION

The research literature in public health and related fields is replete with references to specific mechanisms devoted to bridging the science-politics gap, but it lacks a common language or framework for discussing them. This chapter has conceptually organized the literature on mechanisms to "democratize expertise" and "expertise democracy" (Liberatore & Funtowicz, 2003, p. 146) and identified key dimensions of variation in their goals, orientation, and design. The aim has been to introduce more robustness and consistency in how the field thinks and writes about these mechanisms and greater clarity in how those involved in using them orient their design to specific objectives.

On a practical level, this chapter has highlighted that no single mechanism or category of mechanisms is sufficient to address the science-politics gap in evidence-informed policymaking. Each mechanism has potential advantages and disadvantages for achieving different goals and for different actors involved in the process (e.g., Oliver et al., 2019). In addition, contextual factors affect the feasibility and appropriateness of specific mechanisms in places with different administrative traditions, political cultures, and research system capacities (e.g., Cavazza & Jommi, 2012; Huxley et al., 2016). It is therefore critical for those using these mechanisms to be clear about the goals they are trying to achieve, attentive to the specific environment they are working in, and intentional about issues such as who participates, with what authority, and how this impacts the legitimacy, quality, and relevance of the process and outputs.

Although this chapter has focused on categorizing mechanisms according to their goals and characteristics, it is also critical to consider the overarching components of the good governance of evidence production and utilization in policymaking (Hawkins & Parkhurst, 2016; Parkhurst, 2017). These elements include ensuring that the evidence used in policy decisions is high-quality, rigorous, and appropriate to the question at hand; that the selection of evidence is transparent, involves public deliberation, and is open to contestation; and that the public or its representatives are involved in stewarding the advisory system and making the final evidence-informed decisions (Parkhurst, 2017, pp. 161–162).

Finally, this chapter exists because the past few decades have seen a vast amount of thinking and research on mechanisms to bridge the science-politics gap in public health policymaking. Yet many of the debates happening in the context of the COVID-19 pandemic at the time of writing reflect continuing weaknesses in and dissatisfaction with the mechanisms in place to balance technical considerations with competing values, interests, and goals in government responses around the world. In fact, a perceived battle between science and politics has been one of the defining features of the pandemic discourse. As those concerned with policy, research, and governance begin to scrutinize the pandemic response with an eye to reform, the inventory of mechanisms discussed in this chapter should serve as a roadmap for reconciling technical and political considerations toward more robust and resilient approaches to future crises.

REFERENCES

Abelson, J., Forest, P.-G., Eyles, J., Smith, P., Martin, E., & Gauvin, F.-P. (2003). Deliberations about deliberative methods: Issues in the design and evaluation of public participation processes. *Social Science & Medicine, 57*(2), 239–251. https://doi.org/10.1016/S0277-9536(02)00343-X

Abelson, J., Giacomini, M., Lehoux, P., & Gauvin, F.-P. (2007). Bringing 'the public' into health technology assessment and coverage policy decisions: From principles to practice. *Health Policy, 82*(1), 37–50. https://doi.org/10.1016/j.healthpol.2006.07.009

Anderson, L. M., Brownson, R. C., Fullilove, M. T., Teutsch, S. M., Novick, L. F., Fielding, J., & Land, G. H. (2005). Evidence-based public health policy and practice: Promises and limits. *American Journal of Preventive Medicine, 28*(5), 226–230. https://doi.org/10.1016/j.amepre.2005.02.014

Andresen, S., Baral, P., Hoffman, S. J., & Fafard, P. (2018). What can be learned from experience with scientific advisory committees in the field of international environmental politics? *Global Challenges, 2*(9), 1800055. https://doi.org/10.1002/gch2.201800055

Bailey, K. D. (1994). *Typologies and taxonomies: An introduction to classification techniques*. Sage.

Behdinan, A., Gunn, E., Baral, P., Sritharan, L., Fafard, P., & Hoffman, S. J. (2018). An overview of systematic reviews to inform the institutional design of scientific advisory committees. *Global Challenges, 2*(9), 1800019. https://doi.org/10.1002/gch2.201800019

Bhatia, R., & Corburn, J. (2011). Lessons from San Francisco: Health impact assessments have advanced political conditions for improving population health. *Health Affairs, 30*(12), 2410–2418. https://doi.org/10.1377/hlthaff.2010.1303

Bonell, C., Meiksin, R., Mays, N., Petticrew, M., & McKee, M. (2018). Defending evidence-informed policy making from ideological attack. *BMJ, 362*, k3827. https://doi.org/10.1136/bmj.k3827

Boyko, J. A., Lavis, J. N., Abelson, J., Dobbins, M., & Carter, N. (2012). Deliberative dialogues as a mechanism for knowledge translation and exchange in health systems decision-making. *Social Science & Medicine, 75*(11), 1938–1945. https://doi.org/10.1016/j.socscimed.2012.06.016

Brownson, R. C. (2011). *Evidence-based public health*. Oxford University Press.

Brownson, R. C., Chriqui, J. F., & Stamatakis, K. A. (2009). Understanding evidence-based public health policy. *American Journal of Public Health, 99*(9), 1576–1583. https://doi.org/10.2105/AJPH.2008.156224

Cairney, P. (2016). *The politics of evidence-based policy making*. Springer.

Cairney, P., & Oliver, K. (2017). Evidence-based policymaking is not like evidence-based medicine, so how far should you go to bridge the divide between evidence and policy? *Health Research Policy and Systems, 15*(1), 35. https://doi.org/10.1186/s12961-017-0192-x

Campbell, D. T. (1998). The experimenting society. In W. N. Dunn (Ed.), *The experimenting society: Essays in honor of Donald T. Campbell* (pp. 35–68). Transaction Publishers.

Caplan, N. (1979). The two-communities theory and knowledge utilization. *American Behavioral Scientist, 22*(3), 459–470. https://doi.org/10.1177/000276427902200308

Cashman, S. B., Adeky, S., Allen, A. J., III, Corburn, J., Israel, B. A., Montaño, J., Rafelito, A., Rhodes, S. D., Swanston, S., Wallerstein, N., & Eng, E. (2008). The power and the promise: Working with communities to analyze data, interpret findings, and get to outcomes. *American Journal of Public Health, 98*(8), 1407–1417. https://doi.org/10.2105/AJPH.2007.113571

Catallo, C., Lavis, J. N., & The BRIDGE study team. (2014). Knowledge brokering in public health. In B. Rechel & M. McKee (Eds.), *Facets of public health in Europe* (pp. 301–316). Open University Press.

Cavazza, M., & Jommi, C. (2012). Stakeholders involvement by HTA Organisations: Why is so different? *Health Policy, 105*(2–3), 236–245. https://doi.org/10.1016/j.healthpol.2012.01.012

Choi, B. C. K. (2005). Can scientists and policy makers work together? *Journal of Epidemiology & Community Health, 59*(8), 632–637. https://doi.org/10.1136/jech.2004.031765

Cohen, J. (1997). Deliberation and democratic legitimacy. In J. Bohman & W. Rehg (Eds.), *Deliberative democracy: Essays on reason and politics* (pp. 67–92). MIT Press.

Collier, D., Laporte, J., & Seawright, J. (2011). Putting typologies to work: Concept formation, measurement, and analytic rigor. *Political Research Quarterly, 65*(1), 217–232. https://doi.org/10.1177/1065912912437162

Corburn, J. (2007). Community knowledge in environmental health science: Co-producing policy expertise. *Environmental Science & Policy, 10*(2), 150–161. https://doi.org/10.1016/j.envsci.2006.09.004

Cuppen, E. (2012). Diversity and constructive conflict in stakeholder dialogue: Considerations for design and methods. *Policy Sciences, 45*(1), 23–46. https://doi.org/10.1007/s11077-011-9141-7

de Leeuw, E., Clavier, C., & Breton, E. (2014). Health policy—Why research it and how: Health political science. *Health Research Policy and Systems, 12*(1). https://doi.org/10.1186/1478-4505-12-55

de Leeuw, E., McNess, A., Crisp, B., & Stagnitti, K. (2008). Theoretical reflections on the nexus between research, policy and practice. *Critical Public Health, 18*(1), 5–20. https://doi.org/10.1080/09581590801949924

de Leeuw, E., & Peters, D. (2014). Nine questions to guide development and implementation of health in all policies. *Health Promotion International, 30*(4), 987–997. https://doi.org/10.1093/heapro/dau034

Degeling, C., Carter, S. M., & Rychetnik, L. (2015). Which public and why deliberate?—A scoping review of public deliberation in public health and health policy research. *Social Science & Medicine, 131,* 114–121. https://doi.org/10.1016/j.socscimed.2015.03.009

Degeling, C., Rychetnik, L., Street, J., Thomas, R., & Carter, S. M. (2017). Influencing health policy through public deliberation: Lessons learned from two decades of Citizens'/community juries. *Social Science & Medicine, 179,* 166–171. https://doi.org/10.1016/j.socscimed.2017.03.003

Den Broeder, L., Uiters, E., ten Have, W., Wagemakers, A., & Schuit, A. J. (2017). Community participation in Health Impact Assessment: A scoping review of the literature. *Environmental Impact Assessment Review, 66,* 33–42. https://doi.org/10.1016/j.eiar.2017.06.004

Earwicker, R. (2012). The role of parliaments: The case of a parliamentary scrutiny. In D. V. McQueen, M. Wismar, V. Lin, C. M. Jones, & M. Davies (Eds.), *Intersectoral governance for health in all policies: Structures, actions and experiences* (pp. 69–84). World Health Organization, on behalf of the European Observatory on Health Systems and Policies.

Edwards, A., Zweigenthal, V., & Olivier, J. (2019). Evidence map of knowledge translation strategies, outcomes, facilitators and barriers in African health systems. *Health Research Policy and Systems, 17*(16). https://doi.org/10.1186/s12961-019-0419-0

El-Jardali, F., Lavis, J., Moat, K., Pantoja, T., & Ataya, N. (2014). Capturing lessons learned from evidence-to-policy initiatives through structured reflection. *Health Research Policy and Systems, 12*(2).

Ettelt, S., Mays, N., & Allen, P. (2015a). The multiple purposes of policy piloting and their consequences: Three examples from national health and social care policy in England. *Journal of Social Policy, 44*(2), 319–337. https://doi.org/10.1017/S0047279414000865

Ettelt, S., Mays, N., & Allen, P. (2015b). Policy experiments: Investigating effectiveness or confirming direction? *Evaluation, 21*(3), 292–307. https://doi.org/10.1177/1356389015590737

Fafard, P. (2009). Challenging English-Canadian orthodoxy on democracy and constitutional change. *Review of Constitutional Studies, 14,* 175–203.

Fafard, P. (2015). Beyond the usual suspects: Using political science to enhance public health policy making. *Journal of Epidemiology and Community Health, 69*(11), 1129–1132. https://doi.org/10.1136/jech-2014-204608

Fafard, P., & Cassola, A. (2020). Public health and political science: Challenges and opportunities for a productive partnership. *Public Health, 186,* 107–109. https://doi.org/10.1016/j.puhe.2020.07.004

Fafard, P., & Hoffman, S. J. (2020). Rethinking knowledge translation for public health policy. *Evidence & Policy, 16*(1). https://doi.org/10.1332/174426 418X15212871808802

Fafard, P., McNena, B., Suszek, A., & Hoffman, S. J. (2018). Contested roles of Canada's Chief Medical Officers of Health. *Canadian Journal of Public Health, 109*, 585–589. https://doi.org/10.17269/s41997-018-0080-3

Fielding, J. E., & Briss, P. A. (2006). Promoting evidence-based public health policy: Can we have better evidence and more action? *Health Affairs, 25*(4), 969–978. https://doi.org/10.1377/hlthaff.25.4.969

Fishkin, J., Luskin, R., & Jowell, R. (2000). Deliberative polling and public consultation. *Parliamentary Affairs, 53*(4), 657–666. https://doi.org/10. 1093/pa/53.4.657

French, R. D. (2018). Lessons from the evidence on evidence-based policy. *Canadian Public Administration, 61*(3), 425–442. https://doi.org/10. 1111/capa.12295

Fung, A. (2003). Recipes for public spheres: Eight institutional design choices and their consequences. *The Journal of Political Philosophy, 11*(3), 338–367. https://doi.org/10.1111/1467-9760.00181

Fung, A. (2015). Putting the public back into governance: The challenges of citizen participation and its future. *Public Administration Review, 75*(4), 513–522. https://doi.org/10.1111/puar.12361

Gagnon, M.-P., Desmartis, M., Lepage-Savary, D., Gagnon, J., St-Pierre, M., Rhainds, M., Lemieux, R., Gauvin, F.-P., Pollender, H., & Légaré, F. (2011). Introducing patients' and the public's perspectives to health technology assessment: A systematic review of international experiences. *International Journal of Technology Assessment in Health Care, 27*(1), 31–42. https://doi.org/10. 1017/S0266462310001315

Ganuza, E., & Francés, F. (2012). The deliberative turn in participation: The problem of inclusion and deliberative opportunities in participatory budgeting. *European Political Science Review, 4*(2), 283–302. https://doi. org/10.1017/S1755773911000270

Gelijns, A. C., Brown, L. D., Magnell, C., Ronchi, E., & Moskowitz, A. J. (2005). Evidence, politics, and technological change. *Health Affairs, 24*(1), 29–40. https://doi.org/10.1377/hlthaff.24.1.29

Gopinathan, U., Hoffman, S. J., & Ottersen, T. (2018). Scientific advisory committees at the World Health Organization: A qualitative study of how their design affects quality, relevance, and legitimacy. *Global Challenges, 2*(9), 1700074. https://doi.org/10.1002/gch2.201700074

Greer, S. L., Bekker, M., de Leeuw, E., Wismar, M., Helderman, J.-K., Ribeiro, S., & Stuckler, D. (2017). Policy, politics and public health. *European Journal of Public Health, 27*(suppl_4), 40–43. https://doi.org/10.1093/eurpub/ ckx152

Grimshaw, J. M., Eccles, M. P., Lavis, J. N., Hill, S. J., & Squires, J. E. (2012). Knowledge translation of research findings. *Implementation Science, 7*(1), 50. https://doi.org/10.1186/1748-5908-7-50

Groux, G. M. N., Hoffman, S. J., & Ottersen, T. (2018). A typology of scientific advisory committees. *Global Challenges, 2*(9), 1800004. https://doi.org/10.1002/gch2.201800004

Hagelskamp, C., Schleifer, D., Rinehart, C., & Silliman, R. (2018). Participatory budgeting: Could it diminish health disparities in the United States? *Journal of Urban Health, 95*(5), 766–771. https://doi.org/10.1007/s11524-018-0249-3

Haigh, F., Harris, P., & Haigh, N. (2012). Health impact assessment research and practice: A place for paradigm positioning? *Environmental Impact Assessment Review, 33*(1), 66–72. https://doi.org/10.1016/j.eiar.2011.10.006

Harris-Roxas, B., Viliani, F., Bond, A., Cave, B., Divall, M., Furu, P., Harris, P., Soeberg, M., Wernham, A., & Winkler, M. (2012). Health impact assessment: The state of the art. *Impact Assessment and Project Appraisal, 30*(1), 43–52. https://doi.org/10.1080/14615517.2012.666035

Hawkins, B., & Oliver, K. (2022). Select committee governance and the production of evidence: The case of UK E-Cigarettes policy. In P. Fafard, A. Cassola, & E. de Leeuw (Eds.), *Integrating science and politics for public health.* Palgrave Springer.

Hawkins, B., & Parkhurst, J. (2016). The "good governance" of evidence in health policy. *Evidence & Policy, 12*(4), 575–592. https://doi.org/10.1332/174426415X14430058455412

Hoffman, S. J., Ottersen, T., Tejpar, A., Baral, P., & Fafard, P. (2018). Towards a systematic understanding of how to institutionally design scientific advisory committees: A conceptual framework and introduction to a special journal issue. *Global Challenges, 2*(9), 1800020. https://doi.org/10.1002/gch2.201800020

Huxley, K., Andrews, R., Downe, J., & Guarneros-Meza, V. (2016). Administrative traditions and citizen participation in public policy: A comparative study of France, Germany, the UK and Norway. *Policy & Politics, 44*(3), 383–402. https://doi.org/10.1332/030557315X14298700857974

Jasanoff, S. (Ed.). (2004). *States of knowledge: The co-production of science and social order.* Routledge.

Jensen, P. H. (2020). Experiments and evaluation of public policies: Methods, implementation, and challenges. *Australian Journal of Public Administration, 79*(2), 259–268. https://doi.org/10.1111/1467-8500.12406

Johnson, G. F. (2009). Deliberative democratic practices in Canada: An analysis of institutional empowerment in three cases. *Canadian Journal of Political Science, 42*(3), 679–703. https://doi.org/10.1017/S0008423909990072

Jull, J., Giles, A., & Graham, I. D. (2017). Community-based participatory research and integrated knowledge translation: Advancing the co-creation of knowledge. *Implementation Science, 12*(1). https://doi.org/10.1186/s13012-017-0696-3

Kothari, A., & Wathen, C. N. (2013). A critical second look at integrated knowledge translation. *Health Policy, 109*(2), 187–191. https://doi.org/10.1016/j.healthpol.2012.11.004

Latour, B. (2004). Why has critique run out of steam? From matters of fact to matters of concern. *Critical Inquiry, 30*(2), 225–248. https://doi.org/10.1086/421123

Lavis, J. N., Boyko, J. A., & Gauvin, F.-P. (2014). Evaluating deliberative dialogues focused on healthy public policy. *BMC Public Health, 14*(1). https://doi.org/10.1186/1471-2458-14-1287

Lawrence, L. M., Bishop, A., & Curran, J. (2019). Integrated knowledge translation with public health policy makers: A scoping review. *Healthcare Policy = Politiques de Sante, 14*(3), 55–77. https://doi.org/10.12927/hcpol.2019.25792

Lee, K. (2020). WHO under fire: The need to elevate the quality of politics in global health. *Global Social Policy, 20*(3), 374–377. https://doi.org/10.1177/1468018120966661

Liberatore, A., & Funtowicz, S. (2003). 'Democratising' expertise, 'expertising' democracy: What does this mean, and why bother? *Science and Public Policy, 30*(3), 146–150. https://doi.org/10.3152/147154303781780551

MacAulay, M., Macintyre, A. K., Yashadhana, A., Cassola, A., Harris, P., Woodward, C., Smith, K., de Leeuw, E., Palkovits, M., Hoffman, S. J., & Fafard, P. (2021). Under the spotlight: Understanding the role of the Chief Medical Officer in a pandemic. *Journal of Epidemiology and Community Health.* https://doi.org/10.1136/jech-2021-216850

Maxwell, J., Jackson, K., Legowski, B., Rosell, S., Yankelovich, D., Forest, P.-G., & Lozowchuk, L. (2002). *Report on citizens' dialogue on the future of health care in Canada*. Commission on the Future of Health Care in Canada.

McFadgen, B., & Huitema, D. (2018). Experimentation at the interface of science and policy: A multi-case analysis of how policy experiments influence political decision-makers. *Policy Sciences, 51*(2), 161–187. https://doi.org/10.1007/s11077-017-9276-2

McGann, M., Blomkamp, E., & Lewis, J. M. (2018). The rise of public sector innovation labs: Experiments in design thinking for policy. *Policy Sciences, 51*(3), 249–267. https://doi.org/10.1007/s11077-018-9315-7

Milewa, T. (2006). Health technology adoption and the politics of governance in the UK. *Social Science & Medicine, 63*(12), 3102–3112. https://doi.org/10.1016/j.socscimed.2006.08.009

Mitton, C., Adair, C. E., McKenzie, E., Patten, S. B., & Perry, B. W. (2007). Knowledge transfer and exchange: Review and synthesis of the literature. *Milbank Quarterly, 85*(4), 729–768.

NICE. (2019). *National Institute for Health Care and Excellence: What we do.* National Institute for Health Care and Excellence. Retrieved 18 June, 2019, from https://www.nice.org.uk/about/what-we-do

Nguyen, T., Graham, I. D., Mrklas, K. J., Bowen, S., Cargo, M., Estabrooks, C. A., Kothari, A., Lavis, J., Macaulay, A. C., MacLeod, M., Phipps, D., Ramsden, V. R., Renfrew, M. J., Salsberg, J., & Wallerstein, N. (2020). How does integrated knowledge translation (IKT) compare to other collaborative research approaches to generating and translating knowledge? Learning from experts in the field. *Health Research Policy and Systems, 18*(1), 35. https://doi.org/10.1186/s12961-020-0539-6

Nyström, M. E., Karltun, J., Keller, C., & Andersson Gäre, B. (2018). Collaborative and partnership research for improvement of health and social services: Researcher's experiences from 20 projects. *Health Research Policy and Systems, 16*(1), 46. https://doi.org/10.1186/s12961-018-0322-0

OECD. (2015). *Scientific advice for policy making: The role and responsibility of expert bodies and individual scientists* (OECD Science, Technology and Industry Policy Papers No. 21). https://doi.org/10.1787/5js33l1jcpwb-en

Olejniczak, K., Borkowska-Waszak, S., Domaradzka-Widła, A., & Park, Y. (2020). Policy labs: The next frontier of policy design and evaluation? *Policy & Politics, 48*(1), 89–110. https://doi.org/10.1332/030557319X15579230420108

Oliver, K., & Cairney, P. (2019). The dos and don'ts of influencing policy: A systematic review of advice to academics. *Palgrave Communications, 5*(1), 21. https://doi.org/10.1057/s41599-019-0232-y

Oliver, K., Kothari, A., & Mays, N. (2019). The dark side of coproduction: Do the costs outweigh the benefits for health research? *Health Research Policy and Systems, 17*(1), 33. https://doi.org/10.1186/s12961-019-0432-3

Oxman, A. D., Lavis, J. N., Lewin, S., & Fretheim, A. (2009). SUPPORT Tools for evidence-informed health Policymaking (STP) 1: What is evidence-informed policymaking? *Health Research Policy and Systems, 7*(S1). https://doi.org/10.1186/1478-4505-7-S1-S1

Pantoja, T., Barreto, J., & Panisset, U. (2018). Improving public health and health systems through evidence-informed policy in the Americas. *BMJ,* k2469. https://doi.org/10.1136/bmj.k2469

Parkhurst, J. O. (2017). *The politics of evidence: From evidence-based policy to the good governance of evidence.* Routledge.

Partridge, A. C. R., Mansilla, C., Randhawa, H., Lavis, J. N., El-Jardali, F., & Sewankambo, N. K. (2020). Lessons learned from descriptions and evaluations of knowledge translation platforms supporting evidence-informed policy-making in low- and middle-income countries: A systematic review. *Health Research Policy and Systems, 18*(1), 127. https://doi.org/10.1186/s12961-020-00626-5

Pearce, W., & Raman, S. (2014). The new randomised controlled trials (RCT) movement in public policy: Challenges of epistemic governance. *Policy Sciences, 47*(4), 387–402. https://doi.org/10.1007/s11077-014-9208-3

Petticrew, M. (2013). Public health evaluation: Epistemological challenges to evidence production and use. *Evidence & Policy, 9*(1), 87–95. https://doi.org/10.1332/174426413X663742

Rabeharisoa, V., Moreira, T., & Akrich, M. (2014). Evidence-based activism: Patients', users' and activists' groups in knowledge society. *BioSocieties, 9*(2), 111–128. https://doi.org/10.1057/biosoc.2014.2

Rawlins, M. D. (2015). National Institute for Clinical Excellence: NICE works. *Journal of the Royal Society of Medicine, 108*(6), 211–219. https://doi.org/10.1177/0141076815587658

Richardson, L. (2014). Engaging the public in policy research: Are community researchers the answer? *Politics and Governance, 2*(1), 32–44. https://doi.org/10.17645/pag.v2i1.19

Ritter, A., Lancaster, K., & Diprose, R. (2018). Improving drug policy: The potential of broader democratic participation. *International Journal of Drug Policy, 55*, 1–7. https://doi.org/10.1016/j.drugpo.2018.01.016

Rowe, S., Alexander, N., Weaver, C. M., Dwyer, J. T., Drew, C., Applebaum, R. S., Atkinson, S., Clydesdale, F. M., Hentges, E., Higley, N. A., & Westring, M. E. (2013). How experts are chosen to inform public policy: Can the process be improved? *Health Policy, 112*(3), 172–178. https://doi.org/10.1016/j.healthpol.2013.01.012

Russell, J., Greenhalgh, T., Byrne, E., & Mcdonnell, J. (2008). Recognizing rhetoric in health care policy analysis. *Journal of Health Services Research & Policy, 13*(1), 40–46. https://doi.org/10.1258/jhsrp.2007.006029

Safaei, J. (2015). Deliberative democracy in health care: Current challenges and future prospects. *Journal of Healthcare Leadership*, 123. https://doi.org/10.2147/JHL.S70021

Sanderson, I. (2002). Evaluation, policy learning and evidence-based policy making. *Public Administration, 80*(1), 1–22. https://doi.org/10.1111/1467-9299.00292

Sanderson, I. (2009). Intelligent policy making for a complex world: Pragmatism, evidence and learning. *Political Studies, 57*(4), 699–719. https://doi.org/10.1111/j.1467-9248.2009.00791.x

Sheard, S., & Donaldson, L. J. (2006). *The nation's doctor: The role of the Chief Medical Officer 1855–1998*. Radcliffe.

Smith, E., Ross, F., Donovan, S., Manthorpe, J., Brearley, S., Sitzia, J., & Beresford, P. (2008). Service user involvement in nursing, midwifery and health visiting research: A review of evidence and practice. *International Journal of Nursing Studies, 45*(2), 298–315. https://doi.org/10.1016/j.ijnurstu.2006.09.010

Smith, G., & Wales, C. (2000). Citizens' juries and deliberative democracy. *Political Studies, 48,* 51–65.

Smith, K. (2013). *Beyond evidence based policy in public health.* Palgrave Macmillan.

Stewart, E., & Smith, K. E. (2015). "Black magic" and "gold dust": The epistemic and political uses of evidence tools in public health policy making. *Evidence & Policy, 11*(3), 415–437. https://doi.org/10.1332/174426415X14381786400158

Stobbe, M. (2014). *Surgeon General's warning: How politics crippled the nation's doctor.* University of California Press.

Street, J., Duszynski, K., Krawczyk, S., & Braunack-Mayer, A. (2014). The use of citizens' juries in health policy decision-making: A systematic review. *Social Science & Medicine, 109,* 1–9. https://doi.org/10.1016/j.socscimed.2014.03.005

Viswanathan, M., Ammerman, A., Eng, E., Garlehner, G., Lohr, K. N., Griffith, D., Rhodes, S., Samuel-Hodge, C., Maty, S., Lux, L., Webb, L., Sutton, S. F., Swinson, T., Jackman, A., & Whitener, L. (2004). Community-based participatory research: Assessing the evidence: Summary. In *AHRQ Evidence Report Summaries.* Agency for Healthcare Research and Quality.

Wampler, B. (2007). A guide to participatory budgeting. In A. Shah (Ed.), *Participatory budgeting* (pp. 21–54). The World Bank.

Ward, V., House, A., & Hamer, S. (2009). Knowledge brokering: The missing link in the evidence to action chain? *Evidence & Policy, 5*(3), 267–279. https://doi.org/10.1332/174426409X463811

WHO. (2021). *22nd expert committee on the selection and use of essential medicines.* Retrieved 5 June, 2021, from https://www.who.int/selection_medicines/committees/expert/22/en/

Williams, O., Sarre, S., Papoulias, S. C., Knowles, S., Robert, G., Beresford, P., Rose, D., Carr, S., Kaur, M., & Palmer, V. J. (2020). Lost in the shadows: Reflections on the dark side of co-production. *Health Research Policy and Systems, 18*(1), 43–43. https://doi.org/10.1186/s12961-020-00558-0

Wright, J., Parry, J., & Mathers, J. (2005). Participation in health impact assessment: Objectives, methods and core values. *Bulletin of the World Health Organization, 83*(1), 58–63. https://doi.org//S0042-96862005000100015

Conclusion: The Added Value of Political Science in, of, and with Public Health

Evelyne de Leeuw, Patrick Fafard, and Adèle Cassola

1 Epistemic Trespassing for Better Public Health Policy

An archaeologist wouldn't dare to proffer suggestions to the work of a brain surgeon in theatre. A theoretical astrophysicist would be ridiculed if they were to engage in the design of pharmaceutical clinical trials. Similarly, an immunologist would hesitate to venture an opinion on the structural engineering calculations of skyscrapers or suspension bridges. Cross-disciplinary transgressions have been deemed 'epistemic

E. de Leeuw (✉)
University of New South Wales, Sydney, NSW, Australia
e-mail: e.deleeuw@unsw.edu.au

P. Fafard
Global Strategy Lab; Faculty of Social Sciences, Faculty of Medicine, University of Ottawa, Ottawa, ON, Canada

A. Cassola
Global Strategy Lab, York University, Toronto, ON, Canada

© The Author(s) 2022
P. Fafard et al. (eds.), *Integrating Science and Politics for Public Health*,
Palgrave Studies in Public Health Policy Research,
https://doi.org/10.1007/978-3-030-98985-9_14

329

trespassing'. Ballantyne (2019) identified that 'Epistemic trespassers judge matters outside their field of expertise. Trespassing is ubiquitous in this age of interdisciplinary research and recognizing this will require us to be more intellectually modest' (p. 367). In the case of the potentially life-threatening ontological challenges, epistemic trespassing is clearly dangerous. But in more fuzzily defined domains like public health and public policy, such encroaching moves sometimes seem to have become 'rights of way'. The public discourse around the COVID-19 pandemic has brought the challenges at the interface (or overlap) between health and public policy into never-before-seen sharp focus.

For the public, opinions, beliefs, advocacy, and assessments of the appropriateness of dimensions of the public policy process are also more easily shared with the world than ever before through the proliferation of individualized and social media. In the past, one needed significant capital, political clout, and entrepreneurial skill to start and maintain an influential media outlet (hence the term 'press baron'). The twenty-first century has seen the emergence of 'influencers' on microblogs (e.g. Twitter and Instagram) and micro-syndication (e.g. Substack and Paper.li). Together with the creation and availability of mass accessible databases (some of which are more validated and credible than others, with *Our World In Data* and *GapMinder* setting gold standards for accountability and transparency) the world has turned into a place where billions of people believe epistemic trespassing is a civic duty. Of course, our new social media environment has also allowed another form of such trespassing—the rapid spread of misinformation and disinformation with sometimes tragic consequences.

In academe, there is also an entire debate to be had about the legitimacy of scholarly disciplines and professional boundaries. The hermetic nature of some forms of knowledge has, indeed, rightfully been challenged. These challenges have led to an attempt at the democratization of knowledge and the recognition that some forms of knowledge have been granted privileged status in knowledge hierarchies (Bhattacharya et al., 2020; Gehlert et al., 2010). An Indigenous knowledge systems discourse appropriately argues that the decolonization of the scholarly enterprise is needed. Also, it makes sense, at least analytically, to understand complex systems of public policymaking for public health as exactly that: systems with distinctive components, performances, outcomes, and impacts. Political deliberation is one part of the systems machine, scholarly interrogation another, as is community activism. For some, this calls for use of systems theory (Knai et al., 2018); for others, it means critical population health research (Labonte et al., 2005).

Notwithstanding these challenges, we are strong proponents of epistemic trespassing of all kinds if it is in support of broader shared goals and more than an attempt to argue the merits of one worldview over another or engage in critique for its own sake. More precisely, this book is an attempt to demonstrate what can be gained by political science for public health. Thus, in the introduction to this book, we outlined our ambitions:

- To show how political science perspectives (broadly defined) can inform public health research and practice;
- To demonstrate how much political science can gain from a deeper engagement with public health; and
- To advance the interconnection of public health and political science as scholarly disciplines with a particular view of addressing the apparently irreconcilable ideas between health scientists and policy students about the role of evidence (generation and dissemination) in policy (development and implementation).

We suggested that exploring and exploiting the interfaces and overlaps between the two fields would yield new, and potentially better, insights for public health policymaking. We took the advice from critical colleagues given in conference sessions and workshops, and heeded the call to proactively develop reciprocal epistemic incursions between the public health community and the policy process interested political science community (Bekker et al., 2018).

In this wrap-up of our collection, we will therefore reflect on two issues:

- Did we meet our own aspirations, and
- Did the contributors convincingly demonstrate the added value of applying notions from each field to the other?

Edited volumes, particularly in fuzzy fields like political science and public health, tend to run a risk of being eclectic collections of unique perspectives, a cabinet of curiosities. We claim a degree of coherence that would allow for a programmatic follow-up towards the further evolution of a public health political science where interests intersect.

2   Does Public Health Political Science Add Value?

First, across the chapters in this book, we have witnessed a significant consistency around the quintessential engine room of the field: the realm where facts and evidence production meet with politics and policies. Whether we explored the more conceptual and theoretical underpinnings of the emergent field in Part I; the empirical contributions in Part II describing knowledge production, the processing and percolation of evidence, and mechanisms that move policies through society and interest groups; or Part III where authors acknowledge the complexities and wicked nature of taking into account other players' role in determining health outcomes (and threats), the lessons are that agents in the public health field with particular policy agendas cannot assume a simple mechanical model. Time and again, the authors of the different chapters describe how successful actors and institutions in the public health policy arena achieve better outcomes through the ability to scan dynamics in institutional arrangements and jurisdictional responsibilities, coupled with an astute processing of (assumed) 'facts' in the policy game. Different theories of the policy process privilege particular roles for policy actors: policy entrepreneurs, coalition builders, equilibrium maintainers and watchguards, policy learning drivers, boundary spanners, street-level bureaucrats, or evidence synthesizers. Yet at their core, each of these actors does the same thing: they flexibly map, monitor, and adapt (e.g. by interfacing mental maps of different networks and identifying the critical pressure points) (de Leeuw et al., 2018).

For seasoned policy officers in large policy bureaucracies, this observation will not come as much of a surprise. But what our volume adds is that the authors have pointed out several highly applicable heuristics to guide and make sense of this quintessential dynamic. By moving beyond the tendency towards theoretical monomania, we witness the significant added value of a flexible identification and adaptation of (sometimes combinations of) theoretical models of the policy process. Many of our authors freely borrow from neighbouring disciplines, most notably sociology, as discussed in Chapter 3 (Greer, 2022), and philosophy (see, for example, Chapter 11 [Cairney et al., 2022]), to augment what political science has to offer to make sense of complex public health realities. This, we feel, creates an invitation and opportunity to budding public health political scientists to identify and pragmatically apply theoretical notions that resonate best with their contexts and provide support to the public health enterprise and not merely make public health a case study among many.

Second, we think that the chapters that explicitly deal with the multi-level complexities of the public health (promotion) effort are nothing but a forceful invitation to the political science community. Here is a field that needs analyses of the policy process and the political forces beyond simplistic stakeholder maps. The empirical chapters show how, for instance, local governments, e-cigarette debates, active (public) transport policies, and population-level vaccination development and deployment programmes are delightfully messy. They are worthy of systematic and ongoing inquiry. The empirical chapters also provide some indication of how to manage the tensions between public health policy that reflects the best available scientific evidence but also policy choices that reflect public concerns. An overview is provided in Chapter 13 by Cassola and colleagues. Hawkins and Oliver in Chapter 9 focus on parliamentary committees, and Smith and her colleagues in Chapter 7 focus on experiments with citizen juries. But many public policy gems remain in the locker, and methodologically, there are magnificent opportunities to understand the present and project the future from a political science analysis of the past.

Public health, in this collection, benefits demonstrably from a political science perspective. There are also clearly great opportunities for the political science community to grow by both analysing public health policy challenges (and not just pandemic-related) and benefitting from the rich data and methodical sophistication of public health research (see, for example, Hoffman et al., 2019; Topp et al., 2021). And we have compiled a collection of arguments that consistently show the importance, and efficacy, of flexible multi-level responses of scholars and practitioners at the nexus between our realms.

This is the time to return to epistemic trespassing. Despite the abundant promise of a fruitful evolution of a public health political science that we have documented consistently in this collection, the world is filled with well-meaning self-anointed 'expert' epistemic transgressors. Submissions to public policy inquiries also highlight a baffling arrogance from

sectors and actors that are peripheral to the public health effort in formu-
lating what proper policy ought to do. For instance, the approach used by
Pogrmilovic et al. (2019) demonstrates that much of the physical activity
policy analyses wholly ignore the body of knowledge that *both* public
health and political science could bring to advance the field. Nevertheless, perhaps because it is a systematic review (see Chapter 5 [Oliver,
2022]), this review has been elevated to a global gold standard in physical activity policy research (Whiting et al., 2021). Such studies often do
not amount to more than loose-sand collections of factoids (Greenhalgh
et al., 2014). They do not elevate our level of understanding public health
policymaking. They fail to add sophistication to the applicability and effi-
caciousness (let alone transfer and learning) of policy development in
public health. In contrast, in this book, we have tried to assemble authors
who have come from different disciplines but have all grappled with how
institutional design can help to make sense of some of the public health
trends that we've seen before and during the COVID-19 pandemic (and
will see again), e.g. why predictions regarding pandemic preparedness
didn't pan out; why rules and plans that were in place weren't followed;
why critical public health institutions were unable to perform as intended,
the apparent disregard for the International Health Regulations, etc.

3   A DEVELOPMENT AGENDA

We believe we have achieved our aspirations. The value at the interface between public health and political science is clear. The authors
in this collection describe the intricacies of providing a political science
perspective on how evidence moves through complex systems to shape
public health policies. Yet several additional challenges remain. As Lenin
famously asked, 'What is to be done?' (Lenin, 1952).

First, the global network of colleagues at this disciplinary interface is
growing but remains dispersed, both spatially and conceptually. There is a
need for some sort of 'home'. There is also a need to systematically incorporate the fact that public health policymaking in low- and middle-income
countries is often quite different from what is described in this collection.
Similarly, most of what is presented in this volume assumes democracy
as usual. In authoritarian regimes and in countries where populism is on
the rise, the challenges of public health policymaking are distinct and very
real (Falkenbach & Greer, 2021).

Second, more cross-disciplinary teaching, training, research, and publishing in public health and political science are required (Abuelezam, 2020; Asgary, 2018; Bekker et al., 2018; de Leeuw et al., 2014; Fafard & Cassola, 2020; Greer et al., 2018). At the teaching and training level, this would require more joint programmes, integrated courses, and faculty cross-appointments that would increase exposure to each other's tools and help to develop a common theoretical, conceptual, and methodological language. On the research side, achieving this goal would require more focused interdisciplinary funding for public health political science. Such funding could bridge the rigid disciplinary application and review criteria that typically channel work into one field or another. In the realm of publishing, creating more venues for public health political science would involve an effort on the part of journal editors to solicit and support the publishing of more interdisciplinary work, including special issues jointly convened by experts in both disciplines and by relaxing strict criteria for article formats and word lengths that may reduce the possibility for in-depth, interdisciplinary work.

Third, public health can benefit from the insights of the full range of sub-disciplines in political science (Gagnon et al., 2017, pp. 496–497). This collection emphasizes the insights of policy scholars and students of comparative politics. But there is a great deal of insightful work being done in international relations (see, for example, Davies & Wenham, 2020); various parts of political theory (see, for example, Weinstock, 2011); studies of local government (see, for example, O'Neill et al., 2019); not to mention various forms of political economy (see, for example, Stuckler & Basu, 2013). Moreover, the authors of the various chapters are from democracies in a relatively small number of high-income countries. But public health can also benefit enormously from the burgeoning political science research from researchers based in or from countries of the Global South (Bonnet et al., 2021; Lavis et al., 2012; Parkhurst et al., 2021; Ridde & Dagenais, 2017).

Finally, and perhaps most importantly, we need to follow the advice by our collaborators Cairney and Oliver (Oliver & Cairney, 2019) and leave the ivory towers of academe (whether political science or public health) and more proactively engage with policymaking efforts. This can take many forms. For some, it will be expert advice to governments; for others, it will be working closely with community organizations; and for still others, it will be media commentary. In all cases, if we are to not simply make a point but actually make a difference, drawing on the insights of both public health and political science is not just desirable, it is essential.

REFERENCES

Abuelezam, N. N. (2020). Teaching public health will never be the same. *American Journal of Public Health, 110*(7), 976–977. https://doi.org/10.2105/AJPH.2020.305710

Asgary, R. (2018). A collaborative multidisciplinary and without-walls research curriculum in global health. *The American Journal of Tropical Medicine and Hygiene, 99*(5), 1283–1290. https://doi.org/10.4269/ajtmh.16-0980

Ballantyne, N. (2019). Epistemic trespassing. *Mind, 128*(510), 367–395. https://doi.org/10.1093/mind/fzx042

Bekker, M. P. M., Greer, S. L., Azzopardi-Muscat, N., & McKee, M. (2018). Public health and politics: How political science can help us move forward. *European Journal of Public Health, 28*(suppl_3), 1–2. https://doi.org/10.1093/eurpub/cky194

Bhattacharya, S., Medcalf, A., & Ahmed, A. (2020). Humanities, criticality and transparency: Global health histories and the foundations of intersectoral partnerships for the democratisation of knowledge. *Humanities and Social Sciences Communications, 7*(1), 1–11. https://doi.org/10.1057/s41599-020-0491-7

Bonnet, E., Bodson, O., Le Marcis, F., Faye, A., Sambieni, N. E., Fournet, F., Boyer, F., Coulibaly, A., Kadio, K., Diongue, F. B., & Ridde, V. (2021). The COVID-19 pandemic in francophone West Africa: From the first cases to responses in seven countries. *BMC Public Health, 21*(1), 1490. https://doi.org/10.1186/s12889-021-11529-7

Cairney, P., Mitchell, H., & St Denny, E. (2022). Addressing the Expectations Gap in preventative public health and 'Health in All Policies': How can Policy Theory Help? In P. Fafard, A. Cassola, & E. De Leeuw (Eds.), *Integrating science and politics for public health*. Palgrave Springer.

Davies, S. E., & Wenham, C. (2020). Why the COVID-19 response needs International Relations. *International Affairs, 96*(5), 1227–1251. https://doi.org/10.1093/ia/iiaa135

de Leeuw, E., Browne, J., & Gleeson, D. (2018). Overlaying structure and frames in policy networks to enable effective boundary spanning. *Evidence & Policy: A Journal of Research, Debate and Practice, 14*(3), 537–547. https://doi.org/10.1332/174426418X15299595767891

de Leeuw, E., Clavier, C., & Breton, E. (2014). Health policy—Why research it and how: Health political science. *Health Research Policy and Systems, 12*(1). https://doi.org/10.1186/1478-4505-12-55

Fafard, P., & Cassola, A. (2020). Public health and political science: Challenges and opportunities for a productive partnership. *Public Health, 186,* 107–109. https://doi.org/10.1016/j.puhe.2020.07.004

Falkenbach, M., & Greer, S. L. (2021). *The populist radical right and health: National policies and global trends.*

Gagnon, F., Bergeron, P., Clavier, C., Fafard, P., Martin, E., & Blouin, C. (2017). Why and how political science can contribute to public health? Proposals for collaborative research avenues. *International Journal of Health Policy and Management, 6x,* 1–5.

Gehlert, S., Murray, A., Sohmer, D., McClintock, M., Conzen, S., & Olopade, O. (2010). The importance of transdisciplinary collaborations for understanding and resolving health disparities. *Social Work in Public Health, 25*(3–4), 408–422. https://doi.org/10.1080/19371910903241124

Greenhalgh, T., Howick, J., & Maskrey, N. (2014). Evidence based medicine: A movement in crisis? *BMJ, 348.* https://doi.org/10.1136/bmj.g3725

Greer, S. L., Bekker, M. P. M., Azzopardi-Muscat, N., & McKee, M. (2018). Political analysis in public health: Middle-range concepts to make sense of the politics of health. *European Journal of Public Health, 28*(suppl_3), 3–6. https://doi.org/10.1093/eurpub/cky159

Greer, S. (2022). Professions, data, and political will. In P. Fafard, A. Cassola, & E. De Leeuw (Eds.), *Integrating science and politics for public health.* Palgrave Springer.

Hoffman, S. J., Poirier, M. J. P., Katwyk, S. R. V., Baral, P., & Sritharan, L. (2019). Impact of the WHO Framework Convention on Tobacco Control on global cigarette consumption: Quasi-experimental evaluations using interrupted time series analysis and in-sample forecast event modelling. *BMJ, 365,* l2287. https://doi.org/10.1136/bmj.l2287

Knai, C., Petticrew, M., Mays, N., Capewell, S., Cassidy, R., Cummins, S., Eastmure, E., Fafard, P., Hawkins, B., Jensen, J. D., Katikireddi, S. V., Mwatsama, M., Orford, J., & Weishaar, H. (2018). Systems thinking as a framework for analyzing commercial determinants of health. *The Milbank Quarterly, 96*(3), 472–498. https://doi.org/10.1111/1468-0009.12339

Labonte, R., Polanyi, M., Muhajarine, N., McIntosh, T., & Williams, A. (2005). Beyond the divides: Towards critical population health research. *Critical Public Health, 15*(1), 5–17. https://doi.org/10.1080/09581590500048192

Lavis, J. N., Røttingen, J.-A., Bosch-Capblanch, X., Atun, R., El-Jardali, F., Gilson, L., Lewin, S., Oliver, S., Ongolo-Zogo, P., & Haines, A. (2012). Guidance for evidence-informed policies about health systems: Linking guidance development to policy development. *PLoS Medicine, 9*(3), e1001186. https://doi.org/10.1371/journal.pmed.1001186

Lenin, V. I. (1952). *What is to be done? Burning questions of our movement.* Foreign Languages Publishing House.

Oliver, K. (2022). How policy appetites shape, and are shaped by evidence production and use. In P. Fafard, A. Cassola, & E. De Leeuw (Eds.), *Integrating science and politics for public health*. Palgrave Springer.

Oliver, K., & Cairney, P. (2019). The dos and don'ts of influencing policy: A systematic review of advice to academics. *Palgrave Communications, 5*(1), 21. https://doi.org/10.1057/s41599-019-0232-y

O'Neill, B., Kapoor, T., & McLaren, L. (2019). Politics, science, and termination: A case study of water fluoridation policy in Calgary in 2011. *Review of Policy Research, 36*(1), 99–120. https://doi.org/10.1111/ropr.12318

Parkhurst, J., Ghilardi, L., Webster, J., Snow, R. W., & Lynch, C. A. (2021). Competing interests, clashing ideas and institutionalizing influence: Insights into the political economy of malaria control from seven African countries. *Health Policy and Planning, 36*(1), 35–44. https://doi.org/10.1093/heapol/czaa166

Pogrmilovic, B. K., O'Sullivan, G., Milton, K., Biddle, S. J., & Pedisic, Z. (2019). A systematic review of instruments for the analysis of national-level physical activity and sedentary behaviour policies. *Health Research Policy and Systems, 17*(1), 1–12.

Ridde, V., & Dagenais, C. (2017). What we have learnt (so far) about deliberative dialogue for evidence-based policymaking in West Africa. *BMJ Global Health, 2*(4), e000432. https://doi.org/10.1136/bmjgh-2017-000432

Stuckler, D., & Basu, S. (2013). *The body economic: Why austerity kills: Recessions, budget battles, and the politics of life and death*. Basic Books.

Topp, S. M., Schaaf, M., Sriram, V., Scott, K., Dalglish, S. L., Nelson, E. M., Sr, R., Mishra, A., Asthana, S., Parashar, R., Marten, R., Costa, J. G. Q., Sacks, E., Br, R., Reyes, K. A. V., & Singh, S. (2021). Power analysis in health policy and systems research: A guide to research conceptualisation. *BMJ Global Health, 6*(11), e007268. https://doi.org/10.1136/bmjgh-2021-007268

Weinstock, D. M. (2011). How should political philosophers think of health? *Journal of Medicine and Philosophy, 36*(4), 424–435. https://doi.org/10.1093/jmp/jhr026

Whiting, S., Mendes, R., Morais, S. T., Gelius, P., Abu-Omar, K., Nash, L., Rakovac, I., & Breda, J. (2021). Promoting health-enhancing physical activity in Europe: Surveillance, policy development and implementation 2015–2018. *Health Policy*. https://doi.org/10.1016/j.healthpol.2021.05.011

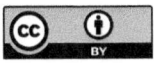

INDEX

A

ACF, 105, 107, 121. *See also* Advocacy Coalition Framework

active transportation, 104, 106–110, 112–118, 122

actor interactions, 105, 106, 108

adverse events, 219, 228–230

Advocacy Coalition Framework, 105, 212. *See also* ACF

agendas, 168, 192, 245, 247, 248, 250, 259, 269, 332

Alberta, 214

antivirals, 10, 213, 214, 216, 218, 221, 226, 228, 231–233

Australia, 128, 130, 159, 251, 254–256, 271, 284

B

boundary spanner(s), 122, 176, 177, 332

bounded rationality, 213, 240, 247, 248

British Columbia, 40, 218

C

CA, 281, 283. *See also* capability approach

capability approach, 24, 281, 282, 283. *See also* CA

CBPR, 303, 315, 317. *See also* community-based participatory research

central governments, 250

Chief Medical Officer, 117–119, 309

Chief Science Advisors, 309

citizens' juries, 10, 128, 129, 131, 134, 137, 139, 147, 149, 298, 299, 305, 307, 315–317

collaborative governance, 252

command-and-control planning, 215

commercial determinants of health, 190, 243

community-based participatory research, 299, 303. *See also* CBPR

community engagement, 178

co-production, 298, 303, 304, 306, 308, 312, 315, 317

© The Editor(s) (if applicable) and The Author(s) 2022
P. Fafard et al. (eds.), *Integrating Science and Politics for Public Health*,
Palgrave Studies in Public Health Policy Research,
https://doi.org/10.1007/978-3-030-98985-9

Coronavirus 2019, 3, 33, 62. *See also* COVID-19
corporations, 90, 130, 171, 189, 194, 196, 202
COVID-19, 3, 5, 11, 15, 23–25, 27, 33–35, 40, 42–46, 48–51, 62, 83, 91, 212, 226, 229–232, 294, 318, 330, 334. *See also* Coronavirus 2019
COVID-19 data, 34, 43, 46
crisis management, 216

D
deliberative approaches, 305
deliberative democracy, 129, 147, 305
deliberative polling, 299, 305, 316

E
EBPM, 240, 249, 259. *See also* evidence-based policymaking; evidence-informed policymaking
emergency measures, 217
England, 10, 38, 130, 132, 245
epidemiological data, 42
evidence-based policymaking, 69, 94, 128, 240, 245
evidence-informed policy, 189, 296, 307, 315. *See also* evidence-informed policymaking
evidence-informed policymaking, 10, 85, 128, 296, 297, 312, 315, 318. *See also* EBPM; evidence-based policymaking; evidence-informed policy
evidence-policy system, 79
evidence production, 9, 86, 87, 94, 202, 299, 303, 318, 332
evidence synthesis, 80
evidence use, 79, 85, 88, 92, 167, 195
expert advisory, 309

expert advisory bodies, 298, 309, 312, 315, 316

F
federalism, 23, 43, 49
First Nations, 218
framing, 38, 78, 86, 94, 108, 110, 120, 164, 167, 174, 175, 178, 192, 199, 200, 203, 231, 244, 255, 280, 281, 311

G
glocal, 157, 171, 174
good governance of evidence, 318

H
H1N1, 10, 213, 214–216, 218–222, 225–229, 231–233. *See also* influenza A
Health Canada, 154, 219, 220, 227, 231
health equity, 9, 21, 27, 60, 153, 156, 160, 162, 240, 241, 243–245, 254, 268, 270–273, 276, 277, 279, 281, 283
health human resources, 217
health impact assessments, 255, 271, 274, 298, 299. *See also* HIAs
health imperialism, 245, 254, 256, 257, 280
Health in All Policies, 10, 63, 240, 244, 267, 270, 272. *See also* HiAP
health inequalities, 10, 128–139, 141, 142, 145–148, 243–245, 252, 275
health policy, v, 4, 7–10, 60, 66, 69, 129, 154–156, 158, 162, 170, 175, 177, 196, 221, 239, 240, 248, 258, 259, 268–270, 273,

276, 279, 284, 293, 308, 310, 329, 331–334
health promotion, 9, 25, 59, 60, 130, 142, 143, 154, 213, 220, 232, 242, 255, 270
health technology assessments, 298, 299. *See also* HTAs
Healthy Cities, 10, 155, 159–162, 170–172, 174
Healthy Public Policy, 120, 154–156, 158, 268, 269, 270, 272. *See also* HPP
HiAP, 10, 240–242, 244, 245, 248, 251–259, 267, 268–280, 283, 284. *See also* Health in All Policies
HIAs, 298, 303. *See also* Health Impact Assessments
history, 35, 38, 120, 160, 195, 198, 218, 268
horizontal collaboration, 215
HPP, 268, 269–273. *See also* Healthy Public Policy
HTAs, 298, 304. *See also* health technology assessments

I
iKT, 303, 308, 315, 316. *See also* integrated knowledge translation
implementation, 62, 79, 104, 106, 120, 163, 164, 167, 172, 196, 198, 201, 211, 212, 220, 222, 246, 251–253, 258, 259, 273, 279, 284, 311, 331
individual responsibility, 144, 145, 243
influenza A, 213. *See also* H1N1
institutional readiness, 215–217
integrated knowledge translation, 298, 300, 303, 308. *See also* iKT
interdisciplinary research, 330

International Health Regulations, 170, 214, 334
intersectoral collaboration, 273, 278–280, 283
Ireland, 49, 129
IT, 178, 217, 219

K
knowledge broker, 317. *See also* knowledge brokering
knowledge brokering, 307. *See also* knowledge broker
knowledge exchange, 193. *See also* knowledge mobilization; knowledge transfer
knowledge mobilization, 88, 298, 300, 303, 304, 307. *See also* knowledge exchange; knowledge transfer
knowledge platforms, 300, 307, 316
knowledge production, 9, 79, 81, 83, 84, 87, 94, 332
knowledge transfer, 191. *See also* knowledge exchange; knowledge mobilization

L
lay perspectives, 132
legislature, 47, 48. *See also* parliament
lifestyles, 241, 243
local government, 39, 44, 69, 155, 158, 162, 170, 171, 178, 333, 335
local public health actors, 9, 104, 105, 108–120

M
Manitoba, 214, 218
meta-ethnography, 132, 141, 146, 149

mini-publics, 127–129, 148
Montréal, 9, 104, 106, 108–116, 118, 119

N
national survey, 131, 138, 139, 142
networks, 63, 116, 121, 122, 155, 159, 161, 162, 171, 173, 174, 177, 179, 197, 250, 300, 332
New South Wales, 255, 284
New Zealand, 49
Nova Scotia, 10, 40, 213, 214, 218, 220, 221, 223–225

O
Ontario, 106, 115, 214, 225, 233

P
paramedics, 217
parliament, 187, 188, 190, 191, 193, 194. See also legislature
participatory budgeting, 299, 306, 316
PHAC, 214, 216, 220–222. See also Public Health Agency of Canada
pharmaceuticals, 219
pharmacists, 217
physicians, 215, 223
planning capacity, 217
policy ambiguity, 247
policy champions, 221, 245, 258
policy experimentation, 298, 310, 315
policy implementation, 79, 163, 212
policy innovation labs, 302, 311, 315
policy learning, 9, 105, 155, 162, 163, 170, 178, 332
policymaking, v, 8, 104, 105, 115, 155, 158, 171, 177, 178, 191, 195, 198, 330, 331, 334, 335
policymaking complexity, 240, 252

policy theory, v, 247, 251, 253. See also public policy
policy transfer, 23, 105, 163, 169, 171–174, 176, 178
political economy of knowledge, 79, 84
political will, 9, 26, 35, 47, 49–51, 65, 240, 243, 244, 247, 252, 259, 294
politics of data, 35, 42, 51. See also politics of surveillance
politics of surveillance, 44. See also politics of data
power, 37, 39–41, 47, 48, 65, 68, 69, 87, 94, 104, 118, 158, 171, 175, 178, 191, 193, 233, 241, 248, 250, 254, 255, 259, 274, 295, 299, 303, 304, 307, 308, 316
prevention policy, 242, 243, 245, 246
Public Health Agency of Canada, 213, 215, 220, 223, 229. See also PHAC
public health policymakers, 35, 65
public health profession, 35, 111, 163
public health scholars, 4, 8, 16, 18, 19, 27, 64–67, 69, 258
public policy, v, 4, 7, 8, 10, 39, 48, 81, 83, 88, 93, 104, 105, 118, 154, 240, 267, 268–270, 280, 330, 333. See also policy theory

Q
Québec, 106, 160, 214, 216, 218, 233

R
randomized control trials, 243, 295, 311. See also RCTs
rationalist model, 78, 79, 81, 82, 85, 86, 88, 92

RCTs, 80, 83, 85, 86, 90, 91. *See also* randomized control trials

S
SARS, 61, 213, 214, 215, 217, 225, 232. *See also* Severe Acute Respiratory Syndrome
Saskatchewan, 218
Science and Technology Studies, 34. *See also* STS
scientific advisory committees, 301, 309
Scotland, 10, 130, 148, 275
Severe Acute Respiratory Syndrome, 61, 213, 214. *See also* SARS
social determinants of health, 63, 129, 162, 240, 241, 243–245, 252, 255, 268, 270, 272, 274, 275, 278, 283
stakeholder dialogues, 299, 306
stalemate, 6, 9, 10, 16, 27, 104, 120, 121, 141, 147, 148
STS, 46, 50. *See also* Science and Technology Studies
surveillance, 39, 42, 43, 45, 46, 51, 60, 213, 219
systematic review, 10, 61, 78, 80, 85–87, 89, 92, 129, 241, 243, 251, 315, 334

T
Tamiflu, 221, 228
tobacco control, 162, 196–198, 243, 268, 269, 275, 276
tobacco industry, 189, 190, 195–198, 201, 202

Toronto, 9, 104, 106–109, 111–113, 115, 117, 118

U
UK, 38, 39, 48, 78, 79, 82, 83, 85, 92, 128, 131–135, 137, 139, 146, 148, 187–190, 192, 197–202, 245, 247, 310. *See also* United Kingdom
United Kingdom, 10, 187. *See also* UK
United States, 43, 49, 174, 230, 309
upstream interventions, 270. *See also* upstream policies
upstream policies, 272. *See also* upstream interventions

V
vaccines, 10, 84, 212–214, 216–219, 221–224, 226–233
values, 17, 61–63, 67, 68, 78, 82, 89, 90, 105, 110, 121, 161, 198, 278, 294–296, 299, 304–306, 310, 318

W
WHO, 115, 154, 155, 161–163, 170, 172, 178, 213–216, 222, 223, 231, 241, 243, 245, 270, 271, 274, 280, 282, 309. *See also* World Health Organization
World Health Organization, v, 154, 159, 196, 213, 241, 270, 309. *See also* WHO